Digital Manufacturing of Bioimplants

The field of biomaterials and bio-manufacturing is undergoing rapid transformation, driven by advancements in material science, additive manufacturing, artificial intelligence, and biomedical engineering. This book provides a comprehensive exploration of cutting-edge developments in biomaterials, bioimplants, and emerging manufacturing techniques that are revolutionizing the healthcare and medical device industries. It explores the latest trends in biomaterials, recent innovations in composite materials, classification and characterization of multifunctional biomaterials, and their impact on biomedical applications. It further explores the role of robotics in surgical planning, the evolution of 2D, 3D, and 4D bioimplant technologies, and the customization of biomaterials for tissue regeneration. Advanced manufacturing approaches such as electrochemical micro-manufacturing and incremental sheet forming are also highlighted, along with their applications in next-generation biomedical implants.

This book:

- Provides in-depth analysis of novel biomaterials and their medical applications.
- Discusses advanced bio-manufacturing techniques including additive and electrochemical manufacturing.
- Highlights the role of AI, IoT, and smart technologies in personalized healthcare solutions.
- Examines sustainable and environmental considerations in biomaterial development.
- Incorporates contributions from leading experts in academia and industry.

Whether you are a researcher exploring biomaterial innovations, a medical professional interested in cutting-edge bioimplants, or an engineer working in biomedical manufacturing, this book provides essential insights into the next generation of biomaterials and healthcare solutions.

Smart Innovations and Technological Advancements in Mechanical and Materials Engineering

Ashwani Kumar, Kishor Gajrani

The book series editors are inviting edited, reference and textbook proposals for consideration in the book series. The main objective of this book series is to invite quality content in the field of smart materials applications, cutting edge manufacturing techniques, innovative designs, and use of advanced computational tools like AI & ML to solve engineering problems. The series includes recent innovative topics in four different sections which are as follows:

TECHNOLOGICAL ADVANCEMENTS: This section covers recent developments in Nanotechnology, Nonlinear dynamics, dynamics of complex systems, MEMS, green and sustainable technologies, vibration control, AI in power station, analog-digital hybrid modulation, advancement in inverter technology, adaptive piezoelectric, pattern recognition, data mining and knowledge discovery, control, robotics, automation and vision, knowledge-based simulation, sensor networks and big data analytics.

BIOINFORMATICS TECHNIQUES: This section covers Bioinformatics & Biomedical Engineering, Biomedical Imaging, Image Processing and Visualization, Biomedical Robotics, Computer-assisted Medical Diagnostic Systems, Biometrics and Bio-measurements, Innovative Technologies in Medicine, Nanoscience and Advanced Computing.

SMART MATERIALS: This section covers bioinspired materials, semiconductor materials, application of phase change materials, biodegradable composites, biomaterials, material synthesis and processing, energy materials, polymers, and biodegradable composites.

DIGITAL MANUFACTURING: This section covers recent developments in additive manufacturing, 3D printing, nanomanufacturing, manufacturing of bioimplants, micromachining, sustainable manufacturing, green manufacturing, environmentally friendly manufacturing, application of soft computing techniques in manufacturing, and adaptive technologies for sustainable growth.

This book series compiled all aspects of manufacturing, design, and computational intelligence techniques from fundamental principles to current advanced concepts. This book series is an effort to address the changes occurring in mechanical and materials engineering and the application of new techniques in this field. The book series covers a variety of topics from conventional to advanced ones.

Digital Manufacturing of Bioimplants: Technology and Applications
Durwesh Jhodkar, Parnika Shrivastava and Puneet Tandon

For more information on this series, please visit: www.routledge.com/Smart-Innovations-and-Technological-Advancements-in-Mechanical-and-Materials/book-series/CRCSITAMME

Digital Manufacturing of Bioimplants

Technology and Applications

Edited by

Durwesh Jhodkar, Parnika Shrivastava and Puneet Tandon

CRC Press
Taylor & Francis Group
Boca Raton London New York

CRC Press is an imprint of the
Taylor & Francis Group, an **informa** business

Designed cover image: Shutterstock

First edition published 2027
by CRC Press
2385 NW Executive Center Drive, Suite 320, Boca Raton FL 33431

and by CRC Press
4 Park Square, Milton Park, Abingdon, Oxon, OX14 4RN

CRC Press is an imprint of Taylor & Francis Group, LLC

ISBN: 9781032946771 (hbk)
ISBN: 9781032946801 (pbk)
ISBN: 9781003581192 (ebk)

DOI: 10.1201/9781003581192

Typeset in Sabon
by Newgen Publishing UK

Contents

Preface

The field of biomaterials and bio-manufacturing technologies is undergoing a transformative evolution, driven by advancements in materials science, additive manufacturing, robotics, and artificial intelligence. This book presents a comprehensive exploration of these innovations, highlighting their impact on biomedical applications, healthcare sustainability, and personalized medicine. By bringing together the latest research and technological developments, this book aims to serve as a valuable reference for researchers, academicians, and industry professionals.

Chapter 1 introduces the current trends in biomaterials and bio-manufacturing technologies, setting the stage for the subsequent discussions on novel material developments and fabrication techniques. Chapter 2 delves into recent advancements in composite materials for biomedical applications, emphasizing their enhanced mechanical and biological properties. Chapter 3 provides insights into the classification and characterization of multifunctional biomaterials, offering a foundation for understanding their biomedical applications.

Chapter 4 explores the transformative role of robotics in surgical planning and navigation, illustrating how precision and automation are reshaping modern surgical procedures. Chapter 5 focuses on the development of bio-implants using 2D, 3D, and 4D additive manufacturing technologies, demonstrating the evolution of personalized medical solutions. Chapter 6 highlights the significance of customized biomaterial architectures for tissue regeneration, showcasing the potential of additive manufacturing in regenerative medicine. Chapter 7 introduces additive electrochemical micro-manufacturing technology and its emerging applications in biomedical device fabrication.

Chapter 8 presents novel bioimplant fabrication strategies, with a focus on incremental sheet forming and additive manufacturing techniques. Chapter 9 discusses advancements in microwave hyperthermia and phased array technology for revolutionizing breast cancer treatment. Chapter 10 examines IoT-based smart health monitoring systems, integrating sensors and electronics for real-time patient care. Chapter 11 emphasizes tailored bioimplants for regenerative medicine, particularly in the domain of bone tissue engineering.

Chapter 12 identifies challenges in bio-implant manufacturing, addressing key limitations related to materials, regulations, and processing techniques. Chapter 13 evaluates the environmental and health impacts of biomaterials and bio-manufacturing, offering a sustainable approach to biomedical research and applications. Chapter 14 concludes the book by discussing AI-powered tailored treatment strategies for PCOS, demonstrating the intersection of artificial intelligence and sustainable healthcare solutions.

This book provides a multidisciplinary perspective on the advancements and challenges in biomaterials and bio-manufacturing technologies, bridging the gap between research and industrial applications. Through its diverse topics and in-depth analysis, it serves as a valuable resource for readers seeking to explore the frontiers of biomedical engineering and healthcare innovation.

Editors
Durwesh Jhodkar
Parnika Shrivastava
Puneet Tandon

Aim and scope

This book aims to provide a comprehensive overview of the latest advancements, challenges, and future directions in biomaterials and biomanufacturing technologies. By integrating cutting-edge research in materials science, additive manufacturing, robotics, artificial intelligence, and biomedical applications, this book serves as a valuable resource for researchers, academicians, and industry professionals. The focus is to explore how emerging technologies are transforming the landscape of biomedical implants, regenerative medicine, surgical planning, and sustainable healthcare solutions.

Chapter 1 discusses the evolution of biomaterials and advancements in bio-manufacturing techniques, highlighting the integration of innovative materials and fabrication processes. Chapter 2 delves into novel composite materials that enhance the mechanical and biological performance of biomedical implants and prostheses. Chapter 3 explores the classification and characterization of various biomaterials based on their functional properties and biocompatibility. Chapter 4 examines the role of robotics and automation in surgical planning and navigation, showcasing their contribution to enhanced precision and minimally invasive procedures. Chapter 5 presents advancements in additive manufacturing, including 2D, 3D, and 4D printing, and their applications in developing next-generation bio-implants. Chapter 6 investigates the fabrication of personalized biomaterials for tissue engineering and regenerative medicine through additive manufacturing. Chapter 7 explores additive electrochemical micro-manufacturing techniques for biomedical applications. Chapter 8 highlights recent developments in bioimplant fabrication using incremental sheet forming and additive manufacturing. Chapter 9 introduces novel therapeutic approaches using microwave hyperthermia for targeted breast cancer treatment. Chapter 10 discusses the integration of IoT-based smart health monitoring systems for real-time patient tracking and disease management. Chapter 11 reviews strategies for designing tailored bioimplants for regenerative medicine, with a focus on bone tissue engineering. Chapter 12 identifies key technical, regulatory, and material challenges faced in bio-implant manufacturing. Chapter 13 evaluates sustainability concerns in biomaterials research, including their environmental and health implications. Chapter 14 examines the role of AI-driven precision medicine in revolutionizing PCOS treatment within a sustainable healthcare framework. By bridging the gap between academia and industry, this book offers valuable insights into innovations and future directions in biomaterials and biomedical manufacturing technologies.

About the editors

Durwesh Jhodkar is an assistant professor in the Mechanical Department at Wainganga College of Engineering in Nagpur, Maharashtra, India. He holds a Ph.D. degree from the Mechanical Engineering Discipline at PDPM IIITDM, Jabalpur, India. His doctoral research likely contributed to the field of machining tool technology. Prior to his Ph.D., Durwesh Jhodkar earned a Master's degree in Industrial Engineering and Management from SGSITS, Indore, India, in the year 2010. This background suggests a strong foundation in both the technical and managerial aspects of industrial engineering. He has a notable academic background with a decade of teaching experience. Additionally, he has post-doctoral experience from the University of Johannesburg, South Africa. Post-doctoral research is typically undertaken after obtaining a Ph.D., allowing researchers to further specialize in a particular area or explore new avenues of research. Durwesh Jhodkar has made significant contributions to the field, evident from his research articles. His publications cover a range of topics, including 3D printing, ergonomics risk assessment, bio-implant machining processes, post-treatment analysis, and cutting tool tribology.

Parnika Shrivastava is currently working as an assistant professor at the Mechanical Engineering Department of the National Institute of Technology Jalandhar (Punjab). She has earned her Doctorate and M.Tech. degree in Mechanical Engineering from PDPM, Indian Institute of Information Technology, Design & Manufacturing Jabalpur, Jabalpur, in 2019. She has completed B.Tech. (Honors) from Mechanical Engineering Discipline of Engineering College Bikaner (E.C.B), Bikaner, Rajasthan. Her research areas of interest are advanced forming operations, hybrid manufacturing, fracture mechanics, rapid product development technologies, and topology optimization. She has been granted a patent on the "Process of analyzing the effect of preheated microstructure vis-à-vis parameters on the orange peel in incremental sheet forming of AA1050 sheets". She has authored various research articles in international journals of repute along with several conference publications and book chapters. She has been recently granted a Core Research Grant funding for undertaking the project “Design and development of an Electrically Assisted Hybrid Double Sided Incremental Forming machine for efficient production of customized biomedical implants with improved surface finish and geometrical accuracy”. She is also the recipient of two national-level awards including the Best Teacher Award 2022 conferred by the Indian Society for Technical Education, New Delhi.

Puneet Tandon, a fellow of IACSIT, is a joint professor of Mechanical Engineering and Design at PDPM Indian Institute of Information Technology, Design and Manufacturing Jabalpur, India. His primary research interests are intelligent and innovative product design, computer-aided design, nature-inspired design, advanced manufacturing technologies, and microfabrication. He graduated in Mechanical Engineering from NIT Kurukshetra. He received his Masters and Doctoral degrees in Mechanical Engineering from IIT Kanpur. He is presently Head, Discipline of Design. He has authored more than 110 papers in referred journals and international conferences. He has been author to one text book titled *Cutting Tool Geometry: 3D Perspective* and a few conference proceedings. Besides, another text book written along with his Japanese collaborators is under production. He was also the organizer of International Conference on Innovations in Design and Manufacturing (InnDeM) 2012 and Design Workshop (DeW) 2010. He is Principal Investigator to a joint Indo-Japan Project and to numerous projects sponsored by Department of Science & Technology, Department of Atomic Energy, Ministry of Human Resource Development, etc. He is a member of the International Programme Committee of CAD Conferences and on advisory committees of various international conferences. He is a co-editor of *International Journal on Manufacturing* and has been a reviewer to several international journals.

Contributors

Aqueel Ahmad
Department of Mechanical Engineering, Graphic Era Deemed to be University, Dehradun, India

Fatima Aksha
Mechanical Engineering Department, National Institute of Technology, Srinagar, Jammu & Kashmir, India

R.S. Banshtu
Department of Civil Engineering, National Institute of Technology Hamirpur, Hamirpur, India

Siddhartha Dan
Biomaterial and Tissue Engineering Research Group, Department of Biotechnology, Dr B R Ambedkar National Institute of Technology, Jalandhar, Punjab, India

Amey Dukle
Department of Mechanical Engineering, Indian Institute of Technology Tirupati, Andhra Pradesh, India

Yatika Gori
ABES Engineering College, Ghaziabad, Uttar Pradesh, India

C. Harsha Vardhan
Mechanical Engineering Department, National Institute of Technology, Srinagar, Jammu Kashmir, India

Ruchin Kacker
School of Mechanical Sciences, Indian institute of Technology, Bhubaneswar, Odisha, India

Nitesh Kashyap
Electronics and Communication Engineering Department, Dr B R Ambedkar National Institute of Technology, Jalandhar, Punjab, India

Ajay Kumar
Electronics and Communication Engineering Department, Dr B R Ambedkar National Institute of Technology, Jalandhar, Punjab, India

Ashwani Kumar
Department of Mechanical Engineering, Raj Kumar Goel Institute of Technology, Ghaziabad, India
ABES Engineering College, Ghaziabad, Uttar Pradesh, India

Ruchin Kacker
School of Mechanical Sciences, Indian Institute of Technology, Bhubaneswar, Odisha, India

Piyush Kumar
Mechanical Engineering Department, National Institute of Technology, Srinagar, Jammu Kashmir, India

Saurabh Kumar
Mechanical Engineering Department, National Institute of Technology, Srinagar, Jammu & Kashmir, India

Neha Kumari
Dept. Electronics and Communication Engineering ABES Engineering College, Ghaziabad, Uttar Pradesh, India

Padmanava Mishra
Biomaterial and Tissue Engineering Research Group, Department of Biotechnology, Dr B R Ambedkar National Institute of Technology, Jalandhar, Punjab, India

Naseeba Mukhtar
Mechanical Engineering Department, National Institute of Technology, Srinagar, Jammu & Kashmir, India

Deepak Kumar Naik
Mechanical Engineering Department, National Institute of Technology, Srinagar, Jammu & Kashmir, India

Divyansh Singh Patel
School of Mechanical Sciences, Indian institute of Technology, Bhubaneswar, Odisha, India

Neha Singh Raghuvanshi
ABES Engineering College, Ghaziabad, Uttar Pradesh, India

Ashish Raman
Electronics and Communication Engineering Department, Dr B R Ambedkar National Institute of Technology, Jalandhar, Punjab, India

Subham Kumar Rana
Mechanical Engineering Department, National Institute of Technology, Srinagar, Jammu & Kashmir, India

Rajeev Ranjan
Department of Mechanical Engineering, Raj Kumar Goel Institute of Technology, Ghaziabad, India

Chandana Rath
School of Materials Science and Technology, Indian Institute of Technology (Banaras Hindu University) Varanasi, India

M. Ravi Sankar
Department of Mechanical Engineering, Indian Institute of Technology Tirupati, Andhra Pradesh, India

Bogala Mallikharjuna Reddy
Center for Research, Innovation, Development, and Applications (CRIDA), Jaiotec Labs (OPC) Private Limited, Amaravati, Andhra Pradesh, India

Mahesh Kumar Sah
Biomaterial and Tissue Engineering Research Group, Department of Biotechnology, Dr B R Ambedkar National Institute of Technology, Jalandhar, Punjab, India

Abhijit Saha
Department of Mechanical Engineering, Raj Kumar Goel Institute of Technology, Ghaziabad, India

Shrishti Sharma
Department of Civil Engineering, National Institute of Technology Hamirpur, Hamirpur, India

Parnika Shrivastava
Mechanical Engineering Department, Dr B R Ambedkar National Institute of Technology, Jalandhar, Punjab, India

Adarsh Singh
Department of Civil Engineering, National Institute of Technology Hamirpur, Hamirpur, India

Navneet Singh
Dept. Electronics and Communication Engineering ABES Engineering College, Ghaziabad, Uttar Pradesh, India

P. Sri Sai Krishna Aditya
Mechanical Engineering Department, National Institute of Technology, Srinagar, Jammu Kashmir, India

Swapnil Shrivastava
Meerut Institute of Engineering and Technology, Meerut, Uttar Pradesh, India

Kshitiz Srivastav
ABES Engineering College, Ghaziabad, Uttar Pradesh, India

Sourabh Tandon
School of Mechanical Sciences, Indian institute of Technology, Bhubaneswar, Odisha, India

Sharad Singh Thakur
Mechanical Engineering Department, Dr B R Ambedkar National Institute of Technology, Jalandhar, Punjab, India

Nikhil Tiwari
Dept. Electronics and Communication Engineering ABES Engineering College, Ghaziabad, Uttar Pradesh, India

Venkatesh Vakucherla
Department of Mechanical Engineering, Annamacharya University, Rajampet, Andhra Pradesh, India

Akhilesh Kumar Yadav
School of Materials Science and Technology, Indian Institute of Technology (Banaras Hindu University) Varanasi, India

Ashok Kumar Yadav
Department of Mechanical Engineering, Raj Kumar Goel Institute of Technology, Ghaziabad, India

Acknowledgment

The successful completion of this book would not have been possible without the invaluable support, guidance, and contributions of many individuals and institutions. First and foremost, we express our sincere gratitude to our academic and research communities for their continuous encouragement and motivation in exploring advancements in biomaterials and biomanufacturing technologies.

We extend our heartfelt appreciation to all the contributing authors whose expertise and dedication have enriched this book with high-quality content. Their relentless efforts in sharing cutting-edge research and insights have played a significant role in shaping the direction of this work. We are also grateful to the reviewers for their constructive feedback and valuable suggestions, which have helped refine the chapters and enhance the overall quality of the book.

Special thanks are due to our respective institutions for providing the necessary resources, facilities, and a conducive research environment that facilitated the successful compilation of this book. We are also indebted to our colleagues, research scholars, and students who have provided constant intellectual support and valuable discussions throughout this journey.

We acknowledge the support of our families and friends, whose patience, understanding, and encouragement have been instrumental in bringing this book to fruition. Their unwavering belief in our efforts has been a source of motivation and strength.

Finally, we would like to express our deep gratitude to the publishers for their cooperation, professionalism, and guidance in making this book a reality. We hope that this work serves as a valuable resource for researchers, academicians, and professionals engaged in the field of biomaterials and biomedical manufacturing technologies.

Chapter 1

Current trends in biomaterial and biomanufacturing technologies

Deepak Kumar Naik, Subham Kumar Rana, Saurabh Kumar, Fatima Aksha, and Naseeba Mukhtar

1.1 INTRODUCTION

Biomaterials play a crucial role in biomedical application. Biomaterials are the substances that are mostly used for medical applications, such as replacing or augmenting tissue. These can be used as tiny particles to deliver or replace conventional drugs. The field of biomaterials gained recognition after the first meeting held on biomaterials at Clemson University, South Carolina in 1969 and continues to receive substantial attention since then. Biomaterials are the natural or artificial substances used in the making of structures or implants to replace the lost or diseased biological structure to restore form and function. Biomaterials are used in different parts of human body; they are used as artificial valves in the heart, replacement implants in shoulders, knees, hips. They are also used for urinary tract reconstruction. The biomaterials are classified into metals, polymers, ceramics and composite biomaterials. Bone biomaterials, also known as bone graft alternatives, have seen a rise in demand in recent years. Every year, more than 2 million procedures are performed in the US to use grafting to heal broken or damaged bones. Consequently, the US market for bone biomaterials surpassed 39 billion dollars in 2013 [1]. Up to 10 million people in China suffer from reduced limb function as a result of bone abnormalities. However, the shortage of available bone biomaterials prevents many patients from receiving successful treatment. The major dominant biomaterials used are cobalt-based (Co) alloys, stainless steel (SS), magnesium-based alloys, and titanium (Ti). These are considered as the superior biomaterials, as they have ability to carry significant stress and go through the plastic deformation prior unit to the fail. These materials ought to have decent mechanical as well as chemical properties; they have a lifespan of 10–15 years only.

In the current era, metals and alloys have emerged as the primary candidates for implant composition owing to their properties: high mechanical strength, minimal risk of rejection, and above all, biological biocompatibility. New compounds with respect to orthopaedics such as synthetically obtained polymers started to be more frequently used in

DOI: 10.1201/9781003581192-1

medical applications after World War II. Synthetic materials have progressed through time from biocompatible and biodegradable materials to the present bioactive materials. The composition of these polymeric compounds can be modulated to emulate the structure of various tissues, while their mechanical properties provide a cytocompatibility scaffold that aids cell growth and attachment.

Furthermore, polymers with the right kind of composition can be designed to elicit a cell response that is conducive to healing/repair. Of the synthetic materials, polyurethane is one of the most versatile, with applications ranging from orthopaedic implants to covering materials to drainage devices but also as a tool for biomechanical testing of various fracture reduction and fixation techniques. What enables such diversity of uses with those polyurethanes is manipulation from chemistry that can give the resulting polyurethanes many structures similar to human tissue. A tremendous amount of old knowledge about the mechanical characteristics of these materials and the biocompatibility is essential for their utilization as orthopaedic surgical implants.

As a matter of fact, human beings used various foreign substances for therapeutic purposes since ancient times, like application of hairs or cellulose as suture material and adoption of wood or horn for osteosynthesis. Nowadays, metals and alloys are considered the major types of used implants, because they have great strength; therefore, they have a lower risk of rejection due to inertness compared with other materials. A new class of compounds, the synthetic polymers, have quickly evolved and have been utilized more in the short time all over the world since World War II. Despite the kind of material utilized in implant devices, they ought to fulfil the general and specific requests—mechanical along with biological features.

3D Printing, also known as additive manufacturing, is a rapidly evolving technology that has the potential to transform the industry of biomaterials. By application of 3D technology, scaffolds, patient-specific implants, and other instruments could be created for use in the regeneration of medicine and tissue engineering [2]. With this 3D printing technology, structures can be designed with the help of obtained images from medical operation like computed tomography (CT) and with magnetic resonance imaging (MRI). In this method, objects are created by using a layer-on-layer process which eventually creates a 3D model of the desired shape and size without any use of tools. Firstly, pictures of a patient are gathered using magnetic resonance imaging (MRI) or computed tomography (CT). These images' data are then converted into a 3D model by use of CAD software and saved in the form of a digital file. Once the file type data have been imported into the 3D printing machine, they complete the model layer by layer. The 3D printer then uses the 2D layer as a guide to layer upon layer of material, living cells, or biomolecules, to create the desired 3D biomedical product. Some of the advantages of 3D Printing for biomedical applications:

- Customization: By using 3D printing, we can make goods that can be for a specific person and can change the dimensions of the same for others.
- Complexity: 3D printing technology is able to generate complex structures that is difficult by using any other techniques.
- Versatility: It can be use to create goods by number of combinations that can be exact replica of the original one.
- Cost-effectiveness: This technology reduces the material waste and increases the production rate, compared to conventional manufacturing techniques.

Nowadays biomaterials are also used for joint and bone replacement which is a severe problem mostly in the people aged 45 years or more. These people are fighting with the problems of bone weakness, inflammation of the human's bone joints, and cartilages weakness, resulting in bone degradation under continuous cyclic loading conditions which is the main cause of degradation of human's bone. The best way to solve these problems is "Total joint replacement "(TJR), where load-bearing joints are replaced with artificial implants.

The advancement of efficient drug-delivery systems is crucial for better patient outcomes across various medical conditions [3]. The quality and access to healthcare significantly influence these outcomes; developed countries generally having better access and thus have better results. Preventive medicine, including routine screenings and vaccinations, plays a vital role in reducing patient side effects. Innovative materials are central to the development of medical technology, enhancing diagnostic tools, implantable devices, and regenerative medicine. Polymers, particularly biocompatible and biodegradable ones, are essential for creating medical devices, tissue engineering scaffolds, and drug-delivery systems, reducing long-term complications, and eliminating the need for additional surgeries. Nanomaterials contribute to advancements in drug delivery, imaging, and diagnostics, while biomimetic polymers enhance tissue compatibility, aiding in organ and tissue engineering. Metamaterials, with their unique properties, offer significant improvements in medical imaging and device functionality. Smart medical devices, utilizing shape memory alloys and conductive polymers, improve patient comfort and monitoring. Regenerative medicine benefits from scaffold materials and hydrogels that support tissue repair, and bioactive materials like glasses and ceramics provide controlled drug release. Overall, the integration of innovative biomaterials in medical technology aims to enhance patient outcomes through a multifaceted approach involving materials science, nanotechnology, and biotechnology.

At present, a lot of synthetic plastic is being used for human convenience. Due to this, there have been serious problems in recent times regarding high toxicity and non-biodegradability. Due to this, the use of plastic has been banned in 2021. Now, we are moving towards 3D printing, and people are paying attention, and the use of its products can be seen soon. At present, it is causing pollution. Polymers or plastics have become a part of society today, because they have a wide range of properties such as being light in weight, their tunable strength and elasticity, ease of modification and dyeing, tunable transparency, thermal/electric insulation, and many more. These properties are responsible for their use in a wide range of applications. Some of these include solid containers and castings, flexible films for packaging, fibers for clothing and ropes, shock-absorbing joints, coatings, adhesive sealants and bonding agents such as elastomers. All of these require different combinations of properties. With production reaching 400.3 million tons, only 9% is recycled, according to 2022 data. The rest breaks down into microplastics, which can be harmful to the environment and pose a threat to human health. Managing plastic waste by burning, landfilling, or recycling, is imperative to curb this growing problem [4–7].

Biodegradable polymers are now proposed to replace plastics, as they are more environmentally sustainable. However, biodegradation depends on factors such as surface area, pH, density, air, temperature, light, and microorganisms. These polymers are easily decomposed into smaller fragments under oxidative conditions— unlike synthetic polymers. Investigation of polyester in seawater, show that temperature and microorganisms affect this process. There are three types of biodegradations: enzyme release to depolymerize the plastic, biofilm formation by microorganisms, and absorption of low molecular weight species by microorganisms. Polymers with aromatic and polyolefin moieties resist biodegradation due to high hydrophobicity and strong C–C bonds, while hydrophilic polymers with easily decomposable bonds are more easily decomposed. Biopolymers such as poly (lactic acid) (PLA) and poly (butylene succinate) (PBS) are being used in medical fields. They can decompose in seawater; studies show that alkali treatment and addition of starch enhance biodegradability. Biodegradable polymers thus reduce plastic waste and pollution, but more research is needed on their decomposition mechanisms and applications [8, 9]. The general mechanism involved in the biodegradation of polymers is shown in Figure 1.1.

1.2 CIRCULAR ECONOMY AND SOCIO-ECONOMIC ASPECTS OF BIOMATERIALS

Circular economy aims to minimize the waste produce and maximize the continual use of resource. 3D printing uses technology to make a replica of a given model by using its software, and biomaterials are the substance that are used to combine with biological system to engage it with medical purpose. If both 3D printing and biomaterials gets combined, then, it can

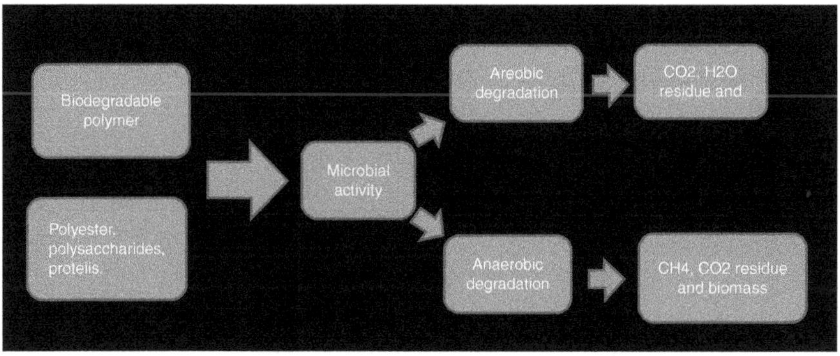

Figure 1.1 General mechanism involved in the biodegradation of polymers.

be a great circular economy, resulting in reuse of the materials and minimizing waste, creating biodegradable and recyclable biomaterials that can reduce the environmental impact, enabling personalized and customized biomedical products that can improve healthcare quality and accessibility, and fostering innovation and collaboration in the biomanufacturing sector. Figure 1.2 shows a brief idea of how 3D printing with biomaterials can be used for the 3R's.

Biomaterials are the products that are obtained via biological systems and converted into products used for medical purpose. They can be collected from natural resources and can also be made artificially with proper shapes and materials as per requirements.

1.3 BIOMATERIALS FOR 3D PRINTING TECHNOLOGY

1.3.1 Materials

Biomaterials are the organic substance that can be used in medical fields to replace, improve, or restore organ tissue. The classification of biomaterial is shown in Figure 1.3.

The main characteristics of biomaterials is that it can be made artificially with help of biomedical implants or can be obtained organically from natural resources. Some common polymeric or synthetic biomaterials include:

1. PLA (polylactic acid): It is a widely used biocompatible and biodegradable synthetic polymer. It is known for being both biocompatible and biodegradable, making it suitable for various biomedical applications. PLA is the leading polymer used in FDM, a popular 3D printing technique.

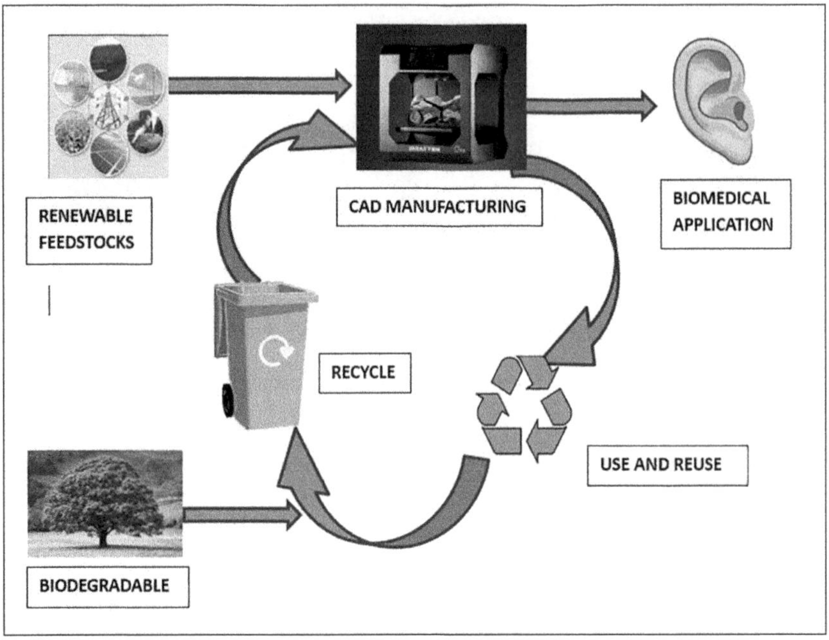

Figure 1.2 Economy of biomaterials for 3D printing.

2. PDLLA (poly-D, L-lactic acid): It is a biodegradable polymer known for its good mechanical strength. PDLLA has been effectively used in a range of biomedical fields, including bone regeneration, wound healing, and tissue engineering, demonstrating its versatility as a biomaterial.
3. PPF (poly (propylene fumarate)): It is a photo-cross linkable and biodegradable polymer widely used in stereolithography (SLA).
4. Poly ether ether ketone (PEEK): It is a high-performance thermoplastic polymer known for its exceptional properties. It is an excellent material for replacing missing bone due to its bio inertness, low heat transfer or conductivity, elasticity, and strength comparable to cortical bone.

1.3.2 Types of biodegradable polymers

Biodegradable polymers are classified as below: -

Natural biodegradable polymers e.g. poly(saccharides), lignin, chitosan, starch, cellulose, guar gum, collagen, albumin, etc. [10–13].

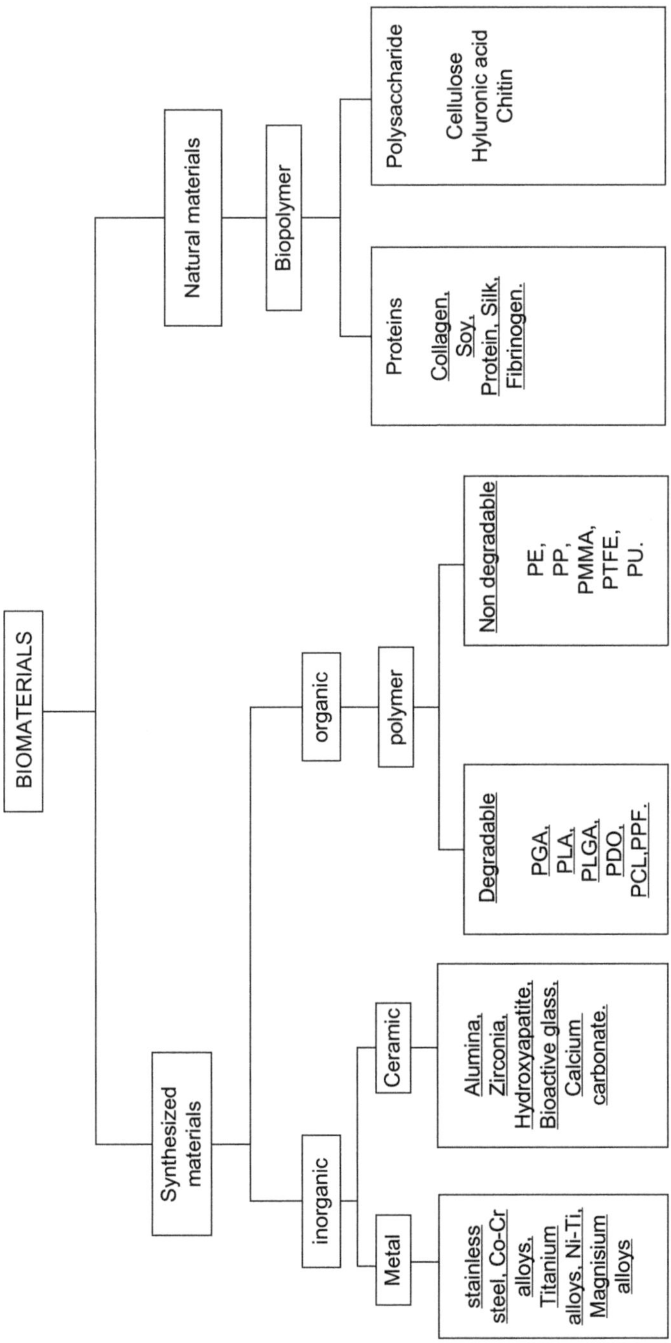

Figure 1.3 Classification of biomaterials.

Synthetic biodegradable polymers e.g. aliphatic polyesters, poly (Ortho esters), poly,(anhydrides), poly(phosphagens), poly (amino acids), vitrine's, BDMPs, etc. [14].

1.3.3 Advances on the toxicity of biodegradable plastics

Biodegradable plastics (BPs) are currently a hot topic of discussion as they have been proposed as a solution, and their environmental impact remains controversial. They make up only a small portion of total plastic production, and their use can lead to microplastics and pollution in the natural environment through their degradation. Biodegradable microplastics (BMPs) can affect human health just as conventional microplastics (CMPs) and also affecting marine life and soil. Biodegradable plastics have been developed to reduce environmental pollution, highlighting the need for careful design and chemical safety. Efforts are underway to better understand and address the ecological challenges posed by BMPs today [15]. The types of biomaterials which are used in the various medical fields is tabulated in Table 1.1.

1.4 SUSTAINABLE MANUFACTURING PRACTICES IN BIOMATERIAL MANUFACTURING

In the present times, industrialization and rapid economic development have led to loss of biodiversity and damage to ecosystems. While economic growth improves employment opportunities, living standards, and

Table 1.1 Types of biomaterials uses in medical industry

Sl no	*Utility*	*Biomaterial uses*
1	Joint replacement	Titanium (Ti) and its alloy Stainless steel (SS) and its alloy Polyethylene (PE)
2	Bone scaffold	Calcium phosphate (Cap) Poly methyl methacrylate (PMMA) Acrylate
3	Oral system	Titanium (Ti) and its alloy Stainless steel (SS) and its alloy Aluminium (Al) and its alloy
4	Cardiovascular stent	Stainless steel (SS) and its alloy Teflon Cobalt-chromium (Co-Cr) alloy
5	Breast implants	Silicone gel Saline solution Composite fillers

healthcare, sustainable manufacturing balances social, ecological, and economic dimensions. Practices such as Lean, Six Sigma, and 6R (Recycle, Reduce, Redesign, Reuse, Recover, Remanufacture) help achieve this balance. These include management support, incentives, knowledge of the circular economy, stakeholder pressure, incentives, and legislation. Markets and organizations adapt unsustainable practices that bring sustainable benefits to the environment and society, thereby gaining a competitive advantage [16–18].

1.4.1 Role of sustainable manufacturing in microwave processing of materials

Mechanical components used in industries such as aerospace engines, power plants, and automotives are exposed to high temperatures, which leads to corrosion and wear. To avoid this, materials are selected for their resistance to these conditions and their surfaces are protected using techniques such as coatings, cladding, and glazing. Surface engineering protects the surface without changing the original properties, which reduces costs. For example, lapping of coatings such as molybdenum disulfide or diamond is done to reduce friction and wear. However, their use has its advantages and disadvantages, and they are expensive for large-scale applications [19–20]. Different areas of life from using sustainable manufacturing is shown in Figure 1.4.

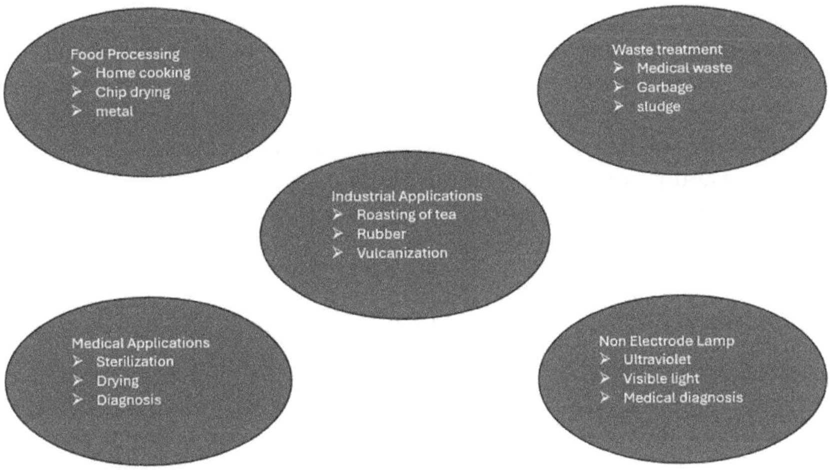

Figure 1.4 Applications of sustainable manufacturing.

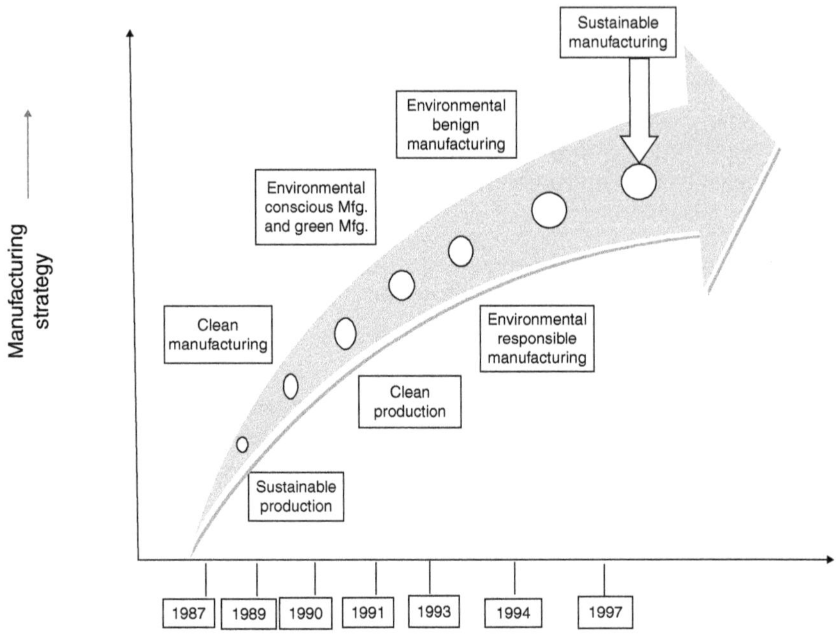

Figure 1.5 Evolution of sustainable manufacturing.

1.4.2 Historical evolution of sustainable manufacturing

Biodiversity and ecological imbalances have become the focus of policy makers, governments, and organizations for development. Sustainable development is defined as "development that meets the needs of the present without compromising the ability of the world to meet its future needs". Securing biodiversity and development requires the focus of organizations, which is achieved through sustainable manufacturing. For example, sustainable production, environmentally conscious, cleaner production, environmentally responsible manufacturing, clean manufacturing, green manufacturing, environmentally friendly manufacturing, and sustainable manufacturing, as shown in Figure 1.5.

1.5 BIOMATERIALS AND THEIR PROPERTIES

Bacterial activity in bone defects can further impair the bone's capacity to heal itself. Chronic viral disorders and high-energy injuries can also lead to infected bone deformities. Injuries are a worldwide public health concern, according to the World Health Organization (WHO). In wealthy nations, between 3 and 9 million injuries are reported each year. As the economy and transportation have grown, over 1.2 million deaths are attributed to high-energy injuries sustained in traffic. In European nations, the number of fatalities from these injuries has increased in the past 30 years. Open comminute fractures can be caused by high-energy traumas to the acuteness. Serious soft tissue injury, bone abnormalities, infections, and eventually non-union, are frequently linked to these types of accidents. A weakened immune system makes it easy for high-energy injuries to progress to severe osteomyelitis when a bacterial infection is introduced. Osteomyelitis is still a serious medical issue that is hard to totally eradicate, especially when it co-occurs with significant bone abnormalities. Since *Staphylococcus aureus* is thought to be responsible for 80% of human osteomyelitis, it is the primary bacterial pathogen [21].

In order to offer a viable therapeutic option for infected bone deformities, novel biomaterials with antibacterial and osteoinductive capabilities were created. Because of their broad bactericidal range and superior biocompatibility, novel antibacterial medications such as quantified chitosan and nanosilver (AgNPs) have promising potential to be used therapeutically . Nonetheless, a variety of growth factors, including vascular endothelial growth factor, insulin-like growth factors, and basic fibroblast growth factor, can also strongly stimulate osteogenesis and angiogenesis.

1.5.1 Orthopedic implant

The mechanical requirements of an implant must be taken into account based on its intended use. Elasticity is linked to shear stress and strength to loading. Implant materials used in orthopedics must withstand a variety of stresses, including shearing, twisting, and bending, during repeated upload/download cycles.

Rigidity is the intrinsic property of a solid body to oppose change in shape or dimension. As the stress rises, micro- fractures developed and additional plastic deformations were observed; ultimately, the material broke up. Instances like implanted materials display constant rigidity, but, in the case of bones, it is not. Bone tissue has been physiologically considered as an anisotropic material. Anisotropy refers to a material being non- homogeneous mechanically depending on the direction their measurement is found. Therefore, the physical properties of the bones are anisotropic depending on the orientation of mechanical loading.

The loading stress is the main factor in the unique background of a pelvic fracture described above. Here, a load deformation curve can be created by transforming the normal load curve. The hardness of an implantation device can now be calculated using this transformed diagram and compared to a healthy bone (as in Young's modulus). Additionally, it can be used in a simulation to assess the stiffness of artificial bones that mimic certain bone disorders, such as osteoporotic bone. The plastic region itself can be used to

Table 1.2 Characteristics of biomaterials and bone

Sl No	*Materials*	*Fracture toughness (Mpa)*	*Ultimate tensile strength (Mpa)*	*Youngs modulus (Mpa)*
1	Titanium	105–125	900	80
2	Stainless steel	200	540–1000	1001
3	Cobalt	240	900–1540	100
4	Cortical bone	10–30	130–150	2–12

determine the ultimate stress that caused the material to fracture. Therefore, the parameters that serve as the foundation for characterizing any mechanical implant material are rigidity and failure-load. The characteristics of biomaterials and bone is illustrated in Table 1.2.

1.5.2 Additive manufacturing of orthopedic implants

Metal additive manufacturing, also known as metal 3D printing, is one of the most successful technologies that dominates a huge space in the field of orthopedics. This method is used to fabricate large numbers of functional medical devices through this technique. This advanced technology can quickly manufacture implants in every dimension and size. In the past, studies on metallic biomaterials were not carried out because polymeric and ceramic biomaterials were successful. But additive manufacturing offers the opportunity to tailor the mechanical properties of metallic biomaterials based on topologically ordered volume-porous biomaterials. Unlike traditional manufacturing methods, which often involve casting or subtractive machining, these machines utilize a layer-by-layer approach to build intricate and highly precise metal structures which can be used in the medical field for designing implants. This could provide biomaterials with a range of mechanical properties, from trabecular bone to cortical bone. Additionally, topologically ordered volume-porous metallic biomaterials also offer the possibility for adjusting other properties, such as fluid flow and mass transport characteristics. This allows the design of metallic biomaterials with new properties so that they are favorable for bone tissue regeneration and bony ingrowth. The third technique is additive manufacturing, which makes fully patient-specific implants a design option. Finally, volume-porous biomaterials allow for large pore spaces, which would be useful for bio-functionalization and infection prevention.

1.5.3 Bio-functionalization of implants

Bio-functionalization is a surface modification technique, where a particular biological functionality, placed on the surface of a material, is utilized without altering its bulk characteristics. This approach enables one to turn materials that are typically non-reactive to biological systems—into active bio-materials. For example, the term bioactivity was first used because of the bonding ability of implanted glasses, known as bio glasses, to living bones or bones made of calcium-based ceramics. Scope of the term bioactivity includes a number of biological activities like adhesion of cells and osteogenesis, localized concentration of growth factors and cytokines, mobilization of stem cells, bactericidal activity as well as pertaining to the immune system. In relation to dental and orthopedic implants, the bioactivity of the materials can be enhanced by a set of different approaches which may be classified into physical, chemical, or combined modifications. These methods involve the alteration of surface contour at the micro- and nano-scale, modification of surface properties such as wettability and chemistry, and application of surface layers. The inorganic modifications focus mainly on the application of superficial implants using biomimetic calcium phosphate coatings. In organic modifications, the materials are coated with (bio)polymers, peptides, and proteins. It also helps in prevention of infection by inhibiting bacterial proliferation, and at the same time, it helps in accommodating the rate at which the implants degrade.

1.5.4 Prevention of infection

Preventing and treating infections linked to implants and biomaterials is of utmost importance in orthopedic surgery. These specific populations include trauma patients who must have lengthy surgery with huge open wounds made for the installation of massive implants, as well as orthopedic oncologic patients whose immune systems were compromised by chemotherapy and/or radiation therapy. Metallic biomaterials that reduce the risk of infection may become extremely important in many of these situations.

Biomaterials that eliminate or drastically lower the risk of infections may be based on physical mechanisms or (bio)chemical antibacterial agents, similar to the case of bio-functionalization approaches intended to improve performance for bone tissue regeneration. Antibiotics, antimicrobial peptides, or inorganic (mostly metallic) antibacterial agents like copper, zinc, or silver, are frequently used in (bio)chemical methods. Furthermore, recent research has demonstrated the potential for synergy with the simultaneous administration of antibiotics and inorganic antibacterial agents at the same site of action. Physically, it has been found that big aspect ratio nano-patterns can both kill bacteria and affect how well they adhere to surfaces.

Numerous natural surfaces with these kinds of nano-patterns, such as cicada and dragonfly wings, have also been shown to exhibit antibacterial properties. Mechanisms that have been proposed include how mechanical stresses and severe deformations may cause bacteria to be killed by nano-patterns. In this way, the physical processes influencing stem cell fate are comparable to those preventing infections. Therefore, it might be feasible to incorporate both kinds of functions into the same kinds of biomaterials. Furthermore, it is difficult to fabricate nano-patterns on metallic surfaces efficiently; therefore, more accurate and efficient methods must be created [22].

1.5.5 Biodegradable metallic biomaterials

Over the past 20 years, biodegradable materials (BMs) have been a top concern for short-term biomedical implants. These substances, which include iron alloys, magnesium, and zinc, are made to gradually disappear in the body after promoting tissue repair. BMs have more mechanical strength and function better as bone implants and cardiovascular stents than their polymer counterparts. In biomedical implants, BMs are preferred over non-biodegradable metals such as titanium alloys and stainless steel. They play a key role in bone tissue replacement and repair in orthopedics, prosthodontics, and other fields. They are a great option because of their special mechanical and physical properties, which include low density, high specific strength, and an elastic modulus comparable to the human cortical bone. After the suggested recovery period, traditional metals need to be surgically removed, which is uncomfortable and expensive. Additionally, these metals are far more rigid than human bone, which can make treating some fractures more difficult. By efficiently addressing these problems, BMs encourage faster bone growth and repair.

Benefits and Uses in Medicine: Because of their special qualities and advantages over conventional materials, biodegradable metals and their alloys have become more and more popular in biomedical applications [23].

Biomaterials in Composite Form: Despite the fact that metallic biomaterials have many beneficial qualities that can be further enhanced through additive manufacturing and logical design, other types of biomaterials, like ceramics and polymers, might provide extra features or even increase the range of potential properties. As a result, biomaterial composites that combine several types of biomaterials may be very valuable. This class of biomaterials has been the subject of continuous research for several years. But with more and more metallic, ceramic, and polymeric elements that can be mixed together, new possibilities open up. More generally, multilateral additive manufacturing and post-additive manufacturing are examples of innovative processing methods that could enable the blending of numerous materials.

1.5.6 Future trends in biomanufacturing of implants

Though much more work needs to be done before the point of practical applicability is achieved, preliminary research indicates that nanoparticles can be used in orthopedic applications. In order to improve bone formation with a shorter treatment duration and a quicker return to function, the main goal of current bone tissue engineering research is to create biocompatible scaffolds that partially replace normal tissues while maintaining interaction with their surroundings, perceiving and responding to environmental cues, and appropriately influencing cellular processes. In order to achieve high performance, design strategies that use nano-materials and nano fabrication techniques will be further developed and purposed. It is necessary to fully comprehend the molecular mechanisms governing the interaction between cells and nano-materials. Because there are legitimate worries about the toxicity of nanoparticles produced as a result of wear and strain, it is also crucial to exercise extreme caution when assessing the biosafety of nano-materials and minimizing any potential consequences. Additionally, the metals' behavior and material characteristics change dramatically from the micro to the nanoscale, so it is necessary to properly study their potential toxicity at the nanoscale. Traditional implants treated by nanotechnology have better qualities than nanostructure implants composed of nanoparticles. This removes the possibility of the nanoparticles to travel throughout the body and cause toxicity. Because of these possible problems, a number of restrictions have been planned.

Businesses are still apprehensive about creating nanostructure implants and prosthetics, mostly because of concerns about their toxicity and therapeutic efficacy, as well as the perceived high cost. Wear and strain cause nanoparticles to develop, which raises questions about their toxicity. In contrast to the micro-scale, the metals exhibit distinct behavior and material characteristics at the nanoscale. Although nanotechnology is still in its infancy, it has the potential to improve orthopedic research, diagnosis, and treatment. Successful companies and services demonstrate that nanotechnology will undoubtedly be used in future medical treatments. It might lower the price of some common medications and enable new applications for medications that would not have been thought of otherwise. More precise therapy is made possible by nanotechnology, which prolongs the life of implants while lowering the risk of infection and promoting better bone and tendon regeneration. The potential advantages of nanomedicine—a word used in science to describe a variety of medical applications utilizing items of the nano size range—have only gradually become evident after extensive investigation, particularly with regard to orthopaedic problems. However, much more investigation is required to fully examine its safety profile and possible utility [24–27].

1.6 CONCLUSION

Biomaterials play a brilliant role in healthcare by providing solutions to injuries, diseases, and disabilities. The purpose of orthopedic implants is to cure bone defects and fractures by reducing the fracture, aligning the pieces, and maintaining the reduction. Manufacturing with 3D printing technology is one of the most efficient processes that can be used in developing the healthcare industry, as it makes easier to access all tissues, organs, and other body part's diseases. The main purpose of biodegradable materials is to minimize pollution in the environment, recycle the waste, and make it environment friendly. And, sustainable manufacturing is used to reduce corrosion and wear in aerospace engines, power plants, automobiles, etc.

REFERENCES

1. C. Gao, S. Peng, P. Feng, C. Shuai, Bone biomaterials and interactions with stem cells. *Bone Res. 5* (2017) 1–33. https://doi.org/10.1038/boneres.2017.59
2. S. S. Bhatti, J. Singh, 3D printing of biomaterials for biomedical applications: a review, *IJIDeM* (2023).
3. P. Trucillo, Biomaterials for drug delivery and human applications, *Materials 17* (2024) 456. https://doi.org/10.3390/ma17020456
4. J.G.B. Derraik, The pollution of the marine environment by plastic debris: a review, *Mar. Pollut. Bull. 44* (9) (2002) 842–852.
5. J.-P. Lange, Towards circular carbo-chemicals: the metamorphosis of petrochemicals, *Energy Environ. Sci. 14* (2021) 4358–4376.
6. Tian, L., van Putten, R.-J., Gruter, M., Dusselier, M., & Lange, J.-P. (2022). *Biodegradable polymers in the circular plastics economy.* In M. Dusselier & J.-P. Lange (Eds.), Biodegradable Polymers in the Circular Plastics Economy, Wiley-VCH, Weinheim, Germany, pp. 58–81.
7. A. Chamas, H. Moon, J. Zheng, Y. Qiu, T. Tabassum, J.H. Jang, M. Abu-Omar, S. L. Scott, S. Suh, Degradation rates of plastics in the environment, *ACS Sustain. Chem. Eng. 8* (2020) 3494–3511.
8. Nakayama, A., Yamano, N., & Kawasaki, N. (2019). *Biodegradation in seawater of aliphatic polyesters.* Polymer Degradation and Stability, 166, 290–299. https://doi.org/10.1016/j.polymdegradstab.2019.06.006.
9. Dilkes-Hoffman, L. S., Lant, P. A., Laycock, B., & Pratt, S. (2019). *The rate of biodegradation of PHA bioplastics in the marine environment: A meta-study.* Marine Pollution Bulletin, 142, 15–24. https://doi.org/10.1016/j.marpolbul.2019.03.020.
10. B. Ghanbarzadeh, H. Almasi, Biodegradation-life of science, InTech Publications, Croatia 1 (2013) 141–186; b) T. D. Moshood, G. Nawanir, F. Mahmud, F. Mohamad, M. H. Ahmad, A. A. Ghani, Green product innovation: a means towards achieving global sustainable product within biodegradable plastic industry, *Curr. Res. Green Sustain. Chem. 5* (2022), 100273.
11. J. E. Weinstein, J. L. Dekle, R. R. Leads, R. A. Hunter, Degradation of bio-based and biodegradable plastics in a salt marsh habitat: another potential source of microplastics in coastal waters, *Mar. Pollut. Bull. 160* (2020) 111518.

12. H. Saygin, A. Baysal, Similarities and discrepancies between bio-based and conventional submicron-sized plastics: in relation to clinically important bacteria, *Bull. Environ. Contam. Toxicol. 105* (2020) 26–35.
13. C. Dussud, C. Hudec, M. George, P. Fabre, P. Higgs, S. Bruzaud, A.-M. Delort, B. Eyheraguibel, A.-L. Meistertzheim, J. Jacquin, Colonization of non-biodegradable and biodegradable plastics by marine microorganisms, *Front. Microbiol. 9* (2018) 1571.
14. Grøndahl, L., Jack, K. S., & Goonasekera, C. S., "Composite materials for bone repair," in *Biomedical Composites*, 2nd ed., ed. L. Ambrosio, Woodhead Publishing (Elsevier), Cambridge, UK, 2017, pp. 83–110.
15. F. Ali, S. N. Kalva, K. H. Mroue, K. S. Keyan, Y. Tong, O. M. Khan, et al., "Degradation assessment of Mg-incorporated 3D printed PLA scaffolds for biomedical applications," *Bioprinting*, vol. 35, 2023, e00302.
16. M. Singh, T. Ohji, R. Asthana, "Green and Sustainable Manufacturing of Advanced Materials—Progress and Prospects," in *Green and Sustainable Manufacturing of Advanced Materials*, eds. M. Singh, T. Ohji, and R. Asthana, Elsevier (Woodhead Publishing), Amsterdam, The Netherlands, 2015, pp. 3–10.
17. H. Zhou, M. Nabiyouni, S.B. Bhaduri, Microwave assisted apatite coating deposition on Ti6Al4V implants, *Mater. Sci. Eng. C. 33* (2013), 4435–4443.
18. R.R. Mishra, A.K. Sharma, A review of research trends in microwave processing of metal-based materials and opportunities in microwave metal casting, *Crit. Rev. Solid State Mate. Sci. 41* (2016) 217–255.
19. R.I. Badiger, S. Narendranath, M. Srinath, A.M. Hebbale, Effect of power input on metallurgical and mechanical characteristics of Inconel-625 welded joints processed through microwave hybrid heating, *Trans. Indian Inst. Met.* 72 (2019) 811–824.
20. N.K. Bhoi, H. Singh, S. Pratap,A study on microwave susceptor material for hybrid heating. *J. Phys. Conf. Ser.* 1240 (2019) 012097.
21. H. Lu, Y. Liu, J. Guo, et al., Biomaterials with antibacterial and osteoinductive properties to repair infected bone defects. *Int. J. Mol. Sci. 17* (2016) 334.
22. Kiradzhiyska, D. D., & Mantcheva, R. D, Mantcheve overview of biocompatible materials and their use in medicine. *Folia Medica (Plovdiv)*, 61(1), 34–40 (2019). https://doi.org/10.2478/folmed-2018-0038.
23. Bobbert, F. S. L., Lietaert, K., Eftekhari, A. A., Pouran, B., Ahmadi, S. M., Weinans, H., & Zadpoor, A. A., "Additively manufactured metallic porous biomaterials based on minimal surfaces: A unique combination of topological, mechanical, and mass transport properties," *Acta Biomaterialia*, 53, 572–584 (2017). https://doi.org/10.1016/j.actbio.2017.02.024.
24. D. Hernandez-Escobar, S. Champagne, H. Yilmazer, B. Dikici, C.J. Boehlert, H. Hermawan, Current status and perspectives of zinc-based absorbable alloys for biomedical applications. *Acta Biomaterialia*, vol. 97, 2019, pp. 1–22.
25. Y. Liu, L. Shi, L. Su, H. C. van der Mei, P. C. Jutte, Y. Ren, H. J. Busscher,"Nanotechnology-based antimicrobials and delivery systems for

biofilm-infection control," *Chemical Society Reviews*, vol. 48, no. 2, pp. 428–446, 2019.https://doi.org/10.1039/C7CS00807D.
26. M. Geetha, A.K. Singh, R. Asokamani, A.K. Gogia AK, Ti-based biomaterials, the ultimate choice for orthopadic implants: a review. *Prog. Mater. Sci. 54*(3) (2009)397–425640
27. C.S. Wong, A.D. Schaffner, *Breast implants*. Statpearls Publishing, Treasure Island, FL.

Chapter 2

Recent developments in composite materials for biomedical applications

Abhijit Saha, Rajeev Ranjan, Ashok Kumar Yadav, Aqueel Ahmad, and Ashwani Kumar

2.1 INTRODUCTION

Wattle and daub, the earliest known composite material, was utilized in ancient times to build walls [1]. However, this material has largely been replaced by concrete, a composite composed of cement and aggregates like gravel. Concrete production now reaches millions of tons annually due to its impressive compressive strength, though its tensile strength is relatively low. To enhance its performance under tension and minimize cracking, steel reinforcements are often embedded [2–9]. Fiber-reinforced composites (FRPs), particularly glass-reinforced plastics (GRP) and carbon fiber-reinforced composites (CFRC), have also gained significant popularity. These composites integrate fibers like glass or carbon into a matrix material, commonly epoxy resin, to achieve strength and flexibility [10–15].

There are several types of composites, including advanced composites, metal matrix composites, ceramic matrix composites, polymer matrix composites, and even wood-based composites [16–22]. The matrix material determines the composite's classification, while the inclusion of high-strength, low-density fibers enhances properties like stiffness and elasticity [23–28]. These materials also offer chemical, thermal, and creep resistance, making them indispensable in industries like construction, automotive, and aerospace [29–30].

In biomedical engineering, composite materials have revolutionized treatment methods. Researchers develop biomaterials to repair or replace damaged tissues, using insights from biology and engineering [31–35]. These materials are tailored for in vitro and in vivo applications by adjusting factors like fiber orientation, particle size, and matrix type [36]. Composite biomaterials are utilized for medical implants, including stents and pacemakers, which address heart and vascular conditions [37]. Stents made from biodegradable composites can dissolve after use, reducing complications, while advanced pacemaker designs now incorporate corrosion-resistant composites instead of traditional metals—improving patient outcomes [38–40].

DOI: 10.1201/9781003581192-2

Dental medicine has also embraced composites for cavity fillings, tooth replacements, and implants [41–44]. Materials like hydroxyapatite and titanium, which mimic natural bone and offer high strength, have replaced older silver amalgams. Similarly, advanced bone repair solutions use composites that promote healing and integrate with the body. These materials can deliver medications or provide structural support while degrading naturally over time.

Composites have even transformed orthopedics, with 3D-printed casts and prosthetics —offering lightweight, durable, and customizable solutions [45–50]. Innovations in joint replacements use composites to mimic the natural movement of hips and knees, ensuring durability and biocompatibility [51]. These advancements highlight the versatility and growing importance of composite materials across medical and engineering applications.

This research explores the potential of composite biomaterials for healthcare, focusing on their role in diagnostics, treatment, and regenerative medicine. As these materials evolve, they continue to improve patient recovery, quality of life, and the performance of medical devices.

2.2 COMPOSITE BIOMATERIALS AND THEIR ROLES

Composite biomaterials have found significant utility in the medical sector, performing a variety of crucial functions, from aiding in diagnostics to interacting with biological systems. These materials hold the potential to, one day, serve as replacements for organs damaged by disease or injury, thanks to their ability to be fine-tuned. The medical industry values composite biomaterials for their large-scale production capabilities and their versatile chemical, mechanical, and physical properties [52–60]. Although synthetic and natural biomaterials have been utilized for decades, composites represent a relatively recent advancement in biomedical engineering. Breakthroughs in developing cutting-edge medical devices and ongoing enhancements to these materials have led to higher survival rates after illnesses or accidents, along with extended lifespan and improved well-being. Composite biomaterials are typically categorized into three main types: particle-reinforced, fiber-reinforced, and structural composites. The unique properties of composite biomaterials often differ significantly from those of their individual components (the matrix and inclusions), as they are composed of a combination of diverse materials.

2.3 CARDIOVASCULAR APPLICATIONS

The heart and blood vessels play a vital role in the body's regulatory functions, forming a physiological network that supports the nourishment and maintenance of various organs. By continuously circulating blood, the heart ensures the removal of metabolic waste through the arterial system.

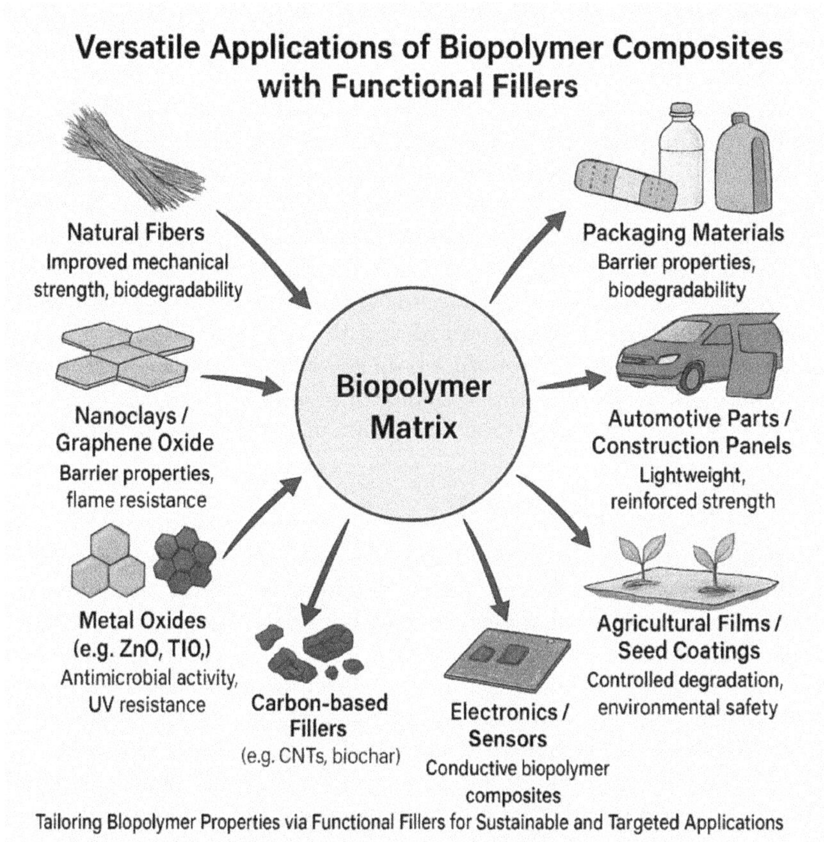

Figure 2.1 Potential application of biopolymers with different fillers [17].

Cardiovascular conditions, including congenital issues, coronary artery disease (CAD), and arrhythmias, often necessitate medical intervention. In some cases, surgical procedures are required to repair or replace damaged components of the cardiovascular system. Biomaterials like stents and pacemakers are widely used in cardiac treatments [61, 5, 63–67]. To treat blockages in blood vessels found in the heart, arteries, veins, and other places, stents are frequently used. These devices, often inserted during angioplasty procedures, help maintain open blood flow and prevent clot formation [68, 45]. Traditional stents are made from materials like stainless steel, titanium, magnesium alloys, and polymers. However, newer composite materials, including metal-polymer matrix composites, are gaining attention due to their advantages. These materials are cost-effective, biodegradable, customizable, and capable of reducing vascular irritation. Composite stents are designed to offer temporary support and can biodegrade over time—minimizing long-term complications. Their biocompatibility stems from research into optimizing interactions between the stent surface and surrounding tissues [69–73].

Similarly, pacemakers represent a groundbreaking development in biomedical engineering. These compact devices regulate abnormal heart rhythms and ensure proper blood circulation. A pacemaker typically comprises a lithium-ion battery, lead, connector block, and protective casing, which houses the pulse generator and other components. It is surgically implanted near the subclavian vein, with a conductive tip positioned in the targeted heart chamber to maintain connectivity. Recently, eco-friendly composite materials are being introduced to replace traditional platinum components in pacemakers, offering both environmental benefits and lightweight designs. These advancements have also extended to replacing heavy metal covers with more adaptable composite materials in medical devices.

2.4 DENTAL APPLICATIONS

The incisors, canines, premolars, and molars—each play unique roles in the process of breaking down food for digestion. While the premolars and molars handle most of the chewing and grinding, the canine teeth specialize in tearing food apart. The incisors, located at the front, are primarily responsible for cutting food into smaller pieces. This intricate dental arrangement has been crucial in the evolution of language and the use of symbols [74]. However, the dental system is vulnerable to various challenges, including diseases, injuries, and congenital abnormalities. Genetic factors can contribute to issues like improper tooth development or loss. Common dental issues include plaque buildup and cavities, with the latter caused by bacterial biofilms producing lactic acid that erodes tooth enamel. Poor nutrition, especially in children, has been linked to the increasing prevalence of cavities. Furthermore, physical trauma to the mouth can damage teeth or heighten the risk of dental infections. The rise in accidents and violence over recent decades has exacerbated head and dental injuries.

Dental implants that replace lost teeth are increasingly using composite biomaterials such as polymer matrix composites. These materials mimic the chemical composition of natural dentine and enamel, offering better biocompatibility compared to traditional metallic biomaterials like silver amalgam. However, acrylic resins lack the strength needed for prosthetic molars, and silver-mercury amalgams pose significant safety risks. Dental implant procedures involve exposing the underlying bone, drilling a hole for the implant screw, and attaching an artificial tooth. Alternatives such as dental bridges and dentures provide long-term solutions but come with their own limitations, including discomfort when removable prostheses are used [75].

To improve performance, advanced materials like high-strength polycarbonates reinforced with glass are used in some dental devices due to their superior corrosion resistance. Durable dental bridges often rely on ultra-high molecular weight polyethylene. Methacrylic matrix composites, infused with fibers and inorganic particles, are superior to conventional polymer composites in both mechanical strength and aesthetics [76]. Titanium-hydroxyapatite has also gained attention as a potential dental material. Hydroxyapatite, known for its bioactive compatibility, is applied to the implant's lower portion, while titanium's exceptional strength makes it suitable for the upper structure.

2.5 ARTIFICIAL CARTILAGE

Cartilage is a softer, more flexible form of tissue compared to bone, found in areas such as the ears, nose, ribs, and joints. In adulthood, its primary role is to support and connect skeletal structures. During early development, cartilage is gradually replaced by harder bone tissue as the skeleton matures. Polymeric composites are often employed to replace cartilage that is either congenitally absent or damaged by injury or illness. One example is poly [2-hydroxyethyl methacrylate] (PHEMA), chemically crosslinked with polyethylene terephthalate (PET), a combination whose performance relies on the interaction between its components. Ultra-high molecular weight polyethylene crosslinked with hyaluronic acid is another often-employed substance that is well-known for its durability in meniscal, intervertebral fibrocartilage, and articular cartilage replication [77].

The primary limitations of artificial cartilage include wear and material degradation caused by repetitive stress. Continuous research is aimed at overcoming these challenges. In some cases, polymeric biomaterials like injectable hydrogels are used alongside composite materials to minimize wear and enhance healing.

2.6 ARTIFICIAL LIGAMENT

Tough, fibrous fibers called ligaments connect cartilage to bones. ACL tears are a common injury, especially in those who are physically active. Composite and polymer-based biomaterials can be used to replace or repair damaged or diseased joints. However, like synthetic cartilage, artificial ligaments are susceptible to deterioration over time as a result of repeated stress. Factors such as synovial membrane inflammation, poor strength under bending and twisting pressures, and inadequate resistance to abrasion are frequently linked to long-term failure [78].

To mitigate these challenges, biocompatible composite biomaterials, such as those made from polylactic acid and hyaluronic acid ester, are employed as prosthetic ligaments. These materials help promote natural ligament healing by reducing reliance on prosthetics. Research has shown that ultra-high-molecular-weight polyethylene (UHMWPE) reinforced with ethylene-butene copolymers exhibits excellent fatigue resistance when optimized for specific copolymer compositions and orientations. Building on this, prosthetic ligaments using such fatigue-resistant materials have been developed.

Animal studies have indicated that using polyethylene terephthalate (PET)-reinforced polyhydroxyethyl methacrylate (PHEMA) in cartilage replacements can lead to synovitis [79]. Despite this, these materials remain widely-used. A high-strength composite material that combines collagen matrix and terephthalate polyester fibers has been created to solve this problem. This substance did not adversely affect the surrounding tissues. However, it was less effective in preventing fibrous tissue growth and infiltration between the prosthesis and adjacent bones, compared to alternative materials. A typical artificial leg system is represented in Figure 2.2.

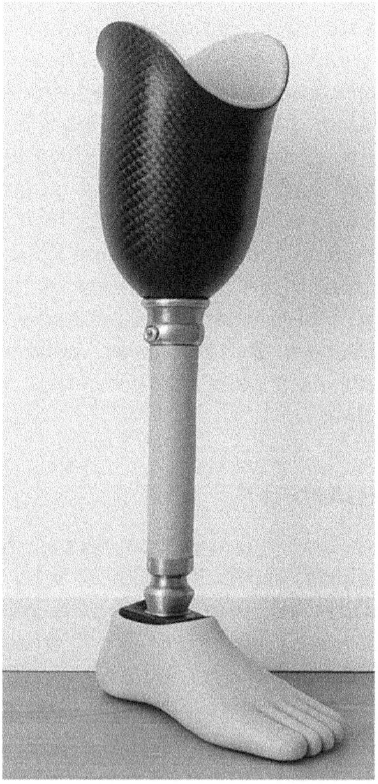

Figure 2.2 Photograph of a typical prosthetic leg showing socket, shaft and foot [26].

2.7 JOINT PROSTHESES

Joints are the points where two or more bones meet, allowing movement and providing structural support for the body. The human body contains around 300 joints, which are constantly in motion, making them susceptible to damage from injuries like fractures or dislocations, as well as conditions such as arthritis. In severe cases of arthritis or physical trauma, total joint replacement may become necessary. However, less severe joint damage can sometimes be treated with medication or therapeutic approaches that encourage natural healing [80].

In joint replacement surgery, specific techniques are employed to attach prosthetic components to the affected bones. For example, in a knee replacement, the prosthetic femur and tibia parts are secured to their respective bones by cutting and preparing the bone surfaces. Once in place, the prosthetic knee provides a similar range of motion to a healthy joint. Similarly, artificial hip joints are used to restore function to damaged hips. The femoral stem and ball are inserted into the femur, while the acetabular cup is anchored to the pelvis using a fixation material.

Metals and metal composites are often used for these prosthetic components due to their durability under high stress and compression. For the hip joint, the ball is commonly made of composite metals, which are more wear-resistant compared to ceramic materials [81]. In cases of minor hip injuries, devices like bone plates, screws, and wires aid in recovery. These components are typically made of metal or composite biomaterials capable of withstanding substantial tensile, compressive, and bending forces. Studies have evaluated the bending properties of bone plates made from various materials, including metals, polymers, and composites.

2.8 BONE REPAIR

Composite materials have shown significant promise in treating bone fractures. Their appearance closely resembles natural bone, and their ability to support bone growth and healing, combined with their interactions with other substances, makes them excellent osteoconductive agents. These materials act as temporary scaffolds that degrade on their own once their function is complete. Furthermore, composites are adaptable for use in internal fixation systems, a role previously dominated by metals [82]. Although metal implants are durable, they can cause discomfort due to their stiffness and potential for corrosion.

Polymer composites offer a solution to these challenges. For instance, carbon fiber-based polymers mimic the strength of natural bone, providing robust support during the healing process. These materials are also resistant to corrosion.

Bone cement, another key material in orthopedics, is utilized for tasks ranging from repairing fractures to securing artificial joints. Functionally similar to adhesive glue [Functionally similar to an adhesive], it creates a strong bond between prosthetics and bone by filling voids and hardening into a permanent state after polymerization. Unlike traditional cotton or plaster casts, those made from fiberglass, polyester fibers, and polyurethane matrices offer superior properties, including greater durability, moisture resistance, and X-ray visibility [83]. Despite being more difficult to remove, these benefits outweigh the drawbacks.

Recent advancements in 3D printing have introduced innovative composite casting techniques. These casts feature a web-like structure that enhances airflow while maintaining the usual advantages of composite materials. Additionally, they enable the creation of personalized ergonomic designs tailored to individual patients. As the technology continues to improve, 3D printing could become widely adopted for orthopedic applications. Composite materials are also revolutionizing external prosthetics, replacing traditional options like wood, metal, and leather. By combining the strengths of these materials, composites provide lightweight, durable, and easily transportable alternatives, making them highly advantageous for modern medical use.

2.9 CONCLUSIONS

Composites are highly versatile materials, making them suitable for a broad spectrum of applications. Their unique combination of properties has played a pivotal role in the development of biomaterials used to repair or replace various human tissues and organs. As a result, they have become integral to the biomedical field. The enhanced physical, mechanical, and chemical characteristics of composite biomaterials often make them superior to traditional metal and polymer alternatives in numerous contexts. As technology develops, more study into new and advanced composites has encouraging potential to influence biomaterial engineering and innovation in the future. The integration of composites into medical applications has revolutionized implant design, enabling the creation of materials with diverse mechanical and biological functionalities.

REFERENCES

1. Egbo, M. K. (2021). A fundamental review on composite materials and some of their applications in biomedical engineering. *J. King Saud Univ.-Eng. Sci.*, 33(8), 557–568.
2. Pelc, M., Vilimkova Kahankova, R., Blaszczyszyn, M., Mikolajewski, D., Konieczny, M., Khoma, V., Kawala-Sterniuk, A. (2023). Initial study on an expert system for spine diseases screening using inertial measurement unit. *Sci. Rep.*, 13(1), 10440.

3. Ahmed, A., Yadav, A. K., Singh, A., Singh, D. K. (2023). Multi-response optimization to improve the performance and emissions characteristics of a VCR engine fueled with microalgae spirulina (L.): A response surface methodology approach coupled with genetic algorithm. *Environ. Dev. Sustain.*, 27, 3313–3341.
4. Yadav, A. K., Khan, M. E., Pal, A., Dubey, A. M. (2016). Performance and emission characteristics of a transportation diesel engine operated with non-edible vegetable oils biodiesel. *Case Stud. Therm. Eng.*, 8, 236–244.
5. Dewangan, A., Ahmad, A., Yadav, A. K. (2024). Innovative research on waste tire recycling for sustainable biofuel production: Assessment of its usability on multi-cylinder diesel engine employing constant injection of oxyhydrogen and biogas through a premixing device. *Int. J. Hydrogen Energy,* 84, 155–163.
6. Dubey, A. M., Ram, R., Yadav, A. K. (2016). Ion cell performance using single particle representation of battery electrode. *J. of Electro Analytical Chemistry*, 768, 11–17.
7. Yadav, A. K., Khan, M. E., Pal, A. (2016). Biodiesel production from Nerium Oleander (Thevetia peruviana) oil through conventional and ultrasonic irradiation methods. *Energy Sources, Part A*, 38(23), 3447–3452.
8. Yadav, A. K., Khan, M. E., Pal, A. (2016). A comparative study on ultrasonic cavitation and mechanical stirring method towards efficient production of biodiesel from non-edible oils and performance testing on a C.I. *Engine, Int. J. of Envt. & Waste Managt.*, 18(4), 349–367.
9. Sharma, G., Dewangan, A. K., Yadav, A. K., Ahmad, A. (2024). Current status of research on hydrogen generation, storage and transportation technologies: A state-of-the-art review towards sustainable energy. *Process Saf. Environ. Prot.*, 191, 1445–1460.
10. Yadav, A. K., Khan, M. E., Pal, A. (2018). Ultrasonic assisted production of biodiesel from karabi oil using heterogeneous catalyst. *Biofuels*, 9(1), 101–112.
11. Ahmad, A., Yadav, A. K., Pal, A., Hasan, S. (2025). A novel intensified anaerobic co-digestion process for high-quality biomethane production using ultrasound energy: Optimization and robustness tests with ML-RSM-TLBO algorithm. *Energy Convers. Manag.*, 325, 119408.
12. Ahmad, A., Yadav, A. K., Hasan, S. (2025). A novel waste-to-energy conversion plant based on catalytic pyrolytic conditions: Modeling and optimization using supervised machine learning and desirability-driven methodologies. *Energy*, 317, 134648.
13. Yadav, A. K., Vinay, Singh, B. (2018). Optimization of biodiesel production from annona squamosa seeds oil using response surface methodology and its characterization. *Energy Sources. Part A: Recovery, Utilization, and Environmental Effects*, 40(9), 1051–1059.
14. Dewangan, A., Yadav, A. K., Mallick, A. (2018). Current scenario of biodiesel development in India: Prospects and challenges. *Energy Sources, Part A*, 40(20), 2494–2501.
15. Yadav, A. K., Khan, M. E., Pal, A. (2018). Performance and emission characteristics of a stationary diesel engine fuelled by Schleichera oleosa oil methyl ester (SOME) produced through hydrodynamic cavitation process. *Egypt. J. of Petroleum*, 27(1), 89–93.

16. Yadav, A. K., Khan, M. E., Pal, A. (2018). Performance, emission and combustion characteristics of an Indica diesel engine operated with yellow oleander (Thevetia peruviana) oil biodiesel produced through hydrodynamic cavitation method. *Int. J. of Ambient Energy*, 39(4), 365–371.
17. Aslam Khan, M. U., Abd Razak, S. I., Al Arjan, W. S., Nazir, S., Sahaya Anand, T. J., Mehboob, H., Amin, R. (2021). Recent advances in biopolymeric composite materials for tissue engineering and regenerative medicines: A review. *Molecules*, 26(3), 619.
18. Khan, I. A., Singh, S. K., Pal, A., Yadav, A. K. (2020). Efficient production of biodiesel from Cannabis sativa oil using intensified transesterication (hydrodynamic cavitation) method. *Energy Sources, Part A*, 42(20), 2461–2470.
19. Dewangan, A., Yadav, A. K., Mallick, A. (2020). Optimization of biodiesel production and engine performance from underutilized Simarouba oil in compression ignition engine. *Int. J. Oil, Gas and Coal Tech.*, 25(3), 357.
20. Vinay, Singh, B., Yadav, A. K. (2020). Optimization of performance and emission characteristics of CI engine fuelled with Mahua oil methyl ester-diesel blend using response surface methodology. *International Journal of Ambient Energy*, 44(6), 674–685.
21. Dubey, A. M., Kumar, A., Yadav, A. K. (2017). Wear behaviour of friction stir weld joint of cast Al (4–10%) Cu alloy welded at different operating parameters. *J. of Materials Processing Tech.*, 240, 87–97.
22. Yadav, A. K., Khan, M. E., Pal, A. (2017). Biodiesel production from oleander (Thevetia peruviana) oil and its performance testing on a diesel engine. *Korean J. Chem. Eng.*, 34(2), 340–345.
23. Khan, O., Khan, M. E., Yadav, A. K., Sharma, D. (2017). The ultrasonic assisted optimization of biodiesel production from Eucalyptus oil. *Energy Sources, Part A*, 39(13), 1323–1331.
24. Dewangan, A., Yadav, A. K. (2017). Wax deposition during production of waxy crude oil and its remediation. *Petroleum Science and Techn.*, 35(18), 1831–1838.
25. Ahmed, A., Yadav, A. K. (2024). Enhanced production of methane enriched biogas through intensified co-digestion process and its effective utilization in a biodiesel/biohydrogen fueled engine with duel injection strategies: ML-RSM based an efficient optimization approach. *Int. J. Hydrogen Energy*, 65, 671–686.
26. Ramakrishna, S., Mayer, J., Wintermantel, E., Leong, K. W. (2001). Biomedical applications of polymer-composite materials: A review. *Compos. Sci. Technol.*, 61(9), 1189–1224.
27. Yadav, A. K., Khan, O., Khan, M. E. (2018). Utilization of high FFA landfill waste (Leachates) as a feedstock for sustainable biodiesel production: Its characterization and engine performance evaluation. *Environ. Sci. Pollut. Res.*, 25(32), 32312–32320.
28. Yadav, A. K., Dewangan, A., Mallick, A. (2018). Effect of n-Butanol and diethyl ether additives on performance and emission characteristics of a diesel engine fuelled with diesel-pongamia biodiesel blends. *J. of Energy Eng.*, 144(6), 04018062.
29. Yadav, A. K., Dewangan, A., Mallick, A. (2018). Synthesis and stability study of biodiesel from Kachnar seed oil. *J. of Energy Eng.*, 144(5), 04018053.

30. Khan, I. A., Singh, S. K., Yadav, A. K., Sharma, D. (2019). Enhancement in the performance of a diesel engine fueled with pongamia methyl ester and n-butanol as oxygenated additive. *Int. J. of Ambient Energy*, 40(8), 842–846.
31. Khan, T. A., Yadav, A. K., Khan, T. A. (2022). A hydrodynamic cavitation-assisted system for optimization of biodiesel production from green microalgae oil using a genetic algorithm and response surface methodology approach. *Environ. Sci. Pollut. Res.*, 29, 49465–49477.
32. Dewangan, A., Yadav, A. K., Mallick, A., Singh, S. (2022). Comparative study of Manilkara zapota and karanja based biodiesel properties and its effect on multi-cylinder diesel engine characteristics. *Energy Sources, Part A*, 44(2), 5143–5153.
33. Yadav, A. K., Khan, T. A., Khan, T. A., Kumar, S. (2021). Methyl ester of Gmelina arborea oil as a substitute for petroleum diesel: An experimental study on its performance and emissions in a diesel engine. *Energy Sources, Part A*, 43(11), 1307–1314.
34. Khan, O., Yadav, A. K., Khan, M. E. (2021). Characterization of bio-ethanol obtained from Eichhornia crassipes plant; Its emission and performance analysis on CI engine. *Energy Sources, Part A*, 43(14), 1793–1803.
35. Dewangan, A., Mallick, A., Yadav, A. K. (2020). Effect of metal oxide nanoparticles and engine parameters on the performance of a diesel engine: A review. *Mater. Today Proc.*, 21, 1722–1727.
36. Dewangan, A., Mallick, A., Yadav, A. K. (2020). Combustion-generated pollutions in CI engine and strategy for its control: A review. *Mater. Today Proc.*, 21, 1728–1733.
37. Yadav, A. K., Khan, M. E., Pal, A. (2019). Custard apple seed (Annona squamosa) oil as a promising feedstock for biodiesel production using advanced techniques and its experimental investigations on an agricultural diesel engine. *Int. J. of Oil, Gas and Coal Tech.*, 20(4), 473–492.
38. Singh, S., Singh, B., Kumar, S., Yadav, A. K. (2019). Temperature-dependent dynamic hysteresis scaling of ferroelectric hysteresis parameters of lead free [(Ba 0.825 + xCa0.175-x) (Ti1- x Snx)O3]ceramics. *Ferroelectrics*, 551(1), 133–142.
39. Das, D. K., Ahmad, A., Singh, A., Singh, D. K., Yadav, A. K. (2023). Numerical simulation of the combustion chamber and performance analysis of microalgae-based biodiesel/diesel-powered CI engine: An axisymmetric flow approach. *Proceedings of the Institution of Mechanical Engineers, Part E: Journal of Process Mechanical Engineering*, 09544089231218121.
40. Dewangan, A., Mallick, A., Yadav, A. K., et.al. (2023). Combined effect of operating parameters and nano particles on performance of a diesel engine: Response surface methodology coupled genetic algorithm approach. *ACS Omega*, 8(27), 24586–24600.
41. Jhariya, M., Dewangan, A. K., Moinuddin, S. Q., Kumar, S., Ahmad, A., Yadav, A. K. (2024). Research progress on efficient battery thermal management system (BTMs) for electric vehicles using composite phase change materials with liquid cooling and nanoadditives. *J. Therm. Anal. Calorim.*, 149, 13653–13680.
42. Sharma, G., Dewangan, A. K., Yadav, A. K., Ahmad, A. (2024). Feasibility of waste-to-hydrogen generation system based on gasification/pyrolysis: A

comprehensive review of experimental studies. *J. Therm. Anal. Calorim.*, 149(23), 13629–13651.
43. Yadav, A. K., Pal, A., Dubey, A. M. (2018). Experimental studies on utilization of Prunus Armeniaca L. (wild apricot) biodiesel as an alternative fuel for CI engine. *Waste Biomass Valor.*, 9(10), 1961–1969.
44. Senger, M. K. S., Dewangan, A. K., Dutt, N., Yadav, A. K. (2024). Research advances in solar dryer technologies integrated with solar air heater: A state-of-the art review on design variations, performance and feasibility assessments. *J. Therm. Anal. Calorim.*, 149(22), 12577–12607.
45. Ahmad, A., Yadav, A. K., Hasan, S. (2024). Enhancing efficiency and environmental impacts of a nano-enhanced oleander biodiesel-biohydrogen dual fuel engine equipped with EGR, through operational parameter optimization using RSM-MOGA technique. *Int. J. Hydrogen Energy*, 78, 1157–1172.
46. Singh, D., Chauhan, A., Yadav, A. K., Samsher, S., Dewangan, A., Ahmad, A. Energy, exergy, energy matrices, exergoeconomic, and enviroeconomic (5E) analysis of active solar distiller using water loaded nanoparticles: A comparative study. *Environ. Prog. Sustain. Energy*, 44(4), e14652.
47. Singh, D., Singh, S., Yadav, A. K., et al., (2023). From theory to practice: A sustainable solution to water scarcity by using a hybrid solar distiller with a heat exchanger and aluminum oxide nanoparticles. *ACS Omega,* 37(8), 33543–33553.
48. Khan, T.A., Khan, T. A., Yadav, A. K., Khan, M. E. (2023). Experimental studies on utilization of neochloris oleoabundans microalgae biodiesel as an alternative fuel for diesel engine. *Int. J. of Ambient Energy*, 44(1), 115–123.
49. Anand, A., Singh, R., Yadav, A. K., et al. (2024). Experimental investigations on the electrochemical machining of D3 die steel material and multi-objective parameters optimization. *J. of Surface Review and Letters*, 31(09).
50. Ahmed, A., Yadav, A. K., Hasan, S. (2024). Biogas as a sustainable and viable alternative fuel for diesel engines: A comprehensive review of production, purification, economic analysis, and performance evaluation. Journal of Process Mechanical Engineering, 240(2), 2306–2318.
51. Khan, F., Karimi, M. N., Khan, O., Yadav, A. K., Alhodaib, A., Gürel, A. E., Ağbulut, Ü. (2024). A hybrid MCDM optimization for utilization of novel set of biosynthesized nanofluids on thermal performance for solar thermal collectors. *Int. J. Thermofluids,* 22, 100686.
52. Alhodaib, A., Yahya, Z., Khan, O. Yadav, A. K., et al. (2024). Sustainable coatings for green solar photovoltaic cells: Performance and environmental impact of recyclable biomass digestate polymers. *Sci. Rep.,* 14, 11221.
53. Singh, B., Yadav, A. K., et al. (2025). Fabrication and characterization of AA6082-T6 produced by friction stir additive manufacturing. *J. of Surf. Rev. Lett.*, 32, 2550022.
54. Equbal, A., Equbal, A., Ahmad, R., Kumar, M., Khan, O., Yadav, A. K. (2024). RSM based statistical approach to enhance the compressive performance of ABS P400 parts fabricated via FDM Technology. *J. of Surf. Rev. Lett., 32*, 2550021.
55. Ahmad, T., Kumari, P., Yadav, A. K. et.al. (2024). Assessing the effectiveness of soft computing techniques in determining optimal welding parameters for

reduced environmental impact in a cold metal transfer welding process-an economic welding approach. *Surf. Rev. Lett. 32*, 2550054.
56. Ahmad, A., Yadav, A. K., Naik, R. T., Hasan, S. (2025). Renewable energy integrated pyrolysis/gasification technologies for hydrogen generation: A bibliometric analysis of decarbonisation strategies for sustainable future. *Therm. Sci. Eng. Prog.*, 65, 103963.
57. Ahmed, A., Yadav, A. K., Singh, A. (2023). Process optimization of spirulina microalgae biodiesel synthesis using RSM coupled GA technique: A performance study of a biogas-powered dual-fuel engine. *Int. J. of Environ Science and Tech.*, 21(1), 169–188.
58. Ahmed, A., Yadav, A. K., Singh, A. (2023). Application of machine learning and genetic algorithm for prediction and optimization of biodiesel yield from waste cooking oil. *Korean J. of Chem. Engg.*, 40, 2941–2956.
59. Yadav, A. K., Khan, M. E., Pal, A. (2017). Kaner biodiesel production through hybrid reactor and its performance testing on a CI engine at different compression ratios. *Egypt. J. of Petroleum*, 26(2), 525–532.
60. Ahmed, A., Yadav, A. K., Singh, A. (2023). Enhancement of biogas yield from dual organic waste using hybrid statistical approach and its effects on ternary fuel blend (Biodiesel/n-butanol /Diesel). *Powered Diesel Engine Environ. Prog. Sustain. Energy*, 43, e14163.
61. Yadav, M., Karimi, M. N., Yadav, A. K. (2023). Effect of graphene oxide nanoparticles dispersed biodiesel on combustion, performance, and emission characteristics of a diesel engine. *J. of Proc. Mech. Eng.: Part E.*, https://doi.org/10.1177/09544089231209139
62. Ahmed, A, Yadav, A. K, Singh, A., Singh, D. K. (2024). A machine learning–genetic algorithm based models for optimization of intensification process through microwave reactor: A new approach for rapid and sustainable synthesis of biodiesel from novel Hiptage benghalensis seed oil. *Fuel*, 374, 132470.
63. Singh, A. K., Kumar, K., Choudhury, U., Yadav, A. K., Ahmad, A., Surender, K. (2024). Applications of artificial intelligence and cell balancing techniques for battery management system (bms) in electric vehicles: A comprehensive review. *Process Saf. Environ. Prot.*.191(Part B), 2247–2265.
64. Ahmad, A., Yadav, A. K., Singh, A. (2025). Predictive modeling and optimization of microalgae chlorella vulgaris biodiesel production: Assessing the performance of a raw biogas-powered diesel engine with diethyl ether blended biodiesel. *J Environ Inform*, 45(1), 42–56.
65. Equbal, M. S., Khan, O., Equbal, A., Parvez, M., Ahmad, S., Yahya, Z., ... Yadav, A. K. (2024). Comparative analysis of machine learning and artificial intelligence models for optimizing mixed refrigerant characteristics in a hydrogen pre-cooling storage system. *J of Energy Storage,* 102, 114101.
66. Ahmed, A, Yadav, A. K. (2024). Parametric analysis of wastewater electrolysis for green hydrogen production: A combined RSM, genetic algorithm, and particle swarm optimization approach. *Int. J. Hydrogen Energy*, 59, 51–62.
67. Ahmed, A, Yadav, A. K, Singh, A., Singh, D. K. (2024). A machine learning-response surface optimization approach to enhance the performance of diesel

engine using novel blends of aloe vera biodiesel with MWCNT nanoparticles and hydrogen. *Process Saf. Environ. Prot.*, 186, 738–755, DOI: 10.1016/j.psep.2024.04.013.

68. Ahmed, A., Yadav, A. K., Singh, D. K., Singh, A. (2024). A comprehensive machine learning-coupled response surface methodology approach for predictive modeling and optimization of biogas potential in anaerobic co-digestion of organic waste. *Biomass and Bioenergy*, 180, 106995.
69. Khan, O, Khan, M. P., Yadav, A. K. (2024). A comparative analysis of various nanocomposites for the remediation of heavy metals from biomass liquid digestate using multi-criteria decision methods. *Biomass and Bioenergy*, 186, 107281.
70. Khan, O., Alsaduni, I, Equbal, A., Parvez, M., Yadav, A. K. (2024). Performance and emission analysis of biodiesel blends enriched with biohydrogen and biogas in internal combustion engines. *Process Saf. Environ. Prot.*, 183, 1013–1037.
71. Ahmed, A., Yadav, A. K., Singh, A., et al. (2024). A hybrid RSM-GA-PSO approach on optimization of process intensification of linseed biodiesel synthesis using an ultrasonication reactor: Enhancing fuel properties and engine characteristics with ternary fuel blends. *Energy*, 288, 129077.
72. Khan, O., Parvez, M., Yahya, Z., Alhodaib, A., Yadav, A. K., Hoang, A. T., Ağbulut, Ü. (2024). Waste-to-energy power plants: Multi-objective analysis and optimization of landfill heat and methane gas by recirculation of leachate. *Process Saf. Environ. Prot.*, 186, 957–968.
73. Khan, O., Ali, V., Parvez, M., Alhodaib, A., Yahya, Z., Yadav, A. K., Agbulut, U. (2024). Exploring the performance of biodiesel-hydrogen blends with diverse nanoparticles in diesel engine: A hybrid machine learning K-means clustering approach with weighted performance metrics. *Int. Journal of Hydrogen Energy*, 78, 547–563.
74. Khan, O., Alsaduni, I., Parvez, M., Yadav, A. K. (2025). Enhancing hydrogen production using solar-driven photocatalysis with biosynthesized nanocomposites: A hybrid machine learning approach towards enhanced performance and sustainable environment. *Int. J. of Hydrogen Energy,* 102, 609–625.
75. Khan, F., Khan, O., Parvez, M., Almujibah, H., Pachauri, P., Yahya, Z., ... Yadav, A. K. (2025). Innovative hydrogen production from waste bio-oil via steam methane reforming: An advanced ANN-AHP-k-means modelling approach using extreme machine learning weighted clustering. *Int. J. Hydrogen Energy,* 105, 1080–1091.
76. Khan, F., Alsaduni, I., Khan, O., Parvez, M., Yadav, A. K., Agbulut, Ü. (2025). Enhancing biogas/biohydrogen utilization in dual-fuel engines using advanced machine learning algorithms. *Int. J. Hydrogen Energy*, 112, 81–90.
77. Ahmad, A., Yadav, A. K., Singh, A., Singh, D. K. (2025). Modeling and optimization of biogas production via ultrasonic pretreatment: Assessment of its usability on dual fuel engine powered by waste plastic oil-hydrogen blends. *Int. J. Hydrogen Energy,* 119, 271–282.
78. Khan, O., Alsaduni, I., Parvez, M., Yahya, Z., Yadav, A. K. (2024). Role of hydrogen-enrichment on performance and emission characteristics of a diesel engine fuelled with metal oxide nanoparticles added biodiesel/diesel

blends: A combined neuro Fuzzy-Gaussian mixture model analysis. *Int. J. Hydrogen Energy,* 93, 1113–1126.
79. Khan, F., Khan, O., Parvez, M., Ahmad, S., Yahya, Z., Alhodaib, A., ... Yadav, A. K. (2024). K-means clustering optimization of various quantum dots and nanoparticles-added biofuels for engine performance, emission, vibration, and noise characteristics. *Therm. Sci. Eng. Prog.,* 54, 102815.
80. Dewangan, A., Mallick, A., Yadav, A. K., et al. (2023). Production of oxy-hydrogen gas and the impact of its usability on CI Engine combustion, performance, and emission behaviors. *Energy*, 278, 127937.
81. Khan, O., Parvez, M., Kumari, P., Yadav, A. K., Akram, W., Ahmad, S., ... Idrisi, M. J. (2023). Modelling of compression ignition engine by soft computing techniques (ANFIS-NSGA-II and RSM) to enhance the performance characteristics for leachate blends with nano-additives. *Sci. Rep.*, 13(1), 15429.
82. Yadav, A. K., Khan, M. E., Pal, A, Dubey, A. M. (2017). Experimental investigations of performance and emissions characteristics of kusum (Schleichera Oleosa) biodiesel in a multi-cylinder transportation diesel engine. *Waste Biomass Valor*, 8(4), 1331–1341.
83. Ahmad, A., Yadav, A. K., Dewangan, A. K. (2025). Synergistic effect of various nanoparticles infused biodiesel/diesel blends on combustion, performance, and environmental characteristics of a CI engine. *J. Energy Inst.*, 120, 102117.

Chapter 3

Classification and characterization of multi-functional biomaterials

Akhilesh Kumar Yadav and Chandana Rath

3.1 INTRODUCTION

Multifunctional biomaterials can be defined as the materials having exceptional physical and mechanical properties with high biocompatibility and chemical stability that can be applied for various biomedical applications without producing any toxicity or adverse effect towards the host tissue [1]. A biomaterial must possess characteristics such as biocompatibility, hemocompatibility, nontoxicity, noncarcinogenic, good physical and mechanical properties, low cost, and wear resistant [2]. The history of biomaterials dates back to ancient civilizations, where materials like wood, bone, and metal were used in rudimentary medical applications. The earliest known surgical operations focused on restoring missing body parts. In 600 BC, the ancient physician *Suśruta* had performed advanced repairs, such as reconstructing noses using patches of living flesh from the cheek. By 1430, Sicilian laymen advanced this technique by creating noses from skin flaps taken from the arms. The 19th century marked a turning point with the development of modern implants for repairing long bones and joints. Between 1893 and 1912, steel plates were designed for fracture treatment, while the 1930s saw the introduction of polymers in surgery. The 1950s brought about heart valve implantation, made possible by advancements in open heart surgery, and in 1944, dialysis for humans was discovered, further revolutionizing medical practices. However, formal recognition and systematic exploration of biomaterials began in the mid-20th century. In the 1950s, the advent of synthetic polymers such as nylon and Teflon, marked a significant step forward. In the 1960s, biocompatible materials like silicone for medical implants, metals for orthopedic implants emerged. The field gained a [omit a] momentum in the late 1960s with the advancement of bioactive ceramics and polymers, followed by the introduction of tissue engineering concepts in the 1980s. In 1969, Larry Hench revolutionized the world by introducing bioactive glasses—a [omit —] bioactive material having capabilities of bonding with the bones directly via the formation of hydroxyapatite [3], [4]. Since then, biomaterials have evolved rapidly,

 DOI: 10.1201/9781003581192-3

with advancements including biodegradable materials, smart implants, and nanotechnology-based applications. Ongoing research continues to expand the possibilities of biomaterials, driving modernization in healthcare and opening the way for personalized medicine. Biomaterials can be divided into broader class, based on their interaction with the host tissue, which are given below [5], [6]:

3.1.1 Bioinert materials

Bioinert materials are the first kind of biomaterials specifically designed for load bearing applications that do not interact directly with biological tissues, aiming to maintain stability and resist degradation when implanted in the body [7]. Commonly used bioinert materials include certain metals and alloys, such as titanium, Ti-6Al-4V, and stainless steel, and some ceramics like alumina and zirconia [8], [9]. Initially, upon implantation, a series of biological events is activated, starting with the immediate development of a protein layer on the surface of the material composed of serum proteins such as fibrinogen and fibronectin, which act as a critical interface between the materials and biological tissue. It also facilitates cellular adhesion and migration, attracting inflammatory cells that help clean the implant site. While the inflammatory response is typically mild due to the bioinert nature of the material, it eventually transitions to a more constructive phase where fibroblasts and other cells migrate to the site, resulting in the formation of a fibrous capsule around the implant. This capsule acts as a protective barrier, minimizing direct contact with the immune system. Over time, the stable protein layer and fibrous capsule provide a favorable environment for tissue remodeling and healing, ensuring that the implant can effectively support biological functions while maintaining its integrity within the host body.

Metals and alloys come in this class of materials and have been used as implants for a very long period of time due to their excellent mechanical, thermal, and electrical conductivity [10]. The primary groups of metallic biomaterials include stainless steel, pure titanium (Ti) and titanium alloys (like Ti-6Al-4V), and cobalt-chromium (Co-Cr) alloys [11]. They face challenges in articulation surfaces due to their lower elasticity and wear resistance. Despite their advantages—such as chemical stability, high mechanical strength, corrosion and wear resistance, ease of sterilization, and shape memory capabilities—metallic biomaterials have drawbacks, including high modulus, potential cytotoxicity, and susceptibility to corrosion, and metal ion sensitivity [12].

3.1.2 Bioactive/Bioresorbable materials

Bioactive/bioresorbable materials are another class of biomaterials that elicit a specific response at the interface between the material and living

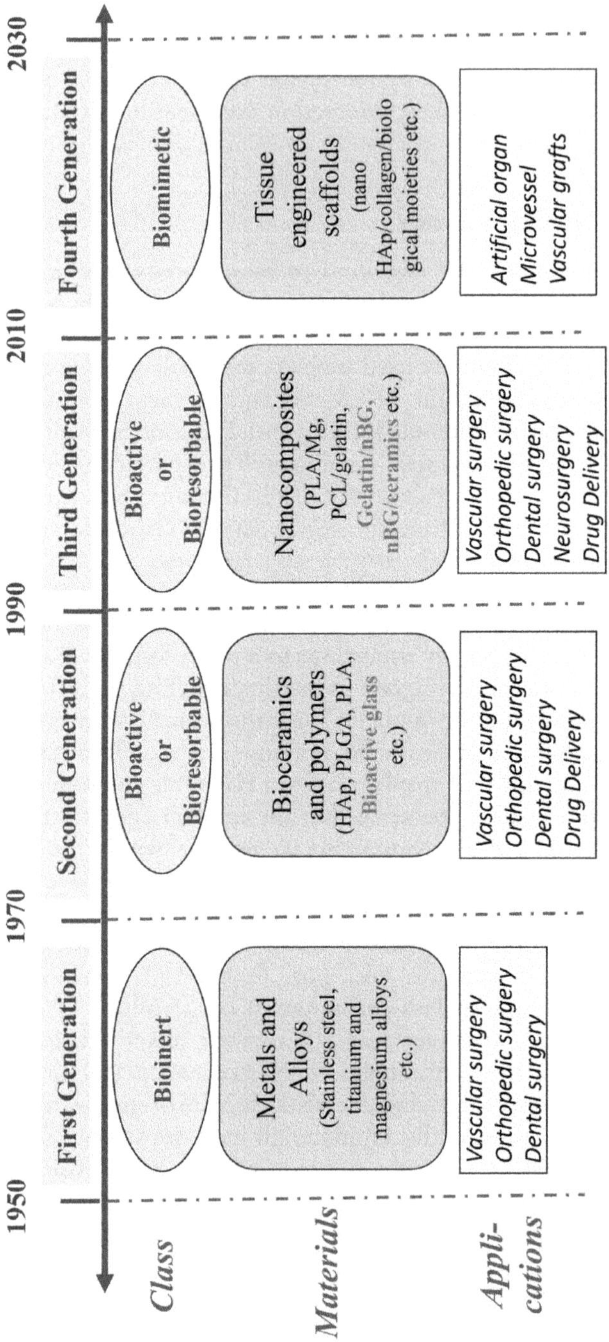

Figure 3.1 Development of biomaterials.

tissues when implanted, that have the ability [when implanted and have the ability] to undergo natural degradation and absorption as the time goes on —eliminating the need for surgical removal. The degradation process typically involves the breakdown of the material without creating any toxic substance which can be metabolized or excreted by the body. These materials find application in different medical devices and implants, such as sutures, stents, and drug delivery systems. One notable example is bioactive glasses, bioresorbable polymers which includes polyglycolic acid (PGA), polylactic acid (PLA), and their copolymers. Unlike bioinert materials, which aim to minimize interaction with the biological environment, bioactive materials actively engage with biological systems, promoting beneficial interactions such as tissue integration and cell adhesion. Bioactive glasses, hydroxyapatite, and certain types of ceramics are examples of bioactive materials.

Bioceramics are basically oxides composed of metallic and non-metallic elements that are bonded together [13], such as alumina (Al_2O_3), magnesium oxide (MgO), and silicon dioxide (SiO_2) that can be used for different applications, i.e., bone grafts, hip prostheses, and artificial tendons. For example, black pyrolytic carbons are used in cardiovascular implants, specifically for blood-contacting devices like heart valves. Bioactive glasses, another class of surface-reactive bioceramics, show a unique characteristic that permit them to interact directly with biological systems [14], [15]. Their composition primarily consists of silica (SiO_2), which forms the structural network, and modifier ions such as calcium (Ca^{2+}) Mg, Na etc. [16], [17], [18]. These modifiers enhance the glass's surface reactivity, promoting integration with living tissue. The most well-known bioglass composition that is being used clinically is 45S5®- $45SiO_2$-$24.5CaO$-$24.5Na_2O$-$6P_2O_5$ (wt%), which was developed by Larry Hench and his colleagues in 1969 [19], [20], [21].

Polymers include both naturally derived and synthetic varieties, which can be classified as biodegradable or non-biodegradable [22]. Starch, chitin, and collagen are natural polymers and are often favored for their biodegradability and accessibility. In contrast, synthetic polymers are commonly used as prosthetics, dental materials, disposable medical supplies, and implants. Current examples of synthetic polymeric materials include polypropylene, polyethylene, polymethylmethacrylate, and polyurethane [22], [23]. Polymers offer several advantages over metals and ceramics as biomaterials, including their versatility in manufacturing different forms—such as fibers, films, and sheets—and their ease of processing, cost-effectiveness and ability to be tailored to achieve specific physical and mechanical properties [24]. However, polymeric biomaterials also have drawbacks, such as their tendency to absorb water and proteins, which can lead to surface contamination and difficulties in sterilization. Furthermore, the extensive use of non-biodegradable polymers raises concerns about environmental pollution and waste management [25], [26].

3.1.3 Biomimetic materials

Biomimetic materials are a class of synthetic materials that draw inspiration from biological systems, attempting to replicate or mimic specific structures, properties, or functions found in nature. The process of developing biomimetic materials involves understanding and replicating the underlying mechanisms that enable certain biological systems to achieve remarkable properties. By incorporating these biomimetic features into synthetic materials, researchers aim to improve the performance and integration of biomaterials in various medical applications, such as implants, prosthetics, drug delivery, and tissue engineering [27]. For instance, self-healing polymers mimic biological healing processes, enabling materials to autonomously repair damage, while synthetic spider silk aims to replicate the strength and elasticity of natural silk for medical and textile applications. The application of biomimetic principles to biomaterials has led to the creation of innovative materials with enhanced biocompatibility, bioactivity, and functionality. For example, biomimetic scaffolds in tissue engineering might replicate the extracellular matrix to provide an ideal environment for cell growth and tissue regeneration. The use of biomimetic materials as biomaterials represents a strategic approach to leverage the remarkable designs and functionalities observed in living organisms. This class of materials also uses the polymers.

3.2 CHARACTERIZATION OF BIOMATERIALS

Before being used, all the materials should be characterized using different techniques to quantify their physical, mechanical, and biological properties. Figure 3.2 shows the different characterization techniques that are discussed below:

3.2.1 Structure and microstructure

3.2.1.1 TGA-DSC

The TGA analysis is a technique employed to check the thermal durability of materials. This method involves measuring the sample's mass as a function temperature, allowing for mass changes (such as absorption or desorption), phase transitions, and thermal decomposition. When the sample's mass remains constant within a specific temperature range, it denotes thermal stability in that range. TGA analysis also aids in determining the calcination temperature, acting as an upper limit where the sample starts degrading; whereas differential scanning calorimetry (DSC) is a thermal analysis technique used to observe changes in thermal behavior during phase transitions within a system. The difference in the heat required to raise the temperature

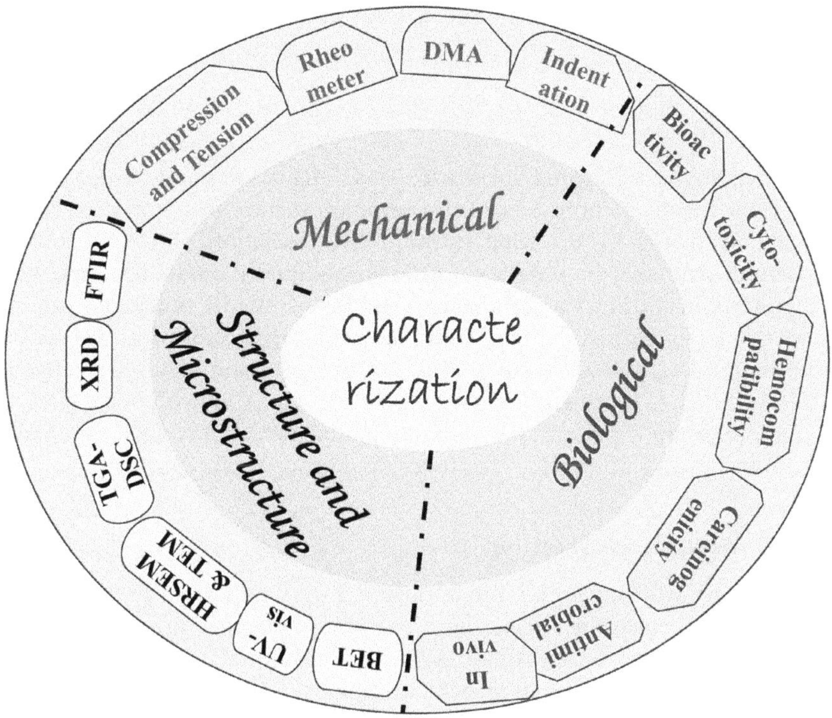

Figure 3.2 Characterization techniques.

of the test sample compared to the reference sample is measured to keep both at the same temperature. The sample material is typically placed in a small capsule made of alumina along with an inert powder like α-Al_2O_3, which doesn't exhibit any heat-related effects [28].

3.2.1.2 XRD

X-Ray Diffraction (XRD) is a powerful analytical technique that helps scientists understand the atomic and molecular arrangement within crystalline materials. It works by directing a focused beam of X-rays onto a sample that rotates at a controlled speed and enables the determination of a material's phase, purity, and crystal structure. This technique relies on Bragg's law of diffraction, which was proposed by W. H. Bragg and his son W. L. Bragg. In case of metals and ceramic biomaterials highly crystalline peak are observed which can be matched with JCPDS data available at Crystallographic open database. This confirms the crystal structure of the material. However, in case of polymers and bioactive glasses, a broad hump-like peak is observed, which shows the amorphous nature of the material, i.e., a very short range or no ordering is present in the sample.

3.2.1.3 FTIR

Fourier-Transform Infrared Spectroscopy (FTIR) is a valuable tool for analyzing the chemical composition of a sample's surface in a non-destructive manner. It works by directing infrared (IR) radiation onto the sample. Molecules with specific functional groups, essentially covalent bonds with a dipole moment, absorb certain wavelengths of this IR radiation. In case of metals or inorganic, the transmittance peaks are observed in the fingerprint region i.e., 400-1200 cm^{-1}, while for organic compounds the range is 1200-4000 cm^{-1}. By observing the spectra, we can confirm which kind of functional group is present. For polymeric biomaterial, it is one of the most crucial techniques after NMR for functional group quantification.

3.2.1.4 Morphological testing

When we are working with biomaterials, it is very important to know their morphology, because it affects the bioactivity and other properties of the materials. For surface morphology, a high-resolution scanning electron microscope (SEM) can be used, which utilizes a focused electron beam to produce images of a sample. Biomaterials can have various kinds of morphologies, such as spherical, sheet-like nanorods, etc. Bioactive glasses are found to have spherical shape and very sharp fine particles of hydroxyapatite are deposited after immersion in simulated body fluid, which is also confirmed via using this technique[29], [30].

However, if we want to quantify the particle size of biomaterials, Transmission Electron Microscopy (TEM) is more precise and can give the specific structure and size of the material. It also consists of a similar assembly like HRSEM. TEM has a remarkable resolution of under 0.2 nm, even with a decent amount of tilting of the specimen. TEM can operate in two modes: diffraction mode and imaging mode. By changing the excitation of the lenses following the objective lens, modern TEM can switch between these two modes. The TEM image displays well-distributed particles that can be analyzed for their shape and size distribution. Using Image J software, a histogram of particle distribution (particles size vs. number of particles) can be plotted. Fitting the data with Lorantzian distribution provides the average particle size. A selective area electron diffraction (SAED) pattern displays well-concentric rings of different radii. The diffraction rings can be indexed by calculating the inverse of their radii and matching them with the interplanar spacing (d) in reciprocal space of XRD data using Win PLOTR software.

3.2.1.5 UV-visible spectroscopy

The UV-Visible spectrophotometer is a tool that utilizes optical principles to analyze the absorption spectra, calculate the concentration and band gap of materials. In the case of a powder sample, a double beam spectrophotometer was used, with one beam directed at the sample and the other at a standard reference material: $BaSO_4$ powder. The device was equipped with a photomultiplier tube (PMT) to capture the spectra, with a light source which can provide ultra-violet as well as visible light. An integrating sphere assembly was employed to facilitate the measurements. Reflectance values were converted to absorbance values in the 200-700 nm range using the Kubelka-Munk function.

3.2.1.6 BET (Brunner-Emmett-Teller) surface area measurement

The BET (Brunner-Emmett-Teller) is used to analyse the surface area and porous structure of the biomaterial which play a very crucial role. The BET technique involves the physical adsorption of nitrogen gas (adsorbate) onto the solid material (adsorbent), which allows us to determine its specific surface area. This physical adsorption relies on the van der Waals force between the gas and the material. After the gas is adsorbed, desorption occurs. The amount of gas adsorbed indicates the specific surface area of the sample. The BET process is typically conducted at a constant temperature, maintained by liquid nitrogen, while the pressure or concentration of the adsorbate gas gradually increases. Therefore, a graph has been plotted between the relative pressure of the gas and the volume adsorbed onto the sample [31], [32]. The BET measurement involves three steps:

i. Standardization of the reference cell.
ii. The sample undergoes pre-treatment through heating at a specific temperature.
iii. The adsorbate is adsorbed onto the adsorbent under isotherm conditions.

3.2.2 Mechanical characterizations

Mechanical characterization of biomaterials can be classified based on handling of the sample post-treatment with the corresponding characterization instruments; Destructive and Non-destructive tests. Destructive tests include Compression-Tensile Testing, Rheology, Dynamic mechanical analysis (DMA), and Cyclic loading, while non-destructive include indentations which are discussed below.

3.2.2.1 Compression-tensile testing

It is very important to quantify the response of a sample when subjected to tension and compression, for material design and performance evaluation. Some standards established by ASTM '(American Society for Testing and Materials)' accomplish the necessities for compressive and tensile strength values along with the corresponding testing methods applicable to various biomaterials. The samples are placed between two plates, and a force is applied by bringing the plates together. The tests assess compressive strength, yield point and strength, and elastic modulus [33]. In these testing, the force applied is orthogonal to the materials' surface under examination. To obtain reliable data, the applied force must be sufficiently low so that the applied stress and the strain maintain a linear relationship for the biomaterial under examination [33].

3.2.2.2 Rheometer

The response of soft materials to shear forces can be measured using Rheometer, which operates basically on the principle of inducing cyclic shear deformations in a sample and measuring the corresponding stress responses. Samples are placed between two plates, keeping the bootom pate stationary and the top plate rotating, which provides a strain curve, depending on time of the sample. If we measure the torque exerted on the sample, we can quantify the time-dependent stress as well.

3.2.2.3 Dynamic mechanical analysis (DMA)

DMA is employed to characterize the viscoelastic properties of materials — primarily polymers. DMA instruments use forced oscillation across many loading modes, such as compression, torsion, uniaxial tension, bending, and in-plane shear, or free oscillation, usually via a torsion pendulum [34]. The Tg (glass transitions) in solid polymers and co-polymers in food products [35], [36] and medications have long been ascertained using DMA [37], [38].

3.2.2.4 Indentation

Indentation methods employ an indenter with a defined geometry that, when subjected to loading and subsequent elastic unloading, results in a lasting indentation in the samples. Consequently, these tests may be omitted from a rigorous classification of nondestructive testing, as they induce confined perpetual deformation that creates a stress concentration, potentially resulting in failure. We can examine the materials' hardness (H), which confirms the materials' resistance towards permanent deformation and can be correlated with the other mechanical properties [35]. Microhardness tests are effective for sampling limited material volumes [34].

3.2.3 Biological characterization

3.2.3.1 *Bioactivity*

The bioactivity of any ceramic is the primary biological characterization to evaluate if it can form calcium hydroxyapatite layer similar to natural bone mineral at the interface or not, and how many days it took when exposed to biological fluids [18], [36]. To assess a bioactivity bone-bonding potential, researchers often utilize simulated body fluid (SBF), an artificially created solution designed to mimic the ion concentrations and pH of human blood plasma [39] following the advised procedures of "Technical Committee 4 (TCO4) of the International Commission on Glass (ICG)" [40]. Further XRD, FTIR, and HRSEM are used to confirm the formation of HAP layer on the sample.

3.2.3.2 *Cytotoxicity*

Cytotoxicity is defined as the compatibility of cells, or if the material is toxic towards the cells, one of the crucial parameters to diagnose. We use different kinds of assays: MTT, XTT, etc. to evaluate the cell viability in presence of the sample. If the material is non toxic, cell viability will remain the same as the control. However, if the viability decrease below 70%, then it is considered to be toxic and will not be used for biomedical applications. Some materials show higher viability than the control, they are considered to be good biomaterials and enhance cell proliferation.

3.2.3.3 *Hemocompatibility*

Since the implantation of a biomaterial, its first interaction is with the blood, so it is very important to quantify the effect of biomaterials on blood components such as platelet, erythrocytes (red blood cells), etc. —defined as hemocompatibility assay [41]. Hemolysis, in this context, denotes the rupture or destruction of erythrocytes (red blood cells), leading to the release of hemoglobin into the surrounding environment [42]. Hemolysis percentage of biomaterials are examined by following the standard protocol ASTM F 756-00 [41].

3.2.3.4 *Antimicrobial study*

The risk of bacterial infection is quite high in the implants, which can cause failure or removal of the implant [43], [44]. Therefore, the materials having inherent antimicrobial properties are crucial, and rigorous research is going on to improve the antimicrobial properties of the biomaterials [45]. It is important to evaluate the efficacy in restricting the growth of bacterial cell in presence of the biomaterials. Different kind of materials have different effects and mechanisms of antimicrobial effect. The primary and the prominent reason is the generation of reactive oxygen species (ROS) which restricts the growth. On the other hand, nanoparticles have the ability to bind with the outer layer of bacterial cell and restrict the important nutrient to reach— leading to the cell death. Antibacterial efficacy can be evaluated using different method such as diffusion method, dilution method, MTT assay, MIC calculation, etc.

3.2.3.5 Carcinogenicity and genotoxicity

Another prominent thing is to monitor the effect of biomaterials on the Genes. Biomaterials are tested to evaluate if they have any genotoxic and carcinogenic effect, i.e., DNA change or rupture, mutation of genes or chromosomes, on living bodies (Ratner et al., 2012; Landsiedel et al. 2009). Ames test, micronucleus and comet assay are few of the tests that can be used to evaluate the genotoxic effect of implants, drugs, chemicals, etc. Ames test is of low cost and simpler to perform as well as quick (seifian).

3.2.3.6 In vivo testing

After confirming the structure, mechanical- and biocompatibility of the materials in the laboratory, they are subjected to in-vivo testing, such as animal modelling. In this test, animals are selected, and the materials are implanted to study their effects. For example, if we have developed a wound healing material, we would select a group of approx. 30–50 mice with similar physical characteristics, such as weight, height, and gender, and divide them into different groups. The material is then applied to the animals, and various parameters are studied, including histopathology, systemic toxicity, inflammation, etc. Following successful in vivo testing, the material can be advanced to preclinical trials.

3.3 CONCLUSION

In this chapter we have discussed the classification of multifunctional biomaterials, based on their interaction with the living body. We provided a brief description about the different class of materials such as metals, alloys, ceramics, and polymers. Further, the characterization techniques are briefly discussed, defining all the properties of biomaterials, such as structural, mechanical, and biological.

REFERENCES

[1] "BIOMATERIALS SCIENCE.Ratner, B. D., Hoffman, A. S., Schoen, F. J., Lemons, J. E. (2013). Biomaterials Science: An Introduction to Materials in Medicine (3rd ed.). Academic Press, Elsevier, Oxford, UK. ISBN: 978-0-12-374626-9."

[2] M. Ebrahimi, "Standardization and regulation of biomaterials," in *Handbook of Biomaterials Biocompatibility*, Elsevier, 2020, pp. 251–265. doi: 10.1016/B978-0-08-102967-1.00013-X.

[3] L. L. Hench, J. W. Hench, and D. C. Greenspan, "Bioglass: A short history and bibliography," *Journal of the Australasian Ceramic Society*, vol. 40, no. 1, pp. 1–42, 2004.

[4] J. R. Jones, "Review of bioactive glass: From Hench to hybrids," *Acta Biomaterialia, 9*(1), 4457–4486. doi: 10.1016/j.actbio.2012.08.023.

[5] M. E. Marquis *et al.*, "Bone cells-biomaterials interactions," *Front Biosci (Landmark Ed)*, vol. 14, no. 3, pp. 1023–1067, Jan. 2009, doi: 10.2741/3293.

[6] **Arjunan, A., Baroutaji, A., Praveen, A. S., Robinson, J., Wang, C.** (2020). *Classification of biomaterial functionality. Reference Module in Materials Science and Materials Engineering* unctionality." pp. 1–31. Elsevier.

[7] R. Agrawal, A. Kumar, M. K. A. Mohammed, and S. Singh, "Biomaterial types, properties, medical applications, and other factors: A recent review," *Zhejiang University, SCIENCE A, 24(11), 1027–1042.*

[8] V. Sharanraj, **V., Rameshkumar, P., Kumar, V. D., et al. (2021).** *Zirconia: As a biocompatible biomaterial used in dental implants. Journal of Biomaterials Science, Polymer Edition, 32*(2), 63–68.

[9] H. Kawahara, M. Hirabayashi, and T. Shikita, "Single crystal alumina for dental implants and bone screws," *J Biomed Mater Res*, vol. 14, no. 5, pp. 597–605, 1980, doi: 10.1002/JBM.820140506.

[10] A. Pandey, A. Awasthi, and K. K. Saxena, "Metallic implants with properties and latest production techniques: A review," *Adv Mater Process Technol*, vol. 6, no. 2, pp. 167–202, Apr. 2020, doi: 10.1080/2374068X.2020.1731236.

[11] C. Morsiya, "A review on parameters affecting properties of biomaterial SS 316L," *Aust J Mech Eng*, vol. 20, no. 3, pp. 803–813, May 2022, doi: 10.1080/14484846.2020.1752975.

[12] L. C. Campanelli, "A review on the recent advances concerning the fatigue performance of titanium alloys for orthopedic applications," *J Mater Res*, vol. 36, no. 1, pp. 151–165, Jan. 2021, doi: 10.1557/S43578-020-00087-0/FIGURES/10.

[13] M. M. Subedi, "Ceramics and its importance," *Himal Phys*, vol. 4, pp. 80–82, Dec. 2013, doi: 10.3126/HJ.V4I0.9433.

[14] A. K. Yadav *et al.*, "Drug kinetics and antimicrobial properties of quaternary bioactive glasses 81S(81SiO2-(16-x)CaO-2P2O5-1Na2O-xMgO); An in-vitro study," *Biomater Adv*, vol. 157, p. 213729, Feb. 2023, doi: 10.1016/J.BIOADV.2023.213729.

[15] A. K. Yadav, H. Tripathi, P. Singh, A. K. Dubey, and C. Rath, "Exploring the physicomechanical properties and biocompatibility traits of CuO

Substituted 45S5 bioactive glass through in-vitro analysis," *Surf Interfaces*, vol. 51,104524, Aug. 2024, doi: 10.1016/j.surfin.2024.104524.
[16] H. Oonishi *et al.*, "Comparative bone growth behavior in granules of bioceramic materials of various sizes," *J Biomed Mater Res*, vol. 44, no. 1, pp. 31–43, Jan. 1999.
[17] S. Mistry, S. Datta, D. Kundu, and D. Basu, "Effects of bioactive glass, hydroxyapatite and bioactive glass – Hydroxyapatite composite graft particles in the treatment of infrabony defects," *J Indian Soc Periodontol*, vol. 16, no. 2, pp. 241–246, Apr. 2012, doi: 10.4103/0972-124X.99269.
[18] J. R. Jones, "Review of bioactive glass: From Hench to hybrids," *Acta Biomater*, vol. 9, no. 1, pp. 4457–4486, Jan. 2013, doi: 10.1016/J.ACTBIO.2012.08.023.
[19] L. L. Hench, R. J. Splinter, W. C. Allen, and T. K. Greenlee, "Bonding mechanisms at the interface of ceramic prosthetic materials," *J Biomed Mater Res*, vol. 5, no. 6, pp. 117–141, 1971, doi: 10.1002/JBM.820050611.
[20] T. K. Greenlee, C. A. Beckham, A. R. Crebo, and J. C. Malmorg, "Glass ceramic bone implants. A light microscopic study," *J Biomed Mater Res*, vol. 6, no. 3, pp. 235–244, May 1972, doi: 10.1002/JBM.820060312.
[21] C. A. Beckham, T. K. Greenlee, and A. R. Crebo, "Bone formation at a ceramic implant interface," *Calcif Tissue Res*, vol. 8, no. 1, pp. 165–171, Dec. 1971, doi: 10.1007/BF02010133/METRICS.
[22] Rohani Shirvan, A., Nouri, A., Wen, C. (2021). Structural polymer biomaterials. In: Wen, C. (Ed.), Structural Biomaterials: Properties, Characteristics, and *Selection*, (pp. 395–439). Woodhead Publishing, Sawston, Cambridge, UK.
[23] A. J. T. Teo, A. Mishra, I. Park, Y. J. Kim, W. T. Park, and Y. J. Yoon, "Polymeric biomaterials for medical implants and devices," *ACS Biomater Sci Eng*, vol. 2, no. 4, pp. 454–472, Apr. 2016, doi: 10.1021/ACSBIOMATERIALS.5B00429/ASSET/IMAGES/LARGE/AB-2015-00429V_0019.JPEG.
[24] P. Parida, A. Behera, and S. C. Mishra, "Classification of biomaterials used in medicine," *International Journal of Advances in Applied Sciences (IJAAS)*, vol. 1, no. 3, pp. 31–35, 2012.
[25] S. Zhang *et al.*, "Non-biodegradable microplastics in soils: A brief review and challenge," *J Hazard Mater*, vol. 409, p. 124525, May 2021, doi: 10.1016/J.JHAZMAT.2020.124525.
[26] "Morganti, P., Morganti, G. (2020). Surgical & beauty facial masks: The new waste problem of post Covid-19. Biomedical Journal of Scientific & Technical Research, 29(5), 22945–22950.", doi: 10.26717/BJSTR.2020.29.004878.
[27] Y. Bar-Cohen, *Biomimetics: Nature-Based Innovation*, 1st ed. USA: CRC Press, Inc., 2011.
[28] Brown, M. E. (1988). *Introduction to Thermal Analysis: Techniques and Applications*. Springer Netherlands, Dordrecht, The Netherlands.1988, doi: 10.1007/978-94-009-1219-9.

[29] Yadav, A. K., Rath, C. (2024). Exploring the impact of silica and modifier ions on bioactivity and antimicrobial characteristics of quaternary 81S and ternary 85S bio-glasses. Bulletin of Materials Science, 47, 214.

[30] A. K. Yadav, H. Tripathi, A. K. Dubey, and C. Rath, "In-vitro assessment of biocompatibility and antimicrobial properties of 85S Bio-glass and SrTiO3 composites," *Mater Chem Phys*, p. 129442, May 2024,320, 129442.

[31] K. S. W. Sing, "Adsorption methods for the characterization of porous materials," *Adv Colloid Interface Sci*, vol. 76–77, pp. 3–11, Jul. 1998, doi: 10.1016/S0001-8686(98)00038-4.

[32] M. D. Donohue and G. L. Aranovich, "Classification of Gibbs adsorption isotherms," *Adv Colloid Interface Sci*, vol. 76–77, pp. 137–152, Jul. 1998, doi: 10.1016/S0001-8686(98)00044-X.

[33] L. L. Hyland, M. B. Taraban, and Y. B. Yu, "Using small-angle scattering techniques to understand mechanical properties of biopolymer-based biomaterials," *Soft Matter*, vol. 9, no. 43, pp. 10218–10228, Oct. 2013, doi: 10.1039/C3SM51209F.

[34] Roeder, R. K. (2013). *Mechanical characterization of biomaterials.* In: Bandyopadhyay, A., Bose, S. (Eds.), *Characterization of Biomaterials* (pp. 49–104).

[35] Herrmann, K. (Ed.). (2011). *Hardness Testing: Principles and* applications, ASM International, Materials Park, Ohio.

[36] L. L. Hench and H. A. Paschall, "Direct chemical bond of bioactive glass-ceramic materials to bone and muscle," *J Biomed Mater Res*, vol. 7, no. 3, pp. 25–42, 1973, doi: 10.1002/JBM.820070304.

[37] J. Gearing, K. P. Malik, and P. Matejtschuk, "Use of dynamic mechanical analysis (DMA) to determine critical transition temperatures in frozen biomaterials intended for lyophilization," *Cryobiology*, vol. 61, no. 1, pp. 27–32, Aug. 2010, doi: 10.1016/J.CRYOBIOL.2010.04.002.

[38] D. S. Jones, "Dynamic mechanical analysis of polymeric systems of pharmaceutical and biomedical significance," *Int J Pharm*, vol. 179, no. 2, pp. 167–178, Mar. 1999, doi: 10.1016/S0378-5173(98)00337-8.

[39] T. Kokubo and H. Takadama, "How useful is SBF in predicting in vivo bone bioactivity?" *Biomaterials*, vol. 27, no. 15, pp. 2907–2915, 2006, doi: 10.1016/J.BIOMATERIALS.2006.01.017.

[40] A. L. B. Maçon *et al.*, "A unified in vitro evaluation for apatite-forming ability of bioactive glasses and their variants," *J Mater Sci Mater Med*, vol. 26, no. 2, pp. 1–10, Feb. 2015, doi: 10.1007/s10856-015-5403-9.

[41] "Standard practice for assessment of hemolytic properties of materials." Accessed: Mar. 28, 2023. [Online]. Available: www.astm.org/f0756-00.html

[42] M. B. Kirschner, J. J. B. Edelman, S. C. H. Kao, M. P. Vallely, N. Van Zandwijk, and G. Reid, "The impact of hemolysis on cell-free microRNA biomarkers," *Front Genet*, vol. 4, 94. May, 2013, doi: 10.3389/FGENE.2013.00094/FULL.

[43] K. Yuan, Y.-J. Chan, K.-C. Kung, and T.-M. Lee, "Comparison of osseointegration on various implant surfaces after bacterial contamination and cleaning: a rabbit study," *Int J Oral Maxillofac Implants*, vol. 29, no. 1, pp. 32–40, 2014, doi: 10.11607/JOMI.2436.

[44] D. Campoccia, L. Montanaro, and C. R. Arciola, "The significance of infection related to orthopedic devices and issues of antibiotic resistance," *Biomaterials*, vol. 27, no. 11, pp. 2331–2339, Apr. 2006, doi: 10.1016/J.BIOMATERIALS.2005.11.044.

[45] D. Campoccia, L. Montanaro, and C. R. Arciola, "A review of the biomaterials technologies for infection-resistant surfaces," *Biomaterials*, vol. 34, no. 34, pp. 8533–8554, Nov. 2013, doi: 10.1016/J.BIOMATERIALS.2013.07.089.

Chapter 4

Transforming surgical planning and navigation through robotics

Neha Singh Raghuvanshi, Kshitiz Srivastav, Yatika Gori, and Ashwani Kumar

4.1 INTRODUCTION

Advancements in surgical technology have transformed the landscape of surgery —with robotics emerging as a game-changing asset in surgical planning and navigation. This article delves into the incorporation of robotics into surgical procedures, emphasizing its capacity to elevate precision, efficiency, and patient outcomes [1]. Robotic-assisted surgery merges the expertise of surgeons with the capabilities of robotic systems to execute intricate procedures with unparalleled accuracy and control. Through the integration of robotics into surgical planning and navigation, healthcare providers can attain a level of precision that surpasses traditional methods. This technology enables meticulous preoperative planning, real-time intraoperative imaging, and precise execution of surgical maneuvers, ultimately leading to enhanced outcomes for patients [2].Surgical planning and navigation with robotics serve diverse roles in modern healthcare. Robotics enables unparalleled precision—vital for delicate procedures or tight spaces. Many systems support minimally invasive surgery, reducing incision size and trauma, easing patient recovery [3]. Enhanced visualization through planning software with robotics allows for patient-specific plans, tailoring treatment to individual anatomy and condition. Robotic surgery improves outcomes by enabling precise, personalized techniques—leading to reduced complications, shorter hospital stays, and faster recoveries. Particularly advantageous for complex procedures like cardiac, neurosurgery, and orthopedics, robotics enhances surgical proficiency through simulation-based training, ensuring safer patient care. Additionally, advanced robotics holds promise for remote surgery, offering access to specialized expertise in distant locations [4].

4.1.1 Fundamentals of robotics

Robotic-assisted surgical planning and navigation enhance the surgeons' visualization and spatial awareness through 3D imaging and virtual

DOI: 10.1201/9781003581192-4

simulations. This technology allows for meticulous preoperative planning, identification of anatomical structures, and anticipation of challenges—resulting in increased confidence and accuracy in the operating room. Advanced sensors and user-friendly interfaces in robotic advanced imaging aids decision-making and procedure execution—an integration of surgical agility and accuracy. Ergonomic benefits also reduce surgeon fatigue during lengthy procedures [3].

Additionally, robotics can streamline workflows and optimize resources by automating tasks like instrument sterilization and equipment setup, reducing procedural times and increasing efficiency. This benefits patients by minimizing anesthesia exposure and maximizing surgical service throughout. Robotic-assisted systems also revolutionize surgical education through virtual reality simulations, allowing trainees to gain hands-on experience safely—expediting their learning curve, and ensuring proficiency. Overall, integrating robotics in surgical planning and navigation promises enhanced outcomes, increased efficiency, and improved patient care globally [3].

4.1.2 Brief history of robot-assisted surgery

The evolution of computer technology since the 1980s, along with advances in computing power systems—has enabled precise instrument control, facilitating delicate maneuvers with improved and miniaturized tracking devices—leading to the rise of Computer Assisted Surgery (CAS). CAS includes various surgical procedures and computational tools designed for planning, guiding, or performing surgery. Its main clinical goal is to help surgeons define and execute optimal surgical strategies for diagnostic or therapeutic purposes. CAS offers two key benefits: it enables minimally invasive surgery, reducing surgical trauma, morbidity, and postoperative hospitalization, and it enhances the accuracy of procedures by providing additional complementary tools. The historical development of surgical robotics, from Archytas of Tarentum's steam-driven wooden bird in 400 $_{\text{CE}}$ to Leonardo da Vinci's Metal-Plated Warrior in 1495, has paved the way for modern robotic-assisted surgery (Figure 4.1). Innovations like telesurgery, exemplified by Dr. Marescaux's 2001 transatlantic cholecystectomy using the ZEUS surgical system, mark significant milestones in surgical robotics [1].

In 1921, Karel Capek introduced the term "robot" in his play "Rossom's Universal Robots," derived from the Czech word "robota," meaning "labor." Inspired by Capek, Isaac Asimov coined "robotics" in 1942 and established the three laws of robotics. The concept of autonomous machines dates back to 400 $_{\text{CE}}$ with Archytas's steam-driven bird and includes significant innovations such as Gianello Torriano's robotic mandolin player in 1540 and Jaquet-Droz's programmable robot, "The Writer," in 1772. Robotics has revolutionized medicine, exemplified by Dr. Marescaux's 2001 transatlantic telerobotic surgery using the ZEUS system.

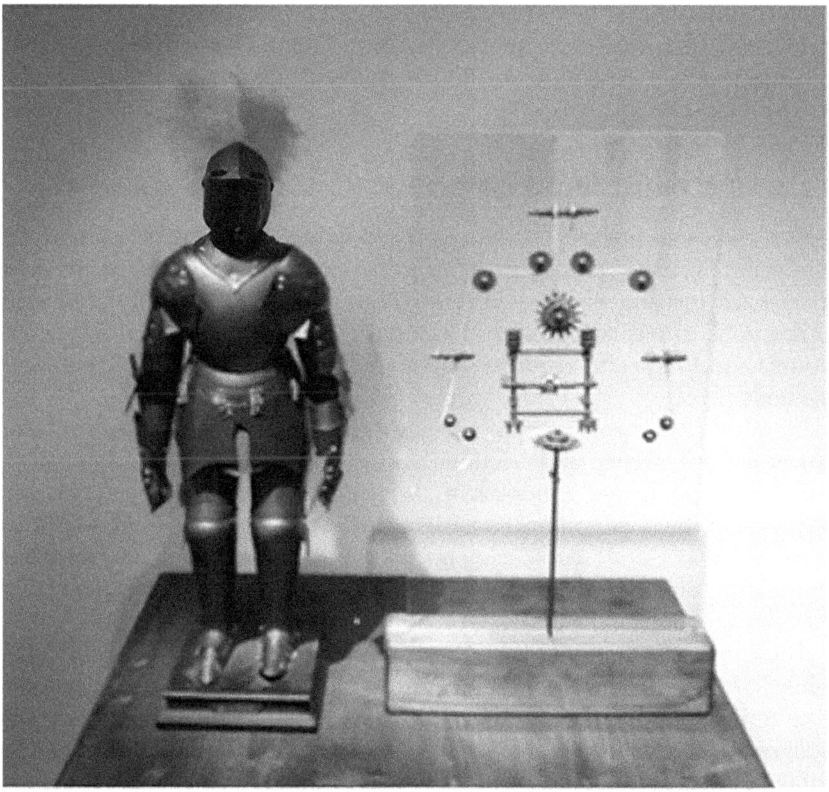

Figure 4.1 Leonardo da Vinci's metallic warrior.

4.1.3 Importance of robotics in modern surgical procedures

Robotics assumes a pivotal role in contemporary surgical procedures, fundamentally transforming patient care. Its precision and accuracy significantly elevate surgical outcomes, particularly in intricate procedures or confined anatomical spaces. Through the facilitation of minimally invasive techniques, robotics diminishes patient trauma, expedites recovery, and mitigates postoperative complications. Advanced imaging modalities accompany robotics, furnishing surgeons with heightened visualization capabilities, thus enabling informed decision-making and precise procedural execution. Furthermore, robotics facilitates patient-specific planning predicated on preoperative imaging, ensuring tailored treatment modalities aligned with individual anatomical nuances and clinical presentations. In intricate surgeries spanning cardiac, neurosurgery, and orthopedics, robotics confers unparalleled advantages, enhancing both surgical proficiency and patient safety. Ultimately, robotics stands as a cornerstone of contemporary surgical practice, reshaping healthcare delivery paradigms and optimizing patient outcomes [2].

4.2 BASIC PRINCIPLES OF ROBOTIC-ASSISTED SURGERY

Robotic-assisted surgery utilizes surgeon-controlled robotic systems for minimally invasive procedures. Surgeons manipulate robotic arms with specialized instruments, providing superior precision, dexterity, and visualization. This technology seeks to enhance surgical results, reduce patient trauma, and expedite recovery, compared to conventional open surgery methods [2].

In robotic surgical systems, a microprocessor enhances precision and dexterity by digitizing and refining the surgeon's console-based movements before relaying them to robotic arms. Surgeons, seated at a console, remotely operate instruments within the patient. Robots provide surgical assistance in several ways: endoscopic cameras on robotic arms follow the surgeon's commands, eliminating guesswork, tremor, and fatigue, allowing focus on the virtual operating field [5].

The camera's zoom and motion-scaling features enable fine procedures, while 3D imaging and full motion control facilitate minimally invasive surgery training and reduce the learning curve. Master-slave robotic systems designed for telesurgery allow remote procedures without direct patient contact; however, latency over 700 milliseconds remains a challenge, requiring high-bandwidth communication [6]. In image-guided therapy, robots use MRI and CT data to guide instruments precisely, integrating pathology, anatomy, and resection margins into the surgical field. This "enhanced reality" concept is used in neurosurgery and orthopedics, and image-guided technology is being developed for surgical training and simulation (Figure 4.2) [5].

4.3 Classification of robotic systems used in surgical procedures

Robotic systems in surgery have revolutionized the way complex procedures are performed: by enhancing precision, reducing invasiveness, and improving patient outcomes. These systems augment the capabilities of surgeons and are categorized based on their functionality, application, and level of autonomy. Below is a detailed classification of robotic systems used in surgical procedures, exploring their unique features, advantages, and limitations [7].

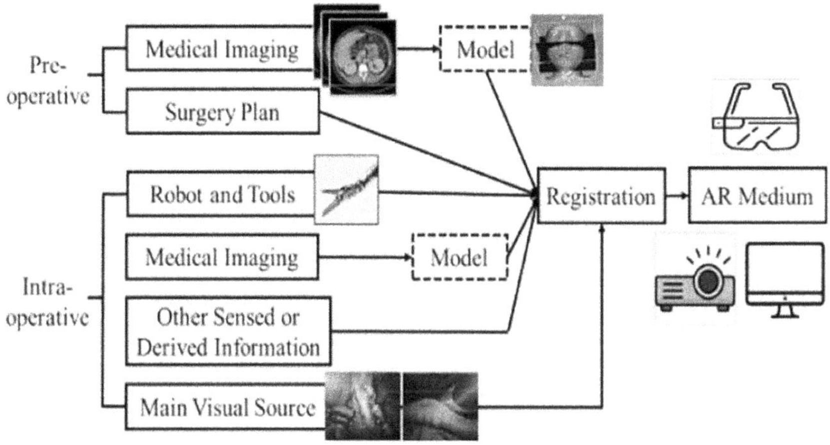

Figure 4.2 Surgeon-controlled robotic systems.

4.3.1 Robotic-assisted surgical systems

These systems are designed to enhance the precision and dexterity of surgeons during minimally invasive procedures. The surgeon controls robotic arms equipped with surgical instruments, offering better maneuverability than conventional laparoscopic tools [8].

Examples:

a. da Vinci Surgical System: The **da Vinci Surgical System**, developed by Intuitive Surgical, is a pioneering robotic platform designed to enhance the precision and control of minimally invasive surgeries. It is one of the most widely used systems globally and has revolutionized procedures in **urology, gynecology, and cardiothoracic surgery**. The system allows surgeons to operate from a console that provides a high-definition, three-dimensional view of the surgical site. From this console, the surgeon controls multiple robotic arms equipped with specialized instruments that can mimic the range of motion of the human wrist, enabling intricate movements with precision that surpasses conventional laparoscopic tools [9, 7].

Key features include **Endo Wrist technology**, which provides the instruments with seven degrees of freedom, offering a range of motion similar to that of a human hand but with greater flexibility. Additionally, the system's **3D HD Vision System** enhances depth perception, allowing for better visualization of complex anatomical structures. Another significant advantage is **tremor filtration**, which eliminates unintentional movements, ensuring smoother and safer operations [9, 7].

The da Vinci system has been particularly transformative in procedures like **prostatectomies, hysterectomies,** and **mitral valve repairs,** offering patients shorter recovery times, reduced pain, and fewer complications compared to traditional open surgeries (Table 4.1) [10].

b. Senhance Surgical System: The **Senhance Surgical System,** developed by Asensus Surgical, is another advanced robotic platform known for its unique ability to provide **haptic feedback,** a feature that distinguishes it from many other robotic systems. Haptic feedback allows surgeons to feel tissue resistance through the controls, which helps them gauge the amount of force being applied, improving surgical precision and safety. This tactile sensation is particularly useful in delicate procedures where excessive force could cause tissue damage (Table 4.1) [10].

In addition to haptic feedback, the Senhance system incorporates **eye-tracking technology,** enabling surgeons to control the camera intuitively with their gaze. This feature enhances efficiency by allowing for seamless adjustments of the visual field during surgery. The system also supports **cost-effective reusable instruments,** making it a more economical option for hospitals compared to systems that rely on disposable tools [10, 11, 4].

The Senhance system is gaining popularity for various laparoscopic procedures and is seen as a promising alternative, especially in settings where cost and tactile feedback are significant considerations. Its innovations in sensory input and control are helping bridge the gap between traditional and robotic surgery, improving outcomes and enhancing the surgeon's experience (Table 4.1) [10, 11, 4].

4.3.1.1 Key features of robotic-assisted surgical systems

Robotic-assisted surgical systems have transformed the landscape of modern surgery by providing surgeons with enhanced precision, better visualization, and improved ergonomics. These technologies are designed to overcome the limitations of traditional surgery and optimize outcomes for both patients and surgeons. Below is a detailed exploration of the key features and their impact, supported by examples [1].

1. Enhanced Precision

Robotic arms are capable of making micro-movements with an accuracy that exceeds human capabilities. This precision is crucial in delicate procedures where even the slightest error can have significant consequences. For example, in **prostatectomies,** where the surgeon must navigate around nerves and blood vessels, robotic systems such as the **da Vinci Surgical System** allow for highly controlled and refined movements. The system's **EndoWrist**

Table 4.1 Comparison between da Vinci Surgical System and Senhance Surgical System

Feature	*da Vinci Surgical System*	*Senhance Surgical System*
Manufacturer	Intuitive Surgical	Asensus Surgical
Control Mechanism	Master-slave system with surgeon at a console remotely controlling robotic arms.	Surgeon at a console with haptic feedback and eye-tracking for control.
Purpose	Minimally invasive surgeries in various fields, including general, urological, gynecological, and cardiac surgeries.	Focuses on minimally invasive surgeries, particularly in general, gynecological, urological, and thoracic fields.
User Interface	3D high-definition visualization with a magnified view.	Enhanced 3D or 2D high-definition visualization with ergonomic support.
Haptic Feedback	Lacks true haptic feedback; relies on visual cues.	Provides haptic feedback for enhanced tactile perception.
Instrument Size and Precision	Offers a wide range of interchangeable instruments with a high degree of precision.	Utilizes standard laparoscopic instruments, reducing costs and offering precise control.
Ergonomics	Focuses on reducing surgeon fatigue through an intuitive console setup.	Incorporates eye-tracking and ergonomic controls for improved surgeon comfort.
Learning Curve	Requires significant training to master complex procedures.	Offers a shorter learning curve due to the familiarity of laparoscopic techniques.
Setup Time	Typically longer due to system complexity and instrument calibration.	Quicker setup time, emphasizing simplicity and efficiency.
Cost	High initial investment, along with significant maintenance and per-use costs.	Lower overall costs due to reusable instruments and a modular design.
Port Size	Utilizes specialized ports with varying sizes, typically larger.	Supports smaller laparoscopic ports for less invasive procedures.
Key Differentiator	Advanced capabilities for complex surgeries with unparalleled precision.	Focus on cost efficiency and integrating tactile feedback with laparoscopic familiarity.
Regulatory Approval	FDA-approved and widely adopted globally.	FDA-approved, gaining popularity, particularly in cost-sensitive markets.
Target Audience	Hospitals and surgeons seeking cutting-edge technology for advanced robotic surgeries.	Institutions aiming to balance advanced robotic capabilities with cost-efficiency.

technology mimics the flexibility of a human wrist but with far greater control, enabling complex suturing and dissection tasks. **Neurosurgery:** Robots like the **Rosa robot** assist in placing electrodes with sub-millimeter precision during brain surgeries [1].

2. Minimally Invasive Procedures

Robotic systems facilitate minimally invasive surgery by allowing surgeons to operate through small incisions. Unlike traditional open surgery, these smaller incisions result in reduced trauma to surrounding tissues, leading to less postoperative pain, minimal scarring, and faster recovery times. The **Senhance Surgical System**, for instance, is designed to enhance laparoscopic procedures, reducing the need for large incisions. **Hysterectomy:** Using the da Vinci system, surgeons can perform complex hysterectomies through small incisions, reducing hospital stays and recovery time [1].

3. Improved Visualization

Robotic surgical systems are equipped with advanced imaging technology, providing surgeons with high-definition, three-dimensional views of the surgical area. This enhanced visualization offers better depth perception and allows surgeons to see anatomical structures in great detail, which is essential for identifying critical structures such as nerves and blood vessels. In procedures like **mitral valve repair**, 3D imaging helps surgeons visualize intricate areas of the heart, ensuring precise suturing and minimal complications [3].

4. Reduced Fatigue

Surgeons often experience fatigue during lengthy procedures, which can compromise their performance. Robotic systems address this issue by taking over repetitive and physically demanding tasks. Surgeons control the robotic arms from a console, allowing them to maintain a comfortable posture throughout the procedure. This ergonomic setup not only reduces fatigue but also enhances focus and precision. In **colorectal surgery**, which can last several hours, robotic assistance helps maintain consistency in performance, reducing the risk of errors caused by fatigue [3].

5. Consistency and Standardization

One of the major advantages of robotic surgery is the consistency it offers. Unlike manual surgery, where outcomes can vary based on the surgeon's experience and fatigue, robotic systems provide standardized procedures. This leads to predictable and reproducible results, improving patient safety and overall outcomes. Systems like **MAKO** assist in orthopedic procedures, ensuring precise placement of implants, thereby reducing variability and improving joint alignment and longevity [7].

Robotic-assisted surgical systems have redefined the possibilities of modern surgery by offering enhanced precision, minimally invasive techniques, improved visualization, reduced surgeon fatigue, and consistent outcomes. Technologies like the **da Vinci Surgical System** and **Senhance Surgical System** continue to push the boundaries of what is possible, benefiting both patients and medical professionals. As these systems evolve, they promise even greater advancements in surgical care, making procedures safer, more effective, and less invasive [10].

4.3.1.2 Limitations of robotic-assisted surgical systems

While robotic-assisted surgical systems have revolutionized modern surgery by enhancing precision, visualization, and outcomes, they also come with notable limitations. These include high costs, the need for specialized training, technical challenges, and restricted accessibility. Below is a detailed discussion of these challenges and their implications for healthcare providers and patients [12].

1. High Cost

One of the most significant barriers to the widespread adoption of robotic surgical systems is their high cost. The initial investment for purchasing a system like the **da Vinci Surgical System** can range from $1 million to $2.5 million, depending on the model and features. In addition to the purchase price, maintenance costs, software updates, and consumable parts such as robotic instruments add to the financial burden. These ongoing expenses can place a strain on hospital budgets, particularly for smaller facilities. The financial burden often translates to increased costs for patients, making robotic surgery less accessible to those without adequate insurance coverage. Hospitals may need to prioritize certain specialties over others to justify the expense, potentially limiting the types of procedures available [12].

2. Training Requirements

Robotic-assisted surgery requires specialized training for surgeons and operating room staff. Unlike traditional surgery, where surgeons rely on direct hand-eye coordination, robotic systems necessitate mastering the use of a console and understanding the system's capabilities and limitations. Training programs can be time-consuming and costly, further adding to the overall expense of implementing these systems. Surgeons must undergo extensive training to gain proficiency, which can take months or even years. This can delay the system's integration into regular clinical practice. Operating room staff, including nurses and technicians, also need to be familiar with the robotic system's setup and troubleshooting, requiring ongoing education. Intuitive Surgical, the manufacturer of the da Vinci system, offers structured training programs, but these can be expensive and time-consuming [12].

3. Technical Challenges

Robotic systems, like any complex technology, are susceptible to technical issues. System malfunctions, software glitches, or hardware failures can occur during surgery, posing risks to patient safety. Although backup systems and fail-safes are typically in place, unexpected technical issues can lead to delays, cancellations, or the need to convert to open surgery mid-procedure. Technical malfunctions can cause significant delays, increasing the duration of anesthesia and associated risks. Maintenance and repairs can lead to system downtime, limiting the availability of robotic surgery and causing scheduling disruptions. If a robotic arm or surgical instrument malfunctions during a procedure, the surgeon may need to quickly revert to manual techniques, which can be challenging in a high-stakes situation. [12].

4. Limited Accessibility

The high costs associated with robotic systems restrict their availability to larger, well-funded hospitals and academic medical centers. Smaller community hospitals and rural healthcare facilities often lack the financial resources to invest in such technology, leading to disparities in access to advanced surgical care. Patients in rural or underserved areas may need to travel long distances to access robotic-assisted surgery, creating barriers to timely care. The concentration of robotic systems in affluent areas contributes to disparities in healthcare outcomes, with patients in less affluent regions missing out on the benefits of minimally invasive robotic procedures. Large urban hospitals may offer a wide range of robotic surgeries, while smaller rural hospitals may not have any robotic capabilities, limiting patient options. While robotic-assisted surgical systems offer significant benefits in terms of precision, minimally invasive techniques, and improved outcomes, their adoption is hindered by several limitations. High costs, the need for specialized training, technical challenges, and limited accessibility present substantial hurdles for healthcare providers. Addressing these challenges will require innovative solutions, such as reducing costs through technological advancements, expanding training opportunities, and developing more affordable systems to ensure equitable access to robotic surgery. Despite these limitations, the potential of robotic surgery remains immense, and ongoing advancements may help mitigate these issues in the future [12].

4.3.2 Image-guided robotic surgery

Image-guided robotic surgery combines advanced imaging technologies with robotic systems to enhance the precision and accuracy of complex surgical procedures. By integrating real-time imaging modalities such as CT scans, MRI, or ultrasound, surgeons can visualize the patient's anatomy in three dimensions, enabling them to navigate complex structures with greater accuracy. This technology is particularly valuable in procedures where precise targeting of tissues or organs is critical, such as neurosurgery, orthopedic surgery, and oncology. In these procedures, imaging systems continuously provide feedback, allowing the surgeon to adjust the robotic instruments based on the patient's unique anatomical features (Figure 4.3). For example, in neurosurgery, image-guided robotic systems help map critical areas of the brain, ensuring that tumors are removed while sparing vital structures [13]. Similarly, in orthopedic procedures such as joint replacements, surgeons can use preoperative imaging to plan the optimal placement of implants and make real-time adjustments during the operation. The integration of imaging also enhances patient safety by reducing the risk of damaging healthy tissues. Surgeons can visualize the exact location of nerves, blood vessels, and other critical structures—minimizing complications and improving outcomes. Moreover, image-guided systems often facilitate minimally invasive approaches, which involve smaller incisions, less tissue trauma, and faster recovery times. A notable example of image-guided robotic surgery is the use of the **Mazor X Stealth Edition** system in spinal surgeries. This platform combines robotic precision with real-time imaging, enabling surgeons to place screws and other implants with exceptional accuracy. Another example is **Cyber Knife**, a robotic system that uses imaging to deliver targeted radiation therapy for cancer treatment, sparing healthy tissues while focusing on tumors. Despite its benefits, image-guided robotic surgery faces challenges, including high costs and the need for specialized training. The complexity of integrating imaging with robotic platforms also requires sophisticated software and robust technical support. However, as technology continues to evolve, these systems are likely to become more accessible and widely adopted, transforming the landscape of precision surgery and improving patient outcomes across various specialties [13].

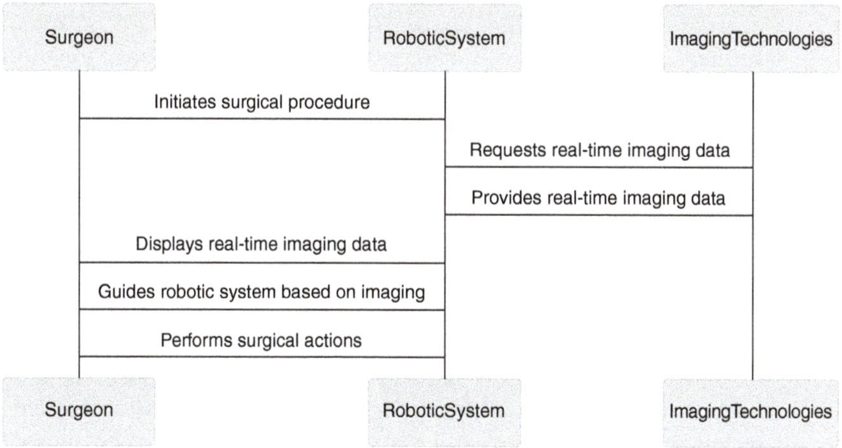

Figure 4.3 Features of image-guided robotic surgery.

4.3.2.1 Key Features:

Image-guided robotic surgery represents a revolutionary advancement in modern medicine by integrating real-time imaging technologies with robotic systems. This combination allows for unparalleled precision, accuracy, and control during surgical procedures, particularly those involving complex or delicate anatomy. The key features of this technology include real-time visualization, enhanced precision, minimally invasive techniques, and greater dexterity, each contributing to improved surgical outcomes and patient care [13].

a. **Real-Time Visualization** is one of the most critical aspects of image-guided robotic surgery. By utilizing advanced imaging modalities such as CT scans, MRI, or fluoroscopy, surgeons gain a dynamic and detailed view of the surgical site as the procedure progresses. Unlike traditional approaches that rely on preoperative images, real-time imaging allows for continuous updates, enabling surgeons to adapt their strategies as needed. This feature is especially vital in procedures where anatomical structures can shift during surgery, such as in neurosurgery or complex spinal operations. For example, real-time visualization in brain surgery helps in mapping functional areas and avoiding damage to critical regions responsible for motor or sensory functions [13].
b. **Enhanced Precision** is another hallmark of image-guided robotic systems, making them indispensable in delicate procedures. The combination of robotic arms and imaging technologies allows surgeons to target specific tissues or structures with micrometer accuracy, reducing the risk of errors. In neurosurgery, for instance, precision is paramount when operating near vital areas of the brain. Robotic systems, guided by imaging, ensure that tumors or other abnormalities can be removed while sparing healthy tissues. Similarly, in spinal surgery, precise placement of screws and implants is crucial to avoid nerve damage and ensure structural stability. The **Mazor X Stealth Edition** system is a notable example, using imaging guidance to assist in the accurate placement of spinal hardware [13].
c. **Minimally Invasive** techniques are a significant advantage of image-guided robotic surgery. Traditional open surgeries often require large incisions, leading to more significant trauma, longer recovery times, and increased risk of complications. In contrast, robotic systems allow for smaller incisions, reducing tissue damage and promoting faster healing. Minimally invasive approaches also result in less post-operative pain and lower rates of infection. In procedures such as robotic-assisted prostatectomy or gynecologic surgeries, patients benefit from shorter hospital stays and quicker returns to normal activities. The ability to visualize the surgical field in detail through

imaging further enhances the safety and effectiveness of these minimally invasive techniques [13].

d. **Greater Dexterity** provided by robotic instruments is another transformative feature. Robotic arms can mimic and even surpass the range of motion of the human hand, allowing for movements that are not possible manually. These instruments can rotate and bend in ways that facilitate access to hard-to-reach areas, making complex procedures more manageable. For example, in cardiac surgery, where space is limited, robotic systems enable surgeons to perform intricate maneuvers with precision. The **da Vinci Surgical System,** widely used in urology, gynecology, and cardiothoracic surgery, exemplifies this capability by offering wristed instruments that enhance dexterity and control. Surgeons operate from a console, using joysticks and foot pedals to guide the robotic arms, translating their movements into fine, precise actions [13].

The combination of these key features results in several benefits for both patients and surgeons. Patients experience fewer complications, reduced pain, and faster recoveries, while surgeons benefit from improved ergonomics, reduced fatigue, and enhanced confidence in performing complex procedures. Additionally, the consistency provided by robotic systems ensures standardized outcomes, minimizing variability in surgical performance. However, it is important to acknowledge the challenges associated with image-guided robotic surgery. The high cost of these systems and the need for specialized training can limit their accessibility, particularly in smaller or resource-constrained healthcare facilities. Despite these barriers, ongoing advancements in technology and increased adoption are likely to drive down costs and expand availability. In conclusion, image-guided robotic surgery represents a significant leap forward in surgical innovation, offering real-time visualization, enhanced precision, minimally invasive approaches, and greater dexterity. These features collectively improve the safety, effectiveness, and outcomes of complex surgical procedures. As technology continues to evolve, the potential for even greater advancements in this field holds promise for transforming patient care and setting new standards in surgical excellence [13].

Advantages:

Image-guided robotic surgery offers numerous advantages that significantly enhance both patient outcomes and the surgeon's experience. The combination of advanced imaging and robotic precision has transformed surgical practice, leading to more effective, safer, and less invasive procedures. Two key benefits are improved patient outcomes and enhanced support for surgeons, which, together, redefine the landscape of modern surgery [13].

a. **Improved patient outcomes:** The ability to visualize and navigate complex anatomy in real time allows for more precise targeting of pathological tissues, reducing the likelihood of complications. For example, in brain surgery, precision is critical to avoid damage to functional areas that control movement, speech, or sensory processing. Image-guided robotic systems help surgeons identify and navigate these regions, enabling safer tumor resections or other interventions. Similarly, in orthopedic procedures, such as joint replacements or spinal surgery, precise placement of implants or screws ensures better alignment, which can lead to improved joint function and longevity of the implant [13].
b. **Reducing postoperative complications:** Moreover, precise targeting minimizes trauma to surrounding healthy tissues, which is a key factor in reducing postoperative complications. Smaller, more accurate incisions result in less blood loss, reduced pain, and lower infection rates. Patients undergoing minimally invasive, image-guided robotic procedures often experience faster recovery times and shorter hospital stays compared to those undergoing traditional open surgery. For instance, in robotic-assisted prostatectomies or gynecological surgeries, patients typically recover more quickly, with fewer long-term side effects, such as incontinence or scarring. This improved recovery trajectory not only enhances the patient's quality of life but also reduces healthcare costs associated with extended hospital stays and postoperative care [13].
c. **Support to surgeons:** Another significant advantage is the support these systems provide to surgeons, particularly in reducing physical strain during long or complex procedures. Traditional surgery often requires surgeons to maintain awkward or uncomfortable positions for extended periods, leading to fatigue and musculoskeletal issues. Robotic systems alleviate this burden by allowing surgeons to operate from an ergonomically designed console. Seated comfortably, surgeons can control the robotic arms using joysticks and pedals, translating their movements into precise actions within the patient's body. This setup significantly reduces physical fatigue, enabling surgeons to maintain focus and precision throughout lengthy operations [13].
d. **Assistance with repetitive tasks:** Additionally, robotic systems automate or assist with repetitive tasks, such as suturing or tissue manipulation, further relieving the surgeon's workload. This support allows surgeons to concentrate on the critical aspects of the procedure, improving accuracy and decision-making. The reduced physical and mental strain also contributes to better performance and consistency, particularly in complex or high-stakes surgeries [13].
e. **Boost surgeon confidence:** Furthermore, the enhanced visualization and precision offered by robotic systems can boost surgeon

confidence, particularly when navigating challenging anatomy. Real-time imaging updates provide continuous feedback, enabling adjustments as needed and reducing the risk of errors. This support is especially beneficial in delicate procedures, such as cardiovascular or neurosurgery, where millimeter-level accuracy can make a significant difference in outcomes [13].

In summary, image-guided robotic surgery offers substantial advantages, including improved patient outcomes through better targeting and reduced complications, as well as critical support for surgeons by minimizing physical strain and enhancing focus. These benefits not only elevate the quality of care but also contribute to the broader goal of making surgery safer, more effective, and less invasive for patients. As technology continues to advance, the potential for further improvements in this field remains promising [13].

Limitations:

a. High Costs

A significant limitation of image-guided robotic surgery is the **high financial investment** required for procurement, maintenance, and upgrades. Robotic systems, along with the integrated imaging technologies such as CT, MRI, or ultrasound, involve substantial initial costs, often exceeding millions of dollars. Beyond the purchase price, the cost of consumables, maintenance contracts, software updates, and repairs adds to the financial burden. For hospitals, especially smaller facilities or those in resource-constrained areas, these costs can be prohibitive, limiting access to this advanced technology. The economic challenge is further compounded by the need for specialized operating rooms designed to accommodate both the robotic system and imaging equipment. Furthermore, insurance reimbursement for robotic-assisted procedures may not always cover the additional expenses associated with the technology, posing financial challenges for both patients and healthcare institutions. These factors restrict the availability of image-guided robotic surgery to well-funded hospitals and academic centers, creating disparities in access to advanced surgical care [13].

b. Training and Complexity

Another critical challenge is the **extensive training** required for surgeons, nurses, and support staff to effectively use image-guided robotic systems. Mastery of these technologies demands a steep learning curve, encompassing not only proficiency in robotic controls but also the ability to interpret and integrate real-time imaging data during surgery. Unlike conventional surgical techniques, where tactile feedback plays a vital role, robotic surgery relies on visual cues, necessitating a shift in how surgeons approach procedures. Training programs often require surgeons to undergo simulated exercises, workshops, and proctored cases before gaining certification to perform robotic-assisted surgeries independently. This process can be time-consuming and expensive. Moreover, surgical teams must remain updated on technological advancements and software upgrades, necessitating ongoing education and practice. The **integration of imaging modalities** such as CT or MRI into the surgical workflow adds another layer of complexity. Surgeons must coordinate with radiologists and imaging technicians to ensure accurate imaging and interpretation. The need for seamless collaboration between different specialties underscores the importance of multidisciplinary training and teamwork. Additionally, operational challenges such as image registration, calibration of robotic systems, and maintenance of sterile fields complicate the workflow, requiring meticulous planning and execution [13].

c. Technical Issues

The **reliability of image-guided robotic systems** is crucial, yet technical issues and malfunctions can pose significant risks. Robotic systems rely on complex hardware and software, and any malfunction during surgery can lead to delays or complications. For instance, issues with robotic arms, imaging equipment, or software glitches can interrupt the procedure, necessitating a shift to conventional surgical techniques. This transition can be challenging, particularly in minimally invasive surgeries where direct access to the surgical site is limited [13].

Power outages or connectivity issues can also disrupt the functionality of robotic systems, highlighting the need for backup systems and contingency plans. In some cases, technical support may be required to troubleshoot problems, which can delay surgery and increase the risk of complications. Moreover, the precision of robotic arms depends on accurate calibration and alignment with imaging data, and any discrepancies can impact surgical outcomes. The reliance on advanced technology also raises concerns about **cybersecurity and data integrity**. Image-guided systems store and transmit sensitive patient data, making them vulnerable to cyberattacks. Ensuring the security of these systems requires robust cybersecurity measures and compliance with data protection regulations [13].

In conclusion, while image-guided robotic surgery offers numerous benefits, it is not without significant limitations. High costs, extensive training requirements, and potential technical issues pose challenges that must be addressed to maximize the technology's impact. Overcoming these barriers will require continued investment in training programs, infrastructure, and system reliability, along with efforts to make the technology more accessible and affordable [13].

4.3.3 Radiotherapy robotic systems

Radiotherapy robotic systems are advanced technologies designed to deliver **precise, targeted radiation** to cancerous cells while minimizing exposure to surrounding healthy tissues. This precision is crucial in cancer treatment, as it helps reduce side effects and improves patient outcomes. By integrating robotics with imaging and computer algorithms, these systems can adapt to tumor movement and complex anatomical structures, ensuring optimal delivery of radiation. One of the key benefits of these systems is their ability to perform **stereotactic body radiotherapy** (SBRT) and **stereotactic radiosurgery** (SRS). These techniques involve delivering high doses of radiation in fewer sessions, enhancing treatment efficiency and reducing the overall burden on patients (Figure 4.4). The robotic arms can move in multiple directions, providing flexibility in beam angles and allowing for non-invasive treatments of tumors in difficult-to-reach areas, such as the brain, lungs, liver, and spine. A prominent example is the **CyberKnife System**, which uses real-time imaging and robotic positioning to continuously track and adjust for tumor motion, such as that caused by breathing. This dynamic tracking capability ensures that radiation is delivered with sub-millimeter accuracy, sparing healthy tissues and critical structures. CyberKnife is particularly effective for treating small, well-defined tumors and those near sensitive organs [14, 15].

Another system, **Versa HD by Elekta**, combines robotic precision with volumetric imaging to tailor treatments for various cancers. It allows for image-guided radiation therapy (IGRT), where imaging is performed immediately before or during treatment to ensure accurate targeting. Despite their advantages, radiotherapy robotic systems face challenges, including **high costs** and the need for specialized training. The equipment and software are expensive to acquire and maintain, limiting accessibility to well-funded institutions. Additionally, clinicians must be trained not only in

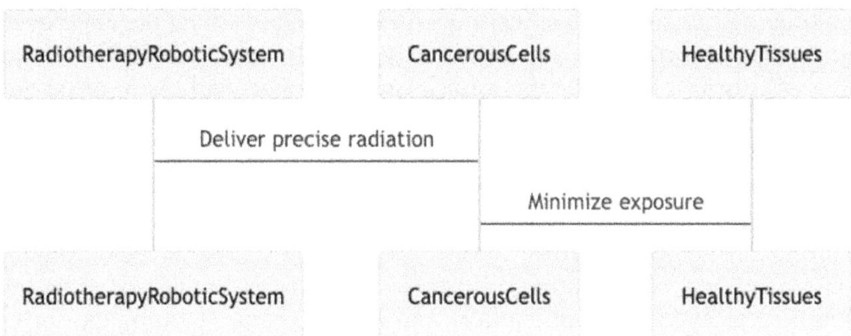

Figure 4.4 Features of radiotherapy robotic systems.

operating the robotic systems but also in understanding complex treatment planning and imaging protocols. In summary, radiotherapy robotic systems represent a significant advancement in cancer care, offering enhanced precision and the ability to treat complex cases. Their ability to protect healthy tissues while delivering effective doses of radiation makes them invaluable tools in modern oncology. However, their widespread adoption depends on addressing cost and training barriers to make this technology accessible to more patients [14, 15].

4.3.3.1 Key Features:

a. Precision: Targets Tumors Accurately, Reducing Collateral Damage
One of the defining features of radiotherapy robotic systems is their **unmatched precision** in targeting cancerous cells. These systems integrate advanced imaging technologies like real-time X-rays, CT scans, and MRI to map the exact location of tumors. This capability ensures that radiation beams are focused solely on cancer cells while sparing healthy tissues and vital organs nearby. For example, the **CyberKnife System** uses robotic arms to deliver high-dose radiation with sub-millimeter accuracy. Its unique ability to track tumor movement, especially in areas prone to motion like the lungs or liver, allows it to adjust in real-time to patient breathing. This dynamic targeting not only improves treatment efficacy but also reduces the risk of complications such as radiation-induced damage to healthy tissues. Similarly, **TrueBeam by Varian** offers image-guided radiotherapy (IGRT), combining imaging and radiation delivery in a single platform. This ensures that any changes in tumor position or size are accounted for, maintaining precise targeting throughout the treatment [14, 15].

b. Patient Comfort: Non-Invasive and Painless
Radiotherapy robotic systems provide a **non-invasive and painless** alternative to traditional cancer treatments like surgery. Patients undergoing robotic radiotherapy do not require incisions or anesthesia, making the experience far more comfortable. The procedure typically involves the patient lying on a treatment table while the robotic arm moves around them, delivering radiation from various angles. The **Gamma Knife** system, used primarily for brain tumors, is a notable example of non-invasive radiotherapy. It delivers focused radiation beams without requiring an open craniotomy. Patients remain awake during the procedure and experience minimal discomfort, significantly improving their overall treatment experience. Additionally, robotic systems often feature custom-designed patient molds or immobilization devices to enhance comfort and ensure precise positioning during treatment. These innovations help reduce anxiety and make the process less daunting for patients [14, 15].

c. Shorter Treatment Times: Advanced Systems Reduce Session Durations
Modern radiotherapy robotic systems are designed to **streamline treatment sessions**, delivering higher doses of radiation in fewer visits. This approach, known as hypofractionation, is especially beneficial for patients who might otherwise need to undergo weeks of daily treatments. For instance, the **Halcyon System** by Varian can complete treatments in as little as five minutes. Its intuitive design and automation capabilities allow for quick patient setup and efficient delivery of radiation. Similarly, Cyber Knife's ability to perform stereotactic body radiotherapy (SBRT) means patients can often complete their entire course of treatment in just one to five sessions, compared to traditional schedules that might require 30 or more sessions. Shorter treatment times not only improve patient convenience but also reduce the workload on healthcare facilities, allowing more patients to access care [14, 15].

d. Versatility: Suitable for Various Cancers and Body Parts
Radiotherapy robotic systems are incredibly **versatile**, making them suitable for treating a wide range of cancers in different parts of the body. Unlike conventional radiotherapy machines that may be limited to specific types of tumors, robotic systems can adapt to complex anatomies and target tumors in challenging locations. The CyberKnife system, for example, is effective for treating tumors in the brain, spine, lungs, liver, pancreas, and even prostate. Its robotic arm can move freely around the patient, delivering radiation from virtually any angle. This flexibility makes it ideal for cases where tumors are located near critical structures or are difficult to reach with traditional methods. Another example is the **MRIdian System** by ViewRay, which integrates MRI imaging with radiation delivery. This system allows continuous visualization of soft tissue during treatment, making it particularly effective for cancers in areas like the abdomen and pelvis, where organ motion can impact accuracy. Robotic systems are also adaptable to various treatment modalities, including stereotactic radiosurgery (SRS) for brain tumors and stereotactic body radiotherapy (SBRT) for other parts of the body. This adaptability ensures that patients receive personalized treatment tailored to their specific condition [14, 15].

Limitations:
While radiotherapy robotic systems offer numerous benefits in cancer treatment, including precision, reduced recovery time, and enhanced patient comfort, they also face several significant limitations. These challenges affect their adoption, accessibility, and overall efficacy in clinical practice [14, 15].

a. Cost: High Initial and Operational Expenses
One of the most significant barriers to the widespread adoption of radiotherapy robotic systems is their **high cost**. The initial investment required to

purchase these systems can range from several million dollars, depending on the technology and manufacturer. For instance, systems like **CyberKnife** and **Gamma Knife** are highly advanced but come with steep price tags. Additionally, operational costs, including maintenance, software updates, and specialized components, add to the financial burden on healthcare institutions. Moreover, the cost of building or retrofitting facilities to accommodate these systems can be substantial. Radiotherapy requires precise shielding to protect patients and staff from radiation exposure, which involves significant infrastructure changes. Hospitals and clinics in low-income or resource-limited settings often find it challenging to justify such investments, especially when budget constraints prioritize more basic healthcare needs [14, 15].

b. Training and Expertise: Need for Specialized Operators
Another critical limitation is the requirement for **highly trained personnel** to operate radiotherapy robotic systems. Unlike conventional radiotherapy machines, these systems demand expertise not only in radiation oncology but also in robotic technology, imaging modalities, and real-time adjustments during treatment. For example, the **MRIdian System** by ViewRay combines MRI imaging with radiation delivery, necessitating proficiency in both MRI operation and radiotherapy planning. Similarly, **CyberKnife** involves complex tumor-tracking algorithms that operators must understand to optimize treatment. This level of complexity means that only experienced radiation oncologists, medical physicists, and dosimetrists can manage these systems effectively. Training programs are often lengthy and expensive, creating additional challenges for healthcare facilities. In regions where skilled personnel are scarce, this requirement further limits access to advanced radiotherapy technologies. Continuous education and certification are also necessary to keep up with technological advancements, adding to the time and cost involved [14, 15].

c. Limited Availability: High Costs Restrict Widespread Use
Due to the financial and training challenges outlined above, radiotherapy robotic systems are primarily found in **large, well-funded hospitals and cancer centers**. Smaller hospitals and clinics, particularly in rural or underserved areas, often cannot afford these systems, leading to disparities in access to advanced cancer treatments. Patients in these regions may need to travel long distances to receive treatment, which can be logistically challenging and financially burdensome. For instance, a patient requiring CyberKnife treatment for a complex brain tumor may have to seek care at a specialized center hundreds of miles away. This not only adds stress but can also delay treatment, potentially affecting outcomes. Furthermore, healthcare systems in developing countries face additional barriers, including limited government funding for high-cost technologies and competing healthcare priorities.

Even when radiotherapy robotic systems are available, patient access may be restricted due to high treatment costs, making these advanced therapies inaccessible to those without adequate insurance coverage or financial resources [14, 15].

d. Technical Challenges and System Malfunctions

Radiotherapy robotic systems, while technologically advanced, are not immune to **technical issues**. Malfunctions, software glitches, or hardware failures can occur, potentially compromising patient safety. For example, a robotic arm delivering radiation may experience calibration errors, leading to inaccurate targeting of tumors. In such cases, immediate intervention by trained personnel is crucial to prevent harm. Moreover, the complexity of these systems means that repairs and maintenance require specialized technicians and parts, which can be costly and time-consuming. Delays in addressing technical issues can disrupt treatment schedules, causing anxiety and inconvenience for patients [14, 15].

e. Patient-Specific Limitations

While radiotherapy robotic systems are versatile, they may not be suitable for all patients. Certain tumors, especially those that are diffuse or located in highly sensitive areas, may not respond well to robotic radiotherapy. Additionally, patients with metal implants or severe claustrophobia may face challenges during imaging and treatment [14, 15].

f. Ethical and Regulatory Considerations

The integration of radiotherapy robotic systems into cancer treatment presents significant ethical and regulatory challenges. These advanced technologies offer precision in targeting tumors and sparing healthy tissues, yet their high costs can lead to disparities in access. Ensuring equitable availability is a critical ethical concern, as patients in underserved regions or with limited financial resources may be excluded from receiving optimal care. Healthcare providers and policymakers must work together to create funding mechanisms or subsidies to bridge this gap. Another ethical consideration is the potential over-reliance on automation. While robotic systems enhance accuracy, they should complement, not replace, human expertise. Clinicians must remain involved in decision-making to ensure that treatments are personalized and patient-centered. Balancing the benefits of automation with the need for human oversight is essential to maintaining ethical standards. On the regulatory front, the development and deployment of radiotherapy robotic systems must comply with stringent quality control and safety standards. Regulatory bodies such as the FDA (in the U.S.) and the European Medicines Agency (EMA) require extensive clinical trials and testing to ensure these systems are safe and effective. This process can be lengthy and complex, delaying the introduction of new technologies to the market. However, these rigorous evaluations are necessary to protect patient safety and build public trust in these innovations. Once approved, ongoing monitoring and quality assurance are crucial. Hospitals and clinics using these systems must adhere to strict operational protocols, conduct regular maintenance, and provide continuous training for staff. This ensures that the equipment functions correctly and that healthcare professionals are well-equipped to manage any technical issues that may arise. In summary, while radiotherapy robotic systems hold immense potential to revolutionize cancer treatment, addressing ethical concerns and navigating regulatory requirements are vital. Equitable access, ethical use, and compliance with safety standards will be key to maximizing their benefits and ensuring they contribute to better health outcomes for all patients [16].

4.3.4 Exoskeleton robotic systems

Exoskeleton robotic systems are wearable devices designed to enhance the physical capabilities of users by providing support, strength, and mobility assistance. These systems are widely used in healthcare, rehabilitation, and industrial settings. They consist of a mechanical framework powered by motors, sensors, and control systems that enable users to perform tasks more efficiently and safely. In healthcare, exoskeletons assist patients with mobility impairments, such as those recovering from spinal cord injuries, strokes, or neurological disorders. They help users regain movement, improve posture, and facilitate physical therapy—by providing controlled, repetitive movements critical for recovery. For instance, the ReWalk system enables paraplegic patients to stand and walk with the aid of motorized leg braces (Figure 4.5). In rehabilitation, exoskeletons ensure consistent therapy by automating precise movements, reducing the workload on therapists, and promoting faster recovery. Devices like the EksoNR guide patients through walking exercises, aiding neurorehabilitation. In industrial settings, exoskeletons reduce physical strain on workers, improve ergonomics, and prevent injuries. They support tasks such as heavy lifting and prolonged standing. The Guardian XO exoskeleton allows users to lift heavy objects with ease, enhancing productivity and minimizing fatigue [17].

Applications of exoskeleton robotic systems

1. Mobility Assistance

Exoskeleton robotic systems have revolutionized mobility support for individuals with physical disabilities, offering life-changing benefits for those with conditions like spinal cord injuries, strokes, and neurological disorders such as multiple sclerosis. These wearable devices provide powered assistance to help patients perform movements that would

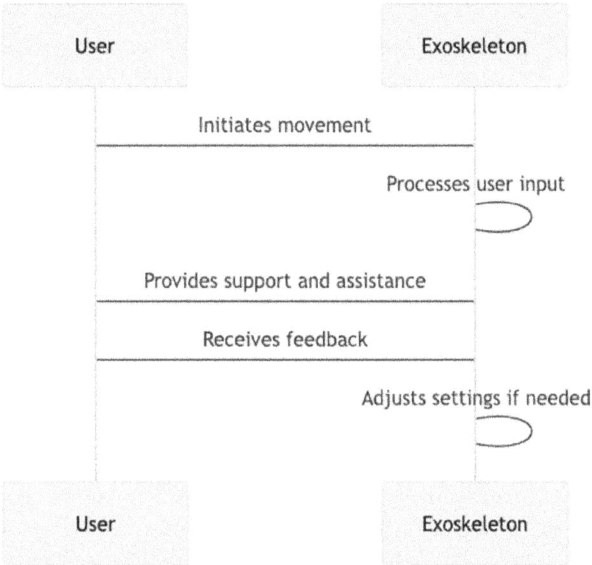

Figure 4.5 Exoskeleton robotic systems.

otherwise be impossible or difficult, such as standing, walking, or climbing stairs. For patients with **spinal cord injuries**, exoskeletons enable upright mobility, which not only improves independence but also has significant health benefits, including enhanced circulation, reduced muscle atrophy, and prevention of pressure sores. Devices like the **ReWalk** exoskeleton allow paraplegic users to walk with the help of motorized joints and crutches, simulating a natural gait. For individuals recovering from **strokes** or dealing with **multiple sclerosis**, exoskeletons assist in regaining mobility by supporting weakened muscles and providing balance. The **EksoNR** exoskeleton, for example, is used in rehabilitation to guide patients through controlled walking exercises, promoting neuroplasticity and motor recovery. Exoskeletons also empower users by fostering a sense of **independence** and improving their **quality of life**. Beyond physical benefits, they enhance psychological well-being by enabling participation in daily activities and social engagements. Innovations in exoskeleton design, such as lighter materials and AI-driven motion control, are making these devices more accessible and comfortable for long-term use. Despite their potential, challenges like cost and training remain barriers to widespread adoption. However, ongoing advancements continue to improve functionality, affordability, and ease of use, offering hope for a future where mobility limitations are significantly reduced [17].

2. Rehabilitation

Exoskeletons play a pivotal role in rehabilitation by facilitating controlled, consistent, and repeatable movements essential for recovery after injuries, surgeries, or neurological conditions. These devices assist patients in performing exercises with a precise **range of motion** and **muscle activation,** critical for rebuilding strength, improving mobility, and retraining motor functions. One significant advantage is the **automation of support**, which reduces the physical demands on therapists. Traditionally, therapists manually guide patients through exercises, often requiring multiple staff members for assistance. Exoskeletons, however, assume this role, allowing therapists to focus on designing and implementing effective treatment strategies rather than providing physical support. This efficiency not only enhances patient outcomes but also improves the overall rehabilitation process by allowing for more intensive and frequent sessions. The **EksoNR exoskeleton** is a prime example of this technology's impact in **neurorehabilitation.** Designed to help stroke survivors and patients with traumatic brain injuries, the EksoNR guides users through walking exercises, promoting proper gait patterns and balance. The system's sensors and adaptive controls adjust to the patient's progress, ensuring optimal challenge and support during therapy. By encouraging neuroplasticity—the brain's ability to rewire and adapt—EksoNR helps patients regain motor control and strength. Additionally, exoskeletons enable **early mobilization**, which is crucial for recovery. Patients can begin walking exercises sooner, even when their strength and stability are limited. This early intervention helps prevent complications like muscle atrophy and joint stiffness, ultimately leading to better long-term outcomes. As technology advances, exoskeletons are becoming more personalized, enhancing comfort and usability, and driving progress in rehabilitation practices [17].

3 Industrial use

In industrial environments, exoskeletons significantly reduce the physical burden on workers tasked with repetitive, strenuous, or awkward movements. These wearable devices enhance strength, endurance, and stability, allowing workers to lift heavy objects, hold tools for extended periods, and maintain uncomfortable postures with minimal effort. By improving **ergonomics** and redistributing the load, exoskeletons help prevent musculoskeletal injuries, which are common in industries like construction, manufacturing, and logistics. A key benefit of industrial exoskeletons is their ability to **enhance worker safety**. Tasks involving heavy lifting, often lead to back injuries and chronic pain. Exoskeletons support the spine, shoulders, and legs, reducing the likelihood of overexertion and repetitive strain injuries. This translates into fewer work-related injuries and lower compensation costs for employers. Exoskeletons also boost **productivity** by enabling workers to perform physically demanding tasks for longer periods without fatigue. For example, workers can handle heavier loads or maintain elevated positions without breaks, improving operational efficiency. Moreover, the reduced fatigue contributes to higher job satisfaction and overall well-being. The **Guardian XO** by Sarcos Robotics exemplifies the potential of powered exoskeletons in industrial applications. This full-body exoskeleton allows users to lift up to 200 pounds with ease while feeling only a fraction of the weight. Its battery-powered hydraulic system provides seamless motion, enabling workers to handle heavy tools and materials without strain. The Guardian XO is designed to be intuitive, requiring minimal training, and enhances both strength and mobility. As industries continue to adopt exoskeletons, they are expected to transform workplace dynamics, creating safer, more efficient environments while protecting the workforce from injury and fatigue [17].

Benefits of exoskeleton robotic systems

1. Enhanced Performance and Precision

Exoskeletons significantly enhance performance and precision across various domains, particularly in **surgical** and **industrial** settings. By providing mechanical support and reducing muscle fatigue, these devices allow users to perform tasks with greater accuracy, stability, and endurance. This is crucial in situations that demand sustained concentration and physical effort. In **surgical applications**, precision is paramount. Surgeons often perform complex, lengthy procedures requiring steady hands and minimal tremors. Exoskeletons, such as the **Levitate AIRFRAME**, offer arm support, alleviating strain and enabling surgeons to maintain a steady posture throughout the operation. By reducing fatigue, the device allows surgeons to focus more on the procedure, enhancing outcomes and reducing the risk of errors. This support is particularly beneficial in microsurgeries and other intricate procedures where even minor hand movements can be critical [18].

In **industrial environments**, exoskeletons improve performance by augmenting workers' strength and endurance. Tasks like welding, overhead assembly, and handling heavy machinery require repetitive motions and awkward postures, leading to fatigue and reduced efficiency. Exoskeletons provide support to key muscle groups, allowing workers to maintain productivity over extended periods without risking injury. The enhanced stability and strength provided by these devices also improve the quality and precision of tasks, such as fitting components in tight spaces or performing detailed work. Overall, exoskeletons empower users to achieve **consistent, high-quality performance** by reducing physical strain, increasing endurance, and enhancing control. Their ability to support precision and efficiency makes them invaluable in demanding environments, ultimately leading to better outcomes in both healthcare and industrial sectors [18].

2. Consistent Therapy and Rehabilitation
Exoskeletons play a pivotal role in delivering **consistent, repeatable movements** during rehabilitation, which is essential for optimal recovery. Unlike manual therapy, which can vary in technique and intensity depending on the therapist's endurance and precision, robotic exoskeletons ensure **uniformity in movement patterns**, providing patients with a standardized therapeutic experience. This consistency helps in retraining the brain and muscles effectively, fostering **neuroplasticity** and improving motor function. One of the key advantages of exoskeleton-assisted therapy is the ability to **tailor treatment** to individual patient needs. Advanced models incorporate **automated adjustments** that customize resistance, speed, and range of motion based on a patient's progress and specific rehabilitation goals. This personalized approach allows for targeted muscle activation and joint mobilization, promoting **faster recovery** and improved functional outcomes. For example, the **Lokomat**, a robotic gait training exoskeleton, is widely used in physical therapy for patients recovering from strokes, spinal cord injuries, or other neurological conditions. By providing controlled, consistent leg movements, the Lokomat assists patients in **relearning how to walk**, improving gait patterns and balance. It also tracks patient performance in real time, enabling therapists to monitor progress and make data-driven adjustments to the therapy regimen. Moreover, exoskeletons reduce the **physical workload on therapists**, allowing them to focus on strategy and patient engagement rather than manual support. This not only improves the efficiency of therapy sessions but also enables therapists to treat more patients. Ultimately, exoskeletons enhance rehabilitation outcomes by ensuring **precise, consistent therapy** that adapts to patient needs [19].

3. Injury Prevention and Ergonomics
Exoskeletons play a critical role in **preventing workplace injuries** by enhancing ergonomics and reducing physical strain during demanding tasks. These wearable devices support the body's natural movements, ensuring that users maintain **proper posture** and avoid awkward or harmful positions that can lead to musculoskeletal disorders (MSDs) and repetitive strain injuries (RSIs). In healthcare, surgeons and medical professionals often endure long hours in static positions, increasing the risk of back and neck pain. Exoskeletons designed for healthcare environments provide **targeted support**, especially for the arms and back, helping to alleviate fatigue and reduce injury risks during complex, prolonged procedures. In industrial settings, exoskeletons offer **essential support** for workers involved in heavy lifting, assembly, and other physically intensive activities. By redistributing the weight and reducing pressure on the lower back and joints, exoskeletons lower the likelihood of strains and sprains. This not only enhances worker safety but also **boosts productivity** by reducing downtime due to injuries. For example, the **SuitX BackX exoskeleton** is specifically designed to support the lower back,

assisting workers in lifting heavy objects with less effort and strain. Studies have shown that devices like the BackX can **reduce spinal loading by up to 60%**, significantly minimizing the risk of back injuries. By promoting **correct ergonomic practices**, exoskeletons help create safer work environments, lower healthcare costs related to workplace injuries, and improve overall job satisfaction by making physically demanding tasks more manageable and sustainable [18].

Challenges of exoskeleton robotic systems

1. High Costs and Maintenance

Exoskeletons are technologically advanced devices, and their **high development and manufacturing costs** make them a significant investment. These systems incorporate sophisticated components such as sensors, actuators, control algorithms, and lightweight yet durable materials. The complexity of designing wearable technology that is both functional and comfortable drives up production costs. As a result, exoskeletons are often priced beyond the reach of smaller organizations, limiting their adoption to **large hospitals, rehabilitation centers, and corporations** with substantial budgets. Beyond the initial purchase, **maintenance and operational costs** add to the financial burden. Regular servicing, software updates, and the replacement of wearable components such as straps or padding, are necessary to ensure optimal performance and user comfort. Maintenance also includes calibrating sensors and adjusting mechanical parts to maintain accuracy and efficiency. These ongoing costs can deter widespread use, especially in resource-constrained settings. For healthcare providers and industries considering exoskeletons, a **cost-benefit analysis** is essential. While the upfront costs are significant, exoskeletons can lead to **long-term savings** by reducing workplace injuries, lowering rehabilitation time, and improving productivity. However, the **return on investment (ROI)** may vary based on usage and efficiency gains. To enhance accessibility, **government subsidies, insurance coverage, or leasing models** could offset costs. Public funding initiatives and partnerships between manufacturers and healthcare providers may also facilitate broader adoption, ensuring that patients and workers can benefit from this transformative technology [18].

2. Training and User Adaptation

Operating exoskeletons effectively requires **extensive training** to ensure users can control and adapt to the technology. Whether the users are **surgeons, patients, or industrial workers**, mastering the complex movements and understanding the system's responsiveness is essential for achieving optimal outcomes. Surgeons need to learn how to integrate the device's support into their workflow, maintaining precision during long, intricate procedures. For **rehabilitation patients**, the challenge lies not only in learning how to move with the exoskeleton but also in adapting both cognitively and physically. The body needs time to adjust to the mechanical support and achieve coordination with the device's movements. This process can be demanding, especially for patients recovering from strokes, spinal cord injuries, or neurological disorders. Therapists must closely guide the training to avoid over-reliance on the device, ensuring that patients continue to build strength and mobility independently. In **industrial settings**, workers need to understand how to use exoskeletons for tasks like heavy lifting or repetitive motion without compromising safety. Improper use or lack of familiarity can lead to discomfort or even injury. To address these challenges, **comprehensive training programs** are critical. Training often includes hands-on sessions, classroom learning, and **user-friendly interfaces** designed to simplify controls and feedback. **Virtual reality (VR) simulations** are increasingly being employed to enhance training, offering immersive experiences that allow users to practice in controlled environments. These simulations help shorten the learning curve and provide a safer, more engaging way to develop the necessary skills before real-world application [18].

3. Comfort and Fit

Long-term use of exoskeletons can pose significant challenges related to **comfort and fit**, particularly if the devices are not tailored to the individual user's body. Poorly fitting exoskeletons may cause **skin irritation, pressure sores, and discomfort**, especially in areas where straps or contact points exert pressure over extended periods. This discomfort can hinder movement and reduce the effectiveness of the device, limiting how long users can wear it. In **rehabilitation and mobility assistance**, patients often need to wear exoskeletons for hours during therapy sessions, making comfort a critical factor. Without proper fit, users may experience restricted movement or increased fatigue, which can slow down recovery and discourage consistent use. For **industrial workers**, discomfort can reduce productivity and increase the risk of improper use, negating the ergonomic benefits of the device. To address these issues, **advances in ergonomic design** are focusing on creating exoskeletons with **customizable components.** Features like **adjustable straps, modular frameworks, and breathable materials** are essential to accommodate diverse body shapes and sizes. **Soft exoskeletons** or hybrid models, which combine rigid support with flexible elements, are gaining popularity for their improved comfort and adaptability. **3D scanning and printing** technologies are also being used to create personalized fits, ensuring that exoskeletons conform to the user's unique anatomy. Additionally, **smart materials** with temperature-regulating properties and enhanced padding can reduce friction and pressure, further improving user comfort. These innovations are essential for encouraging consistent use and maximizing the therapeutic and ergonomic benefits of exoskeletons [18].

4. **Future Directions and Innovations**
The future of exoskeleton robotic systems holds significant potential, driven by advancements in **materials, sensors, and artificial intelligence (AI)**. Emerging technologies focus on the development of **lightweight, flexible materials** that enhance comfort, mobility, and adaptability for users. These materials aim to reduce bulk and weight, making exoskeletons more practical for extended use in both rehabilitation and industrial settings. AI-driven control systems are set to revolutionize user experiences by offering **more intuitive, adaptive interactions**. These systems can learn from user movements and preferences, enabling exoskeletons to respond seamlessly to changes in posture, activity, or physical condition. For instance, AI can help adjust gait patterns or provide targeted support, optimizing therapy outcomes and enhancing efficiency in industrial tasks. **Wireless and battery technologies** are also evolving to improve portability and extend operational durations. Innovations in **energy-efficient power sources** and **wireless connectivity** will allow for untethered, continuous use, making exoskeletons more practical in diverse environments, from hospitals to construction sites. Collaboration between **healthcare providers, industrial manufacturers, and tech companies** is accelerating the development of cost-effective solutions. Joint efforts aim to **reduce costs** and improve accessibility, with a focus on integrating exoskeletons into **insurance coverage and public healthcare systems**. These measures will play a crucial role in expanding adoption, ensuring that exoskeleton technology reaches a broader audience. Future innovations may also explore **biomechanical feedback systems** and **soft robotics**, which mimic natural human movement, further enhancing user comfort and functionality. As these technologies mature, exoskeletons are poised to transform rehabilitation, industrial work, and personal mobility, offering significant benefits across various sectors [20, 18, 21, 19].

Exoskeleton robotic systems are transformative technologies with broad applications in healthcare, rehabilitation, and industrial settings. They enhance human capabilities, promote recovery, and improve safety and productivity. Despite challenges such as high costs, training requirements, and comfort issues, ongoing innovations are addressing these barriers. As these systems become more advanced and accessible, they have the potential to revolutionize how we approach physical assistance, rehabilitation, and labor-intensive tasks, ultimately improving quality of life and workplace efficiency [20, 18, 21, 19].

4.3.5 Teleoperated robotic systems

Teleoperated robotic systems allow surgeons to perform complex medical procedures from a remote location by controlling robotic arms in real-time. This groundbreaking technology bridges geographical gaps, making specialized surgical care accessible to patients in remote or underserved

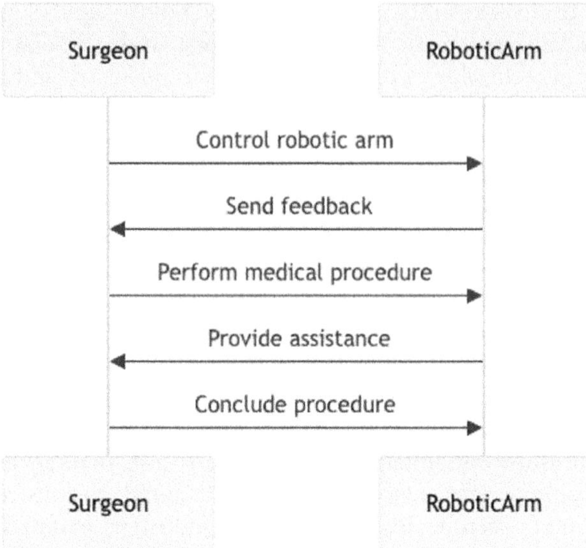

Figure 4.6 Features of teleoperated robotic systems.

areas. It also proves invaluable in disaster scenarios where immediate medical intervention is required but local expertise is unavailable (Figure 4.6) [20, 18, 21, 19].

Key features of teleoperated robotic systems

1. Remote Access

Teleoperated robotic systems revolutionize surgical care by enabling surgeons to perform procedures on patients from virtually any location. Through secure and reliable network connections, these systems bridge geographical barriers, making it possible for specialists to deliver advanced surgical interventions to regions with limited access to skilled medical professionals. This capability is particularly crucial in rural and underserved areas where local expertise may be unavailable. By remotely controlling robotic instruments with precision, surgeons can execute complex, minimally invasive procedures that improve patient outcomes and reduce recovery times. In disaster scenarios, such as earthquakes or hurricanes, teleoperated systems become invaluable tools for life-saving interventions. When local medical infrastructure is compromised, or specialists cannot reach affected areas in time, these systems allow for real-time surgical care. A specialist in a distant city or country can guide robotic arms to perform emergency procedures, stabilizing patients until further care becomes available. This ability to extend the reach of skilled surgeons not only enhances healthcare accessibility but also significantly improves survival rates in critical situations. As telecommunication technologies continue to advance, teleoperated systems will play an even greater role in global healthcare delivery, ensuring that expertise can be mobilized wherever it is needed the most [20, 18, 21, 19].

2. Precision and Control

Teleoperated robotic systems offer remarkable precision and control during surgeries, leveraging advanced robotic arms and imaging technologies to ensure highly accurate movements. These systems are designed to replicate a surgeon's hand movements with an extraordinary degree of precision, eliminating the natural tremors and inconsistencies that can occur during manual surgery. This increased accuracy allows surgeons to perform delicate, minimally invasive procedures with confidence, reducing the risk of human error and improving patient safety. The robotic arms used in these systems are equipped with specialized tools and sensors that enhance the surgeon's ability to maneuver in tight spaces with exceptional control. These instruments can be adjusted to deliver more refined movements than the human hand alone, which is critical for intricate procedures in sensitive areas such as the brain, heart, or spine. Additionally, advanced imaging technologies, such as real-time 3D visualization and augmented reality, are often integrated into the system, providing the surgeon with a clear, enhanced view of the surgical site. This comprehensive combination of robotic precision and imaging support not only minimizes the trauma to surrounding tissues but also speeds up recovery times, as smaller incisions are typically required. Overall, the precision and control offered by teleoperated robotic systems are key to achieving better surgical outcomes, making them indispensable tools in modern medicine [20, 18, 21, 19].

3. Global Reach

Teleoperated robotic systems have a transformative impact on healthcare by extending the reach of specialized surgeons to remote and underserved regions worldwide. Surgeons can operate on patients from virtually any location, using secure, high-speed communication networks to connect with robotic systems in distant locations. This global reach significantly reduces the need for patients to travel long distances to receive specialized care, which can be financially burdensome and logistically challenging, especially for those in rural or impoverished areas [20, 18, 21, 19].

For instance, a surgeon based in New York can remotely control a robotic system to perform a complex procedure on a patient in rural Africa, bringing world-class expertise to a location where local specialists may be scarce. This capability is invaluable in areas with limited access to advanced healthcare services, ensuring that patients receive timely, life-saving treatments without the need to leave their communities. By leveraging teleoperated systems, healthcare can be democratized, breaking down geographical barriers and improving overall access to quality care on a global scale [20, 18, 21, 19].

Advantages of teleoperated robotic systems

1. Accessibility
Teleoperated robotic systems play a critical role in democratizing healthcare by making specialized surgical care more accessible to underserved and remote populations. In many rural or geographically isolated areas, access to highly skilled surgeons is limited due to factors like inadequate healthcare infrastructure, a shortage of medical professionals, or the high cost of specialized care. Teleoperated systems help bridge these gaps by enabling surgeons to remotely perform complex surgeries, ensuring that patients in even the most isolated locations can receive high-quality treatment. For example, in remote islands or mountainous regions with few healthcare facilities, teleoperated systems provide an effective solution for patients who would otherwise have to travel long distances to access care. By connecting local healthcare providers with surgeons in distant cities or even different countries, these systems enable life-saving procedures to be performed in real-time, without the need for the patient to leave their community. This capability not only improves access to specialized care but also reduces the emotional and financial burden associated with traveling for treatment. In areas where healthcare resources are scarce, teleoperated systems can also help train local medical personnel by providing real-time support and guidance during procedures. This further enhances the capacity of local healthcare systems, ensuring that patients benefit from improved care while minimizing the need for them to travel long distances or face extended waiting times for treatment. Through such advancements, teleoperated systems are reshaping the accessibility of healthcare worldwide, particularly for those in rural and underserved regions [22, 23].

2. Disaster Response
Teleoperated robotic systems play a vital role in disaster response, enabling prompt surgical interventions in emergency situations where time and resources are critical. In environments such as war zones or disaster-stricken areas, where access to specialized medical care may be severely limited, these systems allow surgeons to perform life-saving procedures remotely, minimizing the need for physical presence. For example, military surgeons can use teleoperated systems to provide medical care to soldiers injured in combat zones. By connecting to robotic systems located in field hospitals, surgeons can remotely guide robotic arms to perform surgeries on critically injured patients, even while being located far from the scene. This ability to operate remotely helps save lives when immediate access to skilled surgeons

is unavailable, ensuring that soldiers or civilians in conflict areas receive timely and high-quality care, regardless of the geographical constraints. Teleoperated systems are equally beneficial in natural disaster situations, such as earthquakes, hurricanes, or floods, where the destruction of local infrastructure hampers access to medical resources. In these cases, surgeons can remotely assist medical teams on the ground, providing expertise for complex procedures or guiding local healthcare workers through surgeries. This approach significantly enhances the capacity to address medical needs in emergencies and ensures that critical care is delivered as swiftly as possible, even in the most challenging circumstances [22, 23].

By enabling remote surgical interventions, teleoperated systems contribute to improving the effectiveness and efficiency of disaster response, potentially saving countless lives in situations where medical resources are limited [22, 23].

3. Reduced Travel Costs

Teleoperated robotic systems significantly reduce the travel costs associated with accessing specialized healthcare services, benefiting both patients and healthcare providers. Traditionally, patients in need of specialized surgeries would have to travel to large medical centers, often incurring substantial costs for transportation, accommodation, and time away from work or family. However, with teleoperated systems, patients can remain in their local hospitals while skilled surgeons perform complex procedures remotely. For example, a patient requiring a rare cardiac surgery typically would need to travel to a hospital with a specialist on hand to perform the procedure. With teleoperated robotic systems, this patient can undergo the surgery at their local healthcare facility. The specialized surgeon, potentially located in a different city or even country, can control the robotic surgical system remotely, ensuring high-precision operations while the patient is treated closer to home. This not only reduces the financial burden on the patient but also eliminates the logistical challenges and stress of travel during a medical emergency. From the healthcare provider's perspective, these systems save significant costs as well. Surgeons no longer need to travel to remote locations or specialized centers for consultations or surgeries, which reduces time spent away from their home hospitals and decreases operational costs. This also allows hospitals to tap into a broader pool of expertise without geographic limitations, improving access to specialized care in underserved areas. Overall, the ability to conduct surgeries remotely minimizes travel expenses for both patients and medical professionals, making specialized healthcare more accessible and cost-effective. This benefit is particularly important in regions where specialized care is scarce or where patients face financial or logistical barriers to travel [24].

Limitations of teleoperated robotic systems

1. Latency Issues

Latency issues are a significant challenge in teleoperated surgeries, as they rely heavily on real-time data transmission between the surgeon and the robotic system. Any delay in the communication signal, known as latency, can disrupt the precision and timing of the surgeon's movements, which is critical during surgery. A delay in the robotic system's response could lead to inaccurate movements, potentially causing complications or affecting the safety of the patient. For instance, in delicate surgeries such as neurosurgery or cardiac procedures, even a slight delay in the robotic arm's response can have serious consequences. Surgeons depend on real-time feedback and precise control over the robotic instruments to navigate the procedure effectively. Any lag between the surgeon's input and the system's action could lead to incorrect incision placements or the failure to respond to a patient's physiological changes during the procedure. To mitigate these latency issues, advanced communication technologies such as 5G networks are being explored. These high-speed, low-latency networks are capable of providing the near-instantaneous data transfer necessary for remote surgeries. 5G technology offers the potential for faster transmission speeds and reduced delay, making it more suitable for critical applications like teleoperated surgery. In addition, dedicated bandwidth for medical use can prioritize surgical data, ensuring that signals are transmitted without interruption and maintaining a stable connection even in remote locations. By leveraging these advanced communication technologies, latency issues in teleoperated surgeries can be minimized, ensuring a more reliable and safe surgical experience for patients. As the infrastructure for 5G and dedicated networks for medical use continues to improve, the potential for teleoperated robotic surgeries to become more widespread and effective increases, bringing advanced surgical care to even the most remote regions [22, 23].

2. Technical Failures

Technical failures pose a significant risk to teleoperated robotic systems, as these systems rely heavily on stable internet connections, consistent power supplies, and advanced hardware to perform complex surgeries. A malfunction in any of these components could disrupt the surgery and potentially lead to serious complications for the patient. For example, if the internet connection fails or becomes unstable during a procedure, the surgeon might lose control over the robotic instruments, which could result in delayed movements, inaccurate surgical actions, or even the complete loss of communication with the robotic system. Similarly, if the power supply is interrupted or the robotic arm's components fail, it could render the system inoperable, leaving the surgeon unable to continue the surgery. In such cases, the risk of complications or injury increases significantly, as immediate corrective action may not be possible without the proper functioning of the robotic system. To mitigate these risks, it is crucial that teleoperated systems have backup systems and fail-safe mechanisms in place. One consideration is the implementation of redundant power supplies, such as backup generators or battery systems, which can kick in if there is an interruption in the main power source. In addition, redundant internet connections, such as satellite or 4G/5G backup links, can ensure that communication remains stable even if the primary internet connection is compromised. Another important consideration is the incorporation of fail-safe mechanisms within the robotic system itself. These systems can be programmed to recognize potential malfunctions and alert the surgeon immediately, while also providing a backup control system that allows for manual intervention in case of technical failure. This ensures that the surgeon can continue the procedure safely, even if the robotic system encounters a problem. By integrating these precautions, teleoperated systems can minimize the risk of technical failures and enhance their reliability, helping to ensure that surgeries proceed smoothly and safely, even in remote or challenging environments [22, 23].

3. High Costs

High costs present a significant barrier to the widespread adoption of teleoperated robotic systems, particularly in low-resource settings. The initial investment required for these systems is substantial, often involving millions of dollars for state-of-the-art robotic equipment, advanced imaging technologies, and secure networking infrastructure. This financial burden is further compounded by the recurring costs of maintenance, software updates, and repairs, which are essential to ensure the system's reliability and precision over time. Additionally, implementing teleoperated systems requires extensive training for surgeons and support staff. Surgeons must learn to operate the robotic controls effectively, while technicians and nurses need to become proficient in maintaining and troubleshooting the system. These training programs often involve significant time and financial investment, as they require access to simulation platforms, experienced trainers, and certification processes. For example, a hospital seeking to integrate a teleoperated surgical system like the da Vinci or a comparable platform would need to allocate a large portion of its budget not only for the equipment but also for staff training and the establishment of robust IT and communication networks. In resource-constrained healthcare settings, such investments can be prohibitive, often making these systems accessible only to well-funded hospitals or research institutions. To address these challenges, strategies such as government subsidies, public-private partnerships, and inclusion of teleoperated systems in insurance coverage can help lower costs and expand access. Innovations in design and manufacturing, aimed at reducing production costs, could also make these systems more affordable over time. These measures are critical to bridging the gap between high-cost technology and the need for equitable healthcare access worldwide [22, 23].

Applications of teleoperated robotic systems

Teleoperated robotic systems have revolutionized modern medicine by enabling specialists to provide care in scenarios where direct access is limited. These systems expand the reach of skilled healthcare professionals, ensuring that even the most remote or extreme environments benefit from advanced surgical interventions. Teleoperated robotic systems are transforming healthcare by extending the reach of specialized care to areas previously thought inaccessible. Whether addressing the needs of rural populations, providing medical care in extreme environments, or supporting astronauts in space, these systems represent a convergence of technology and medicine, paving the way for a future where geography is no longer a barrier to high-quality healthcare. Continued innovation and investment in these systems will be crucial to realizing their full potential. Key applications include rural healthcare, military and disaster scenarios, and space exploration [22, 23].

1. Rural Healthcare

In rural and underserved regions, access to advanced medical care is often hindered by a lack of infrastructure and specialized personnel. Teleoperated systems bridge this gap by allowing surgeons in urban centers or specialized hospitals to perform procedures remotely. For instance, a patient in a remote village with no local surgical expertise can undergo a life-saving procedure, such as a complex orthopedic or cardiac surgery, performed by a specialist operating from a distant location. These systems utilize secure, high-speed communication networks to transmit data in real time, ensuring precision and safety. This approach eliminates the need for patients to travel long distances for treatment, reducing costs and logistical challenges. By democratizing access to specialized care, teleoperated robotic systems have the potential to significantly improve health outcomes in underserved populations [22, 23].

2. Military and Disaster Scenarios

In conflict zones and areas struck by natural disasters, the presence of on-site surgeons may be impractical or unsafe. Teleoperated robotic systems provide a critical solution in these situations, enabling timely and precise medical interventions. Military applications are particularly noteworthy, as surgeons located in safe zones can remotely operate on injured soldiers in combat areas using these systems. For instance, battlefield injuries that require immediate surgical attention, such as hemorrhages or shrapnel removal, can be addressed remotely, saving lives and reducing long-term complications. Similarly, in disaster scenarios like earthquakes or hurricanes, where local healthcare facilities are overwhelmed or destroyed, teleoperated systems allow surgeons to provide care without delays, ensuring a swift and efficient response [22, 23].

3. Space Exploration
Space missions, especially those of long durations, present unique medical challenges due to the absence of immediate access to Earth-based healthcare. Astronauts on missions to the Moon, Mars, or beyond are exposed to risks such as injuries, organ dysfunctions, or emergencies requiring surgical intervention. Teleoperated robotic systems offer a groundbreaking solution by enabling Earth-based specialists to perform surgeries remotely on astronauts. Advanced imaging technologies and robotic precision ensure that procedures are conducted with minimal risk. For example, a robotic system could perform an emergency appendectomy on a Mars-bound astronaut, with a specialist on Earth controlling the operation in real time. This application not only enhances the safety of space missions but also represents a crucial step in supporting human exploration of deep space [22, 23].

Future directions and innovations

Teleoperated robotic systems are at the forefront of transforming healthcare delivery, offering unparalleled opportunities to extend the reach of specialized care. As the technology evolves, several advancements and innovations are expected to address current limitations and expand the scope of applications. Key areas of development include connectivity, artificial intelligence integration, cost reduction, and training enhancements [22, 23].

1. Advancements in Connectivity
A critical factor for the success of teleoperated systems is reliable and fast communication. The development of ultra-low-latency networks, such as 5G, and the increasing accessibility of satellite-based internet are poised to revolutionize connectivity. These technologies ensure that data transmission between the surgeon's controls and the robotic system occurs in real time, eliminating delays that could compromise surgical precision. For instance, 5G networks offer latency as low as 1 millisecond, enabling smooth and precise movements of robotic arms, even across continents. In disaster-stricken areas or remote regions without traditional infrastructure, satellite-based connectivity can provide consistent performance, making teleoperated surgeries feasible under challenging conditions. These advancements will make remote operations more practical, reliable, and safe, ultimately broadening their adoption [22, 23].

2. Artificial Intelligence Integration
Artificial intelligence (AI) is set to play a transformative role in teleoperated robotic systems. AI-powered decision support tools can analyze real-time

data from imaging systems and sensors, offering surgeons insights during procedures. For example, AI can highlight anomalies, recommend optimal incision points, or predict potential complications based on patient data and surgical progress. Additionally, AI algorithms can automate routine tasks, such as suturing or tissue manipulation, allowing surgeons to focus on the critical aspects of surgery. Machine learning models, trained on vast datasets of past procedures, can also enhance the system's adaptability—improving precision and reducing errors. These capabilities not only increase surgical efficiency but also ensure better outcomes, particularly in complex or high-risk cases [22, 23].

3. Cost Reduction and Accessibility
The high costs associated with teleoperated systems currently limit their widespread adoption, especially in low-resource settings. However, ongoing innovations in hardware design, manufacturing, and software development are paving the way for more cost-effective solutions. Lightweight materials, simplified robotic designs, and modular components are reducing production expenses, while open-source software platforms are decreasing development costs. Collaborative efforts between governments, healthcare providers, and tech companies are also essential in addressing cost barriers. Subsidies, public-private partnerships, and the integration of teleoperated systems into insurance coverage are critical to ensuring that this technology becomes accessible to a broader population. As affordability improves, rural hospitals, small clinics, and disaster relief organizations can incorporate these systems into their operations, democratizing access to advanced surgical care [22, 23].

4. VR/AR-Based Surgical Training
Effective training is vital for the successful implementation of teleoperated systems. The integration of virtual reality (VR) and augmented reality (AR) into training programs offers surgeons an immersive and interactive environment to gain proficiency. These technologies simulate real-world scenarios, allowing surgeons to practice complex procedures without the need for live patients. For instance, VR-based simulators can recreate specific surgical cases, providing a safe platform to refine skills and build confidence. AR, on the other hand, can overlay guidance and annotations onto the surgeon's field of view during both training and live procedures, enhancing accuracy and decision-making. These tools not only shorten the learning curve for teleoperated systems but also ensure that surgeons are well-prepared to handle a wide range of situations, from routine surgeries to emergencies. The future of teleoperated robotic systems is incredibly promising, driven by rapid advancements in technology and a growing recognition of their potential to address healthcare disparities. By leveraging improved connectivity, AI capabilities, cost-effective designs, and cutting-edge training

methods, these systems are poised to overcome current limitations and redefine surgical care. As these innovations mature, teleoperated systems will become more accessible, reliable, and versatile, enabling specialists to deliver high-quality care to patients, regardless of location or circumstances. Collaboration among stakeholders, including governments, healthcare providers, and technology developers, will be crucial in realizing this vision and ensuring that the benefits of teleoperated robotic systems reach their full global potential [22, 23].

5. **Advanced VR/AR Surgical Simulation**
The integration of **virtual reality** (**VR**) and **augmented reality** (**AR**) technologies into training programs for teleoperated robotic systems is revolutionizing how surgeons gain proficiency with these advanced tools. These technologies provide immersive, interactive environments where surgeons can practice intricate procedures without relying on live patients, ensuring a safe and controlled learning experience. VR-based simulations allow surgeons to navigate complex surgical scenarios, replicate real-world challenges, and refine their skills in a risk-free setting. For instance, trainees can virtually manipulate robotic arms, experiment with various techniques, and experience the tactile feedback and visual precision needed for teleoperated procedures. These simulations can recreate rare or high-risk surgeries, offering a depth of training that is difficult to achieve through traditional methods. AR complements VR by enhancing the surgeon's training environment with real-time overlays and annotations. During practice sessions, AR can project guidance, such as highlighting anatomical landmarks or suggesting optimal tool placements, directly onto the surgical field. This technology not only aids in learning but can also be used during live surgeries to boost accuracy and confidence. By combining VR and AR, training programs are becoming more accessible and efficient. Surgeons can gain hands-on experience remotely, eliminating the need for costly and time-consuming in-person workshops. Furthermore, these tools enable continuous skill enhancement, allowing experienced professionals to stay updated on the latest robotic systems and surgical techniques. As teleoperated systems become more prevalent, VR and AR training will be instrumental in addressing the learning curve associated with this technology. These advancements ensure that surgeons are well-prepared to harness the full potential of teleoperated systems, ultimately improving surgical outcomes and expanding access to specialized care worldwide [22, 23].

4.3.6 Nanorobotics in surgery

Nanorobotics, an emerging field at the intersection of nanotechnology and medicine, holds transformative potential in surgical and therapeutic

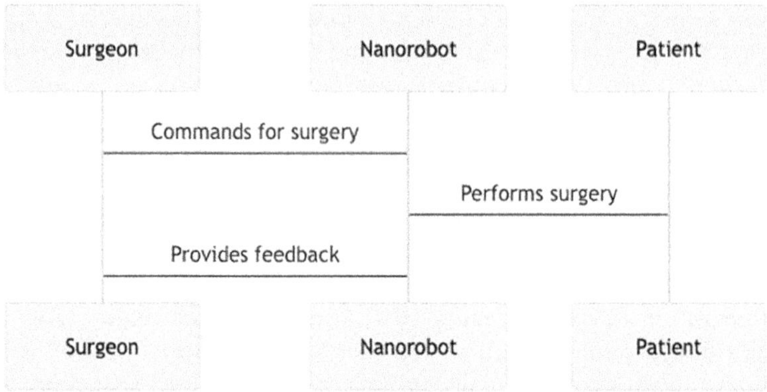

Figure 4.7 Key features of nanorobotics in surgery.

applications. Operating at the molecular or cellular level, nanorobots offer unprecedented precision, enabling interventions that were previously unimaginable. Though still largely in the developmental stage, nanorobots are poised to revolutionize healthcare by improving the efficacy, safety, and personalization of medical treatments (Figure 4.7) [25, 26].

Applications of nanorobotics in surgery

1. Targeted Drug Delivery

One of the most promising applications of nanorobots is **targeted drug delivery**. Traditional methods of administering drugs often result in systemic side effects due to their inability to specifically target diseased tissues. Nanorobots, however, can be engineered to navigate directly to the affected area, ensuring the precise release of therapeutic agents. This approach minimizes damage to healthy tissues and enhances the effectiveness of treatment. For instance, in cancer therapy, nanorobots can deliver chemotherapy drugs directly to tumor cells, significantly reducing side effects like nausea, hair loss, and immune suppression. This precise targeting also allows for smaller doses, lowering the risk of drug toxicity [25, 26].

2. Medical Diagnostics

Nanorobots are equally promising in the realm of **diagnostics**. They can be programmed to detect and monitor biomarkers associated with diseases at an early stage, often before symptoms appear. Nanorobots introduced into the bloodstream can identify abnormal cellular changes, such as the presence of cancer cells or inflammatory markers, providing real-time diagnostic data. This capability supports early intervention, which is crucial in improving treatment outcomes. Moreover, nanorobots can continuously monitor a patient's physiological state, offering valuable insights for personalized medical care [25, 26].

3. **Surgical Interventions**
Nanorobots have the potential to perform minimally invasive surgical procedures with unparalleled accuracy. They can repair damaged tissues, remove blockages in blood vessels, or eliminate harmful deposits, such as plaque in arteries, without the need for traditional surgical incisions. Their ability to manipulate structures at the cellular level opens new possibilities for treating conditions like aneurysms, organ dysfunctions, or even neurodegenerative diseases [25, 26].

Advantages

1. **Precision**
One of the most significant advantages of nanorobotics is the precision with which these tiny machines operate. Unlike traditional treatments, which often have systemic effects, nanorobots can target only the affected areas, significantly reducing side effects [25, 26].

For instance, in chemotherapy, conventional drugs attack both cancerous and healthy cells, leading to severe side effects such as fatigue, nausea, and immune suppression. Nanorobots, however, can be programmed to identify specific tumor markers, delivering drugs directly to cancer cells while sparing healthy tissues. This level of precision ensures that the therapeutic benefits are maximized, while adverse effects are minimized [25, 26].

2. **Controlled Release**
Nanorobots can be designed to deliver therapeutic agents in a **controlled and sustained manner**. This capability ensures that the drug concentration remains within an optimal therapeutic window for longer durations, enhancing treatment efficacy. [25, 26]

For example, in chronic conditions like diabetes or cardiovascular diseases, nanorobots can release medication in response to specific triggers, such as changes in blood sugar or blood pressure levels. This eliminates the need for frequent dosing, improving patient compliance and outcomes. Controlled release mechanisms also allow for multi-phase drug delivery, where different drugs are released sequentially to achieve a synergistic therapeutic effect [25, 26].

3. **Early Diagnostics and Real-Time Monitoring**
Another key advantage of nanorobots is their potential in diagnostics. They can detect diseases at a molecular level, often before symptoms manifest, enabling earlier and more effective interventions. Additionally, nanorobots equipped with biosensors can provide real-time monitoring of a patient's

physiological conditions, such as blood sugar, oxygen levels, or inflammation markers. This continuous feedback allows for dynamic adjustments in treatment, ensuring optimal outcomes [25, 26].

Challenges

1. Complexity and Scalability

The development of nanorobots is a highly complex process requiring precision engineering at the atomic or molecular scale. Achieving consistent functionality across a large number of nanorobots is a significant challenge. Even minor deviations in their structure or programming can result in variability, potentially compromising their effectiveness [25, 26].

Moreover, scaling up production to meet clinical demands while maintaining strict quality control is another significant hurdle. The intricate processes involved in designing, assembling, and testing nanorobots are time-intensive and require specialized facilities. This complexity limits their widespread adoption and delays the transition from research to real-world applications [25, 26].

2. High Costs

The financial burden associated with nanorobotics development is a major barrier. Research in nanotechnology requires substantial investment in advanced materials, state-of-the-art equipment, and highly skilled personnel. Additionally, clinical trials for nanorobots involve extensive safety testing to ensure they are biocompatible and do not provoke immune responses or toxic effects. Even after commercialization, the costs of producing and deploying nanorobots remain high, making them inaccessible to low-resource settings. For instance, while developed nations might integrate nanorobotics into their healthcare systems, developing countries may struggle to afford this technology, exacerbating global health disparities [25, 26].

3. Surgical Planning and Preoperative Imaging

Surgical planning is a critical step in ensuring the success of any procedure. It involves a thorough assessment of the patient's condition, comprehensive imaging, and meticulous strategy formulation. With the advent of advanced technologies, surgical planning has evolved significantly, offering enhanced precision, reduced risks, and better patient outcomes. Among these innovations, **3D printing** stands out as a transformative tool that is redefining preoperative preparation (Figure 4.8) [25, 26].

3D Printing in Surgical Planning: 3D printing has dramatically transformed the field of surgical planning by allowing the creation of precise, patient-specific models, tools, and implants. Using digital imaging data, such as CT

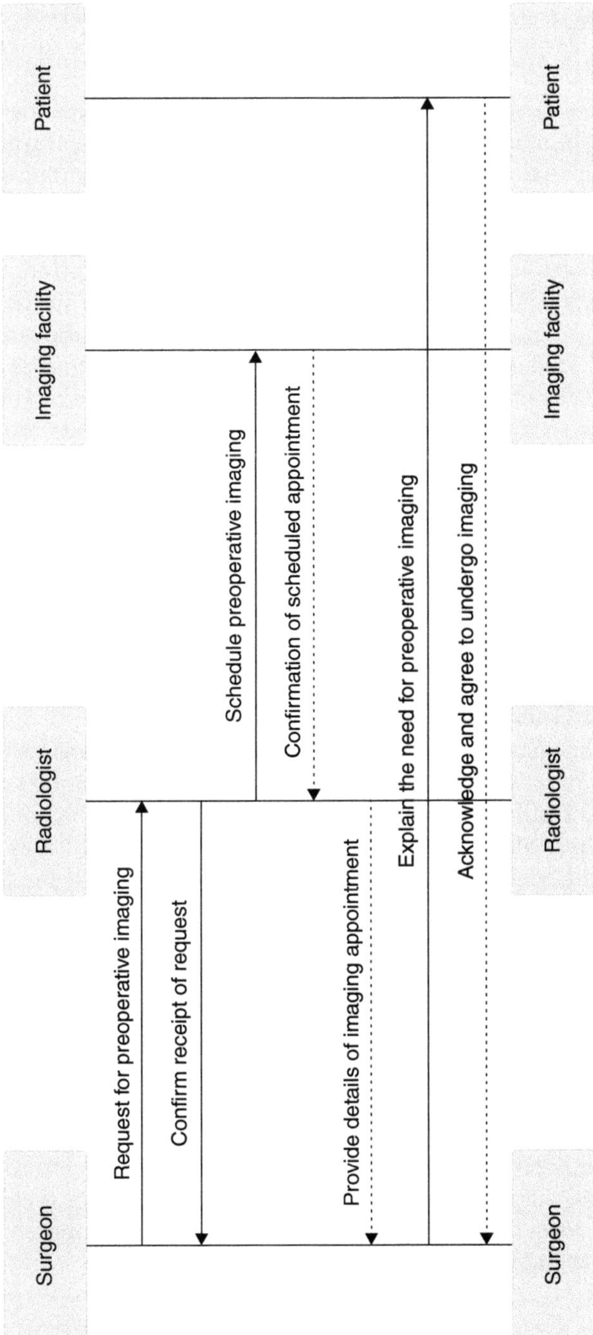

Figure 4.8 Features of surgical planning and preoperative imaging.

or MRI scans, this technology generates highly accurate, three-dimensional physical replicas of a patient's anatomical structures. These 3D-printed models provide surgeons with an unparalleled opportunity to visualize and physically interact with the patient's anatomy before the surgery, which is especially valuable for complex cases involving irregularities or rare conditions. Surgeons can carefully assess the anatomical features, understand their spatial relationships, and develop a tailored surgical approach that minimizes risk and enhances precision. Additionally, these models allow for better preoperative planning and rehearsal, reducing the time spent in the operating room. Surgeons can also use 3D printing to create customized surgical tools, implants, or prosthetics, which further enhances the precision of interventions, particularly in fields like orthopedics, neurosurgery, and cardiovascular surgery. This ability to plan and practice on a tangible model not only improves the safety and efficacy of surgeries but also shortens recovery times and reduces complications, as the surgery is performed with a deeper understanding of the patient's unique anatomy. Furthermore, 3D printing is increasingly integrated with other technologies like augmented reality and virtual reality, which further enhance its potential to revolutionize surgical planning and improve patient outcomes [25, 26].

Benefits of 3D printing

1. Enhanced Visualization
Traditional imaging techniques, such as CT and MRI scans, provide valuable insights into the patient's anatomy. However, 3D printing takes visualization a step further by converting these scans into tangible models. These physical replicas allow surgeons to examine complex structures from multiple angles, offering a clearer understanding of the surgical site [24].

2. Improved Precision and Reduced Operating Time
By allowing surgeons to practice and plan procedures on patient-specific models, 3D printing helps refine surgical techniques. This preoperative rehearsal minimizes, uncertainties during the actual surgery, leading to shorter operating times and reduced risks of complications [24].

3. Patient Education and Communication
3D-printed models are not only beneficial for surgeons but also help in explaining the surgical procedure to patients. Visualizing their condition in a tangible form helps patients better understand the proposed treatment, fostering trust and collaboration [25, 26].

Applications of 3D printing in surgery

1. Cardiovascular Surgery
In cardiovascular procedures, particularly those involving congenital heart defects, 3D models provide a detailed representation of complex cardiac anatomy. Surgeons can plan the most effective approach for correcting structural abnormalities, significantly improving surgical precision and outcomes. In the case of congenital heart defects, 3D-printed models allow surgeons to identify anatomical nuances, such as unusual blood vessel arrangements, ensuring precise surgical interventions [25, 26].

2. Neurosurgery
Neurosurgery often deals with highly delicate and intricate structures. 3D printing aids in visualizing tumors, aneurysms, or other abnormalities in the brain and spinal cord, enabling safer surgical planning [25, 26].

3. Orthopedic Surgery
Custom 3D-printed implants and guides are increasingly used in orthopedic surgeries, such as joint replacements or complex fracture repairs. These personalized tools align perfectly with the patient's anatomy, ensuring better surgical outcomes [25, 26].

3. Radiology and Oncology
Radiologists and oncologists use 3D printing to map tumors and plan their surgical removal with precision. Models of cancerous growths help surgeons determine the exact margins, ensuring complete tumor excision while sparing healthy tissues. [25, 26]

Robotic systems have transformed surgical procedures by enhancing precision, reducing invasiveness, and improving patient outcomes. Each system, from image-guided robots to teleoperated and nanorobotic systems, offers unique advantages and challenges. As technology advances, these systems will become more accessible, leading to further innovations in surgical care and patient outcomes [25, 26].

4.4 CONCLUSION

The integration of robotics into surgical planning and navigation is revolutionizing the healthcare landscape by providing advanced solutions that enhance precision, reduce human error, and optimize patient outcomes. The use of robotic systems, combined with technologies such as 3D printing, augmented reality (AR), and artificial intelligence (AI), is significantly reshaping the way surgeries are planned and executed. In surgical planning, robotics enables surgeons to interact with highly accurate, patient-specific models that provide a better understanding of complex anatomy. These models, often created using 3D printing, allow for more precise preoperative assessments, helping surgeons visualize anatomical structures in three dimensions. This visualization enhances the surgical approach, reduces operating time, and lowers the risk of complications. Additionally, the ability to simulate the surgical procedure before the actual operation allows for more efficient and safer interventions, with a decreased likelihood of unexpected issues arising during the procedure.

Robotic navigation systems, equipped with advanced imaging technologies, guide surgeons with real-time feedback during the operation. These systems ensure that surgical instruments are positioned accurately, and they enable continuous monitoring of the patient's progress throughout the procedure. Such precision reduces the need for invasive techniques, lowers the risk of tissue damage, and ultimately improves the overall quality of patient care. The combination of robotic assistance and navigation ensures that the surgical path is as minimally invasive as possible while maintaining accuracy and reducing variability, even in the most delicate and complex procedures. Moreover, the advancements in robotic technology have expanded the potential for surgery across various specialties, including orthopedics, neurosurgery, cardiovascular surgery, and even minimally invasive procedures. The capacity for real-time adjustments and refinements during surgeries not only ensures better surgical outcomes but also contributes to faster recovery times and fewer complications. With the ability to make highly precise, micro-adjustments in real time, robotic systems allow for minimally invasive techniques that require smaller incisions, reducing patient trauma and speeding up recovery. Despite the numerous benefits, the widespread adoption of robotic surgery and planning systems still faces challenges, including high costs, technical limitations, and the need for specialized training. The equipment is expensive to purchase and maintain, making it difficult for many healthcare institutions, especially those in lower-resource settings, to adopt these technologies. Additionally, the learning curve associated with using robotic systems means that surgeons must undergo extensive training to use them effectively, which can also be a barrier to implementation. Looking ahead, advancements in AI, machine learning, and robotic materials are likely to further enhance the capabilities of surgical planning and navigation systems. The integration of AI can allow for more intelligent and adaptive navigation, potentially learning from each surgery to provide better predictive insights and real-time adjustments. Moreover, the development of lighter, more affordable robotic systems and the increasing availability of telemedicine may help reduce costs and make robotic surgery more accessible to a broader range of healthcare providers and patients. In conclusion, robotic systems in planning and navigation are redefining the field of surgery by providing surgeons with innovative tools that enhance precision, reduce risk, and improve patient outcomes. As technology continues to evolve, we can expect even greater advancements that will expand the role of robotics in healthcare, making surgeries safer, more effective, and accessible to patients around the world. The future of surgical planning and navigation is undoubtedly one that is closely intertwined with robotics, promising even more remarkable improvements in surgical practices and patient care.

REFERENCES

1. Camarillo, D. B., Krummel, T. M., & Salisbury Jr, J. K. (2004). Robotic technology in surgery: Past, present, and future. *The American Journal of Surgery*, 188(4), 2–15.
2. Howe, R. D., & Matsuoka, Y. (1999). Robotics for surgery. *Annual Review of Biomedical Engineering*, 1(1), 211–240.
3. Satava, R. M. (1999). Emerging technologies for surgery in the 21st century. *Archives of Surgery*, 134(11), 1197–1202.
4. Falk, V., Mourgues, F., Adhami, L., Jacobs, S., Thiele, H., Nitzsche, S., ... & Coste-Manière, È. (2005). Cardio navigation: Planning, simulation, and augmented reality in robotic assisted endoscopic bypass grafting. *The Annals of Thoracic Surgery*, 79(6), 2040–2047.
5. Gomes, P. (2011). Surgical robotics: Reviewing the past, analysing the present, imagining the future. *Robotics and Computer-Integrated Manufacturing*, 27(2), 261–266.
6. Yang, L., & Etsuko, K. (2020). Review on vision-based tracking in surgical navigation. *IET Cyber-Systems and Robotics*, 2(3), 107–121.
7. Han, J., Davids, J., Ashrafian, H., Darzi, A., Elson, D. S., & Sodergren, M. (2022). A systematic review of robotic surgery: From supervised paradigms to fully autonomous robotic approaches. *The International Journal of Medical Robotics and Computer Assisted Surgery*, 18(2), e2358.
8. Bell, R. B. (2011). Computer planning and intraoperative navigation in orthognathic surgery. *Journal of Oral and Maxillofacial Surgery*, 69(3), 592–605.
9. Dagnino, G., Georgilas, I., Köhler, P., Morad, S., Atkins, R., & Dogramadzi, S. (2016). Navigation system for robot-assisted intra-articular lower-limb fracture surgery. *International Journal of Computer Assisted Radiology and Surgery*, 11, 1831–1843.
10. Taylor, R. H., Menciassi, A., Fichtinger, G., Fiorini, P., & Dario, P. (2016). Medical robotics and computer-integrated surgery. *Springer Handbook of Robotics*, 1657–1684.
11. Xia, T., Baird, C., Jallo, G., Hayes, K., Nakajima, N., Hata, N., & Kazanzides, P. (2008). An integrated system for planning, navigation and robotic assistance for skull base surgery. *The International Journal of Medical Robotics and Computer Assisted Surgery*, 4(4), 321–330.

12. Liu, Y., Wu, X., Sang, Y., Zhao, C., Wang, Y., Shi, B., & Fan, Y. (2024). Evolution of surgical robot systems enhanced by artificial intelligence: A review. *Advanced Intelligent Systems*, 6(5), 2300268.
13. Marcus, H., Nandi, D., Darzi, A., & Yang, G. Z. (2013). Surgical robotics through a keyhole: From today's translational barriers to tomorrow's "disappearing" robots. *IEEE Transactions on Biomedical Engineering,* 60(3), 674–681.
14. Ashrafian, H., Clancy, O., Grover, V., & Darzi, A. (2017). The evolution of robotic surgery: Surgical and anaesthetic aspects. *BJA: British Journal of Anaesthesia*, 119(suppl_1), i72–i84.
15. Chapuis, J., Schramm, A., Pappas, I., Hallermann, W., Schwenzer-Zimmerer, K., Langlotz, F., & Caversaccio, M. (2007). A new system for computer-aided preoperative planning and intraoperative navigation during corrective jaw surgery. *IEEE Transactions on Information Technology in Biomedicine,* 11(3), 274–287.
16. Bell, R. B. (2010). Computer planning and intraoperative navigation in cranio-maxillofacial surgery. *Oral and Maxillofacial Surgery Clinics*, 22(1), 135–156.
17. Gavriilidis, P., Edwin, B., Pelanis, E., Hidalgo, E., de'Angelis, N., Memeo, R., ... & Sutcliffe, R. P. (2022). Navigated liver surgery: State of the art and future perspectives. *Hepatobiliary & Pancreatic Diseases International,* 21(3), 226–233.
18. Kobayashi, S., Cho, B., Huaulmé, A., Tatsugami, K., Honda, H., Jannin, P., ... & Eto, M. (2019). Assessment of surgical skills by using surgical navigation in robot-assisted partial nephrectomy. *International Journal of Computer Assisted Radiology and Surgery,* 14, 1449–1459.
19. Yip, M., & Das, N. (2019). Robot autonomy for surgery. In J. P. Desai, R. V. Patel, A. Ferreira, & S. K. Agrawal (Eds.), The Encyclopedia of MEDICAL ROBOTICS*: Volume 1: Minimally Invasive Surgical Robotics* (pp. 281–313). World Scientific Publishing Co. Pte. Ltd., Singapore.
20. Andras, I., Mazzone, E., van Leeuwen, F. W., De Naeyer, G., van Oosterom, M. N., Beato, S., ... & Mottrie, A. (2020). Artificial intelligence and robotics: A combination that is changing the operating room. *World Journal of Urology,* 38, 2359–2366.
21. Volonté, F., Pugin, F., Bucher, P., Sugimoto, M., Ratib, O., & Morel, P. (2011). Augmented reality and image overlay navigation with OsiriX in laparoscopic and robotic surgery: Not only a matter of fashion. *Journal of Hepato-Biliary-Pancreatic Sciences*, 18(4), 506–509.
22. Yu, L., Wang, Z., Sun, L., Wang, W., Wang, L., & Du, Z. (2017). A new forecasting kinematic algorithm of automatic navigation for a laparoscopic minimally invasive surgical robotic system. *Robotica*, 35(5), 1192–1222.
23. Gu, L., Yin, C., Jia, T., He, K., Ma, X., & Zhang, X. (2023). Robotic surgery in China. *The Innovation*, 4(5), 100499.
24. Pradhan, B., Bharti, D., Chakravarty, S., Ray, S. S., Voinova, V. V., Bonartsev, A. P., & Pal, K. (2021). Internet of things and robotics in transforming

current-day healthcare services. *Journal of Healthcare Engineering*, 2021(1), 9999504.
25. Low, S. C., & Phee, L. (2004). *A Review of Master-Slave Robotic Systems for Surgery*. In Proceedings of the IEEE Conference on Robotics, Automation and Mechatronics (pp. 37–42), Singapore.
26. Tang, R., Ma, L. F., Rong, Z. X., Li, M. D., Zeng, J. P., Wang, X. D., ... & Dong, J. H. (2018). Augmented reality technology for preoperative planning and intraoperative navigation during hepatobiliary surgery: A review of current methods. *Hepatobiliary & Pancreatic Diseases International*, 17(2), 101–112.

Chapter 5

Bioimplants with 2D, 3D, and 4D additive manufacturing technology

Bogala Mallikharjuna Reddy

5.1 INTRODUCTION

Bioimplants are implants used in clinical therapy or medicine, such as medication delivery systems, prostheses, wearable biosensors, and porous bone implants. Typically, they are inserted into the body for a duration exceeding thirty days [1], [2]. They are designed to imitate, sustain, repair, or improve the functions of human tissues by fusing the human body, material characteristics, and bioimplant integrity. An aging population and a lack of donor organs for medical treatment have resulted in a sharp rise in the demand for bioimplants in recent years [3]. With the study and expansion of the biomaterials field, various bioimplants, such as brain/neural implants, bone/cartilage implants, dental implants, and other structural implants, have been developed [4]. The main difficulty with bioimplants is choosing the right biomaterials, manufacturing process, surface treatment, and biological assessments [1], [4]. Many bioinert materials are used as biologized implants, such as titanium (Ti), tantalum, gold, cobalt-chromium (Co–Cr) alloys, stainless steel (SS; 316L), and nitinol [5].

Technologies such as additive manufacturing (AM), which involve adding materials to the substrate instead of deleting them as in traditional manufacturing, offer greater opportunities for the highly efficient creation of bioimplants with complicated geometry or specific needs [3]. Figure 5.1 represents the historical timeline of AM technologies. Two fascinating studies on the 3D bioprinting of organs or tissues were just released. Based on suspended hydrogels, Lee et al. demonstrated a technique for printing human heart components at different scales [6]. Using photopolymerizable hydrogels, Grigoryan et al. created intravascular and multivascular structures for an alveolar model, which was then applied to a mouse model of chronic liver injury [7]. Currently, bioimplants, such as cortical bone, cranium, cartilage, and surgical instruments, are being effectively manufactured using fused deposition modeling (FDM), selective laser melting (SLM), stereolithography (SLA), and other AM technologies [1], [8]. This book chapter reviews AM materials for bioimplants in two and three dimensions (2D

 DOI: 10.1201/9781003581192-5

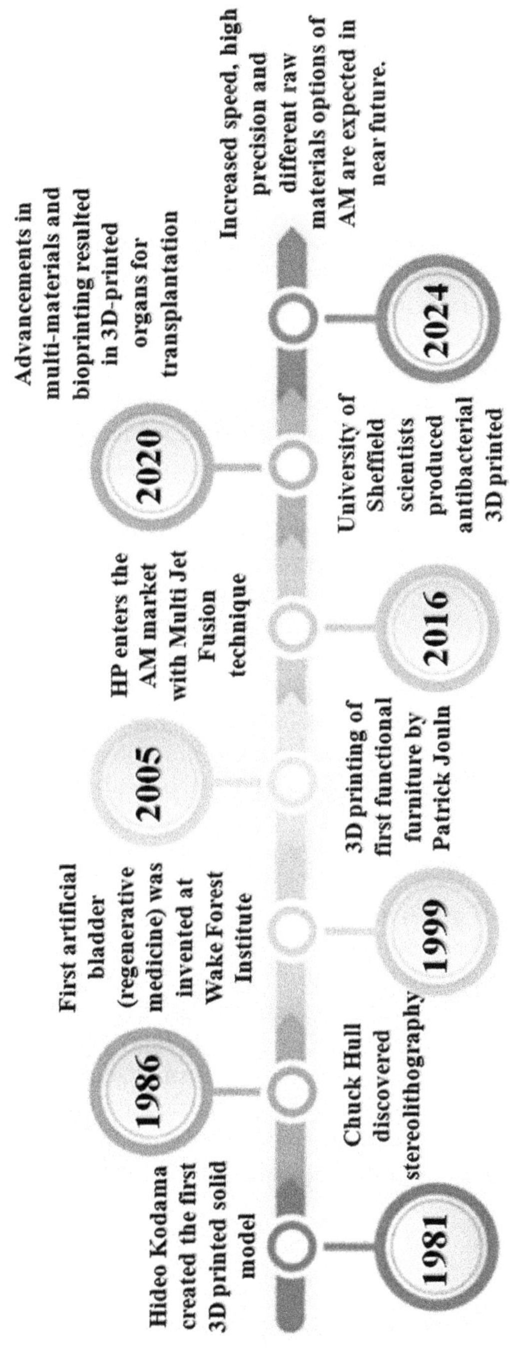

Figure 5.1 History timeline of some key inventions of additive manufacturing technologies.

and 3D). Moreover, both hard and soft bioimplants have been successfully created using innovative ceramic inks as four-dimensional (4D) AM materials and are promising for biomedical implant research.

5.2 AM MATERIALS FOR BIOIMPLANTS

5.2.1 2D materials

Applying materials to an object's surface, usually by coating or other surface-treatment methods, is considered 2D AM. 2D AM materials are widely used in biological sectors, as seen in Figure 5.1 [1], [9]. The physical topography and surface chemistry are important factors [10]. In order to improve the mechanical characteristics, biofunctionality, and biocompatibility of biomaterials like bioceramics, bioglasses, biopolymers, and metal alloys, as well as the functionality of bioimplants or other medical devices, a variety of coating and surface-treatment techniques, such as plasma spraying, sputter coating, and ion-beam-assisted deposition, have been used [4], [10]. Because of their long-term structural and mechanical stability, biodegradable magnesium (Mg) and titanium (Ti) alloys are common bioimplant materials [1]. Two examples are an ultrathin film coating of hydroxyapatite (HAp) on a magnesium–calcium (Mg–Ca) alloy and a pulse-potential coating of calcium phosphate on the surface of a magnesium alloy (AZ91) [1], [11]. To improve the corrosion-resistance qualities, Ti alloy coatings have also been created using the magnetron sputtering technique on commercial purity (CP)-Ti substrates [12]. Studies reveal that magnesium in bioimplants can enhance bone-fracture repair in rats and encourage osteogenic differentiation [13].

5.2.2 3D materials

Not all biomaterials are suitable for 3D printing bioimplants, despite the fact that many have been documented. First and foremost, materials used to make bioimplants should be low in toxicity and have good biocompatibility. The application environment should also be taken into account in order to satisfy the needs of various areas of the human body [14]. The load sharing during implant use may be impacted by a mismatch in the stiffness of the implants and the surrounding tissue. High mechanical strength is a requirement for materials used in load-bearing implants, such as bone implants [1], [14]. The discussion that follows introduces a number of materials that have been utilized in bioimplants.

5.2.2.1 Polymers

Several polymers, including polyetheretherketone (PEEK), polycaprolactone (PCL), poly(vinyl alcohol) (PVA), and poly(L-lactic acid) (PLLA), are frequently utilized in 3D printing scaffolds [3]. PEEK, a thermoplastic biomaterial having mechanical qualities that have been emphasized for use in artificial bone implants, particularly at human load-bearing areas, has been approved by the US Food and Drug Administration (FDA). Because of its high melting and glass-transition temperatures (143 and 343°C, respectively), PEEK presents a substantial processability problem [15]. Additionally, IHaleem and Javaid examined the encouraging use of 3D-printed PEEK in dental implants [15]. Zhang et al. used FDM to create a novel technique for creating costal cartilage replacements with a wavy elastic structure. The most widely utilized thermoplastic polymer for 3D printing bone scaffolds is PCL because of its slow biodegradation, strong biocompatibility, and previous FDA approval [16]. In addition to the polymers listed above, 3D-printed implants frequently use poly(lactic-co-glycolic acid) (PLGA), poly(methyl methacrylate) (PMMA), and PVA.

5.2.2.2 Metals

Metals or their alloys are often 3D printed using SLM or electron beam melting (EBM) [1].

5.2.2.2.1 Titanium-based alloys

Ti alloys' low modulus, corrosion resistance, and superior biocompatibility have made them useful as biomaterials. Ti-6Al-4V is utilized in the fabrication of mandibular and clavicular implants, as well as in foot osteotomy, flanged acetabular cups, and other focal zones, including hip and dental implants [17]. But the release of Al and V causes neurological problems such as osteomalacia and Alzheimer's disease [1]. Presently, femoral prosthesis stems are made of Ti–6Al–7Nb and Ti–5Al–2.5Fe without V [1].

5.2.2.2.2 Stainless steel

The most widely utilized implant materials for creating internal fixation devices (stents, bone plates, and artificial joints) are austenitic 316L SS alloys, which contain 2% to 3% molybdenum (Mo) [1]. Hao et al. introduced a combination material consisting of 316L SS and HAp bioceramic for the production of load-bearing and bioactive composite implants by SLM since 316L SS is unable to stimulate the formation of new tissue [18]. Compared to 316L, 317L SS alloys with 3%–4% Mo has superior pitting and overall corrosion resistance [18, 19]. Chai et al. investigated the antibacterial activity and biocompatibility of 317L SS-Cu both in vitro and in vivo—to lower bacterial infections of bone implants [19].

5.2.2.2.3 Iron-based alloys

Because of their low hemolysis ratio and superior anticoagulant capabilities, iron and its alloys—which do not encourage hydrogen evolution—are another class of biodegradable metal that can be utilized as bone implants or cardiovascular stents. They also offer higher mechanical qualities than alloys based on magnesium [1]. Pure Fe has a larger elastic modulus (211.4 GPa) than either pure Mg (41 GPa) or 316L SS (190 GPa) [20]. In order to increase the pace at which pure iron material degrades (0.16 mma1 in an osteogenic environment) and decrease its magnetic susceptibility in clinical applications, Mn, carbon (C), Si, and palladium (Pd) elements are frequently alloyed with iron [20].

5.2.2.2.4 Cobalt-based alloys

Orthopedic implants frequently use Co–Cr alloys, which are biomaterials made of Co, Cr, Ni, and Mo. Co-based alloys are superior to SS in terms of mechanical strength, abrasion resistance, corrosion resistance, and biocompatibility [1]. Co-Cr–Mo alloys and Co-Ni–Cr–Mo alloys are the two primary varieties of Co–Cr alloys. Co–Cr–Mo alloys, which contain element levels of 27%–30% Co, 2.5% Ni, and 5%–7% Mo, have been utilized in dental implants and artificial alloy joints [21]. Co-Ni-Cr-Mo alloys, which are made up of 19%–21% Cr, 33%–37% Ni, and 9%–11% Mo, have been utilized for large joints [21].

5.2.2.2.5 Magnesium-based alloys

By using EBM, Xiang et al. produced a Co–Cr–Mo alloy with mechanical properties and an anisotropic microstructure [22]. Because magnesium's elastic modulus (45 GPa) is comparable to that of cortical bone, it may be a suitable candidate for bone implants if researchers can regulate its rate of corrosion. Magnesium alloys (Mg–Zn-, Mg–Ca-, Mg–Si-, and Mg–Sr-based alloys) have demonstrated significant promise in the domains of tissue engineering, orthopedics, and cardiovascular medicine [1].

5.2.2.2.6 Zinc-based alloys

Zn-based alloys' high biodegradability and biocompatibility make them extremely promising materials for tissue implants [23]. According to Bowen et al. (2013), zinc is an excellent candidate material for stent production [24]. The ultimate tensile strength of pure zinc is 20 MPa when cast and 120 MPa when wrought [1]. Nevertheless, it lacks the strength necessary for use in stents (a vascular stent requires 300 MPa). For biomedical uses, zinc must therefore be mixed with other metals to create alloys. Some articles have reviewed Zn–Mg, Zn–Ca/Sr, Zn–Al, Zn–Li, Zn–Ag, Zn–Cu, and Zn–Mn systems [23].

5.2.2.3 *Ceramics*

Because natural bone is made up of collagen and ceramic (HAp, about 80% of the wet weight of bone), ceramics are favored for preparing bone implants. In addition to being biocompatible, desirable bioceramics should be osteoconductive and osteoinductive and should not release any harmful substances when applied. At first, zirconia (ZrO_2) and alumina (Al_2O_3) were used as bioinert bioceramics to produce the femoral heads of total hip replacement prostheses [1]. In 2019, Chen et al. studied ceramic 3D printing technologies, including bulk solid, powder, and slurry-based techniques [25].

5.2.2.4 *Bulk metallic glasses*

A type of metallic material known as bulk metallic glasses (BMGs) has a Young's modulus of 50–100 GPa, a strength of ~2 GPa, and an elasticity of ~2% [1]. Their distinct disordering atomic structure gives them a great resilience to wear and corrosion. Consequently, compared to its crystalline bulk, BMGs have superior biocompatibility and can be utilized as innovative implant materials. $Zr_{44}Ti_{11}Cu_{10}Ni_{10}Be_{25}$ BMG better supports attachment and promotes cell development [26].

5.3 3D AM TECHNOLOGIES FOR BIOIMPLANTS

Figure 5.2 depicts the schematic of some AM methods discussed in the following sections. Table 5.1 summarizes a number of exemplary 3D AM technologies that are frequently utilized for bioimplant manufacture, along with their benefits, drawbacks, and uses [1].

5.3.1 Fused deposition modeling

FDM is an AM technique where a thin polymer filament is created—following extrusion and melting [41]. Polycarbonate (PC), acrylonitrile butadiene styrene (ABS), PCL, polyamide (PA), and PLA are examples of thermoplastic polymers that are frequently utilized. Using FDM technology, Zeng et al. created an artificial human ear. Polyurethane was used to create the auricular framework because of its high degree of flexibility and biocompatibility [42]. In orthopedic surgery, this trial demonstrated an effective method for reconstructing macrotia and mitigating other cartilage abnormalities. For two patients, Gronet et al. created acrylic cranial implants that made it easier to restore significant or intricate cranial abnormalities [43].

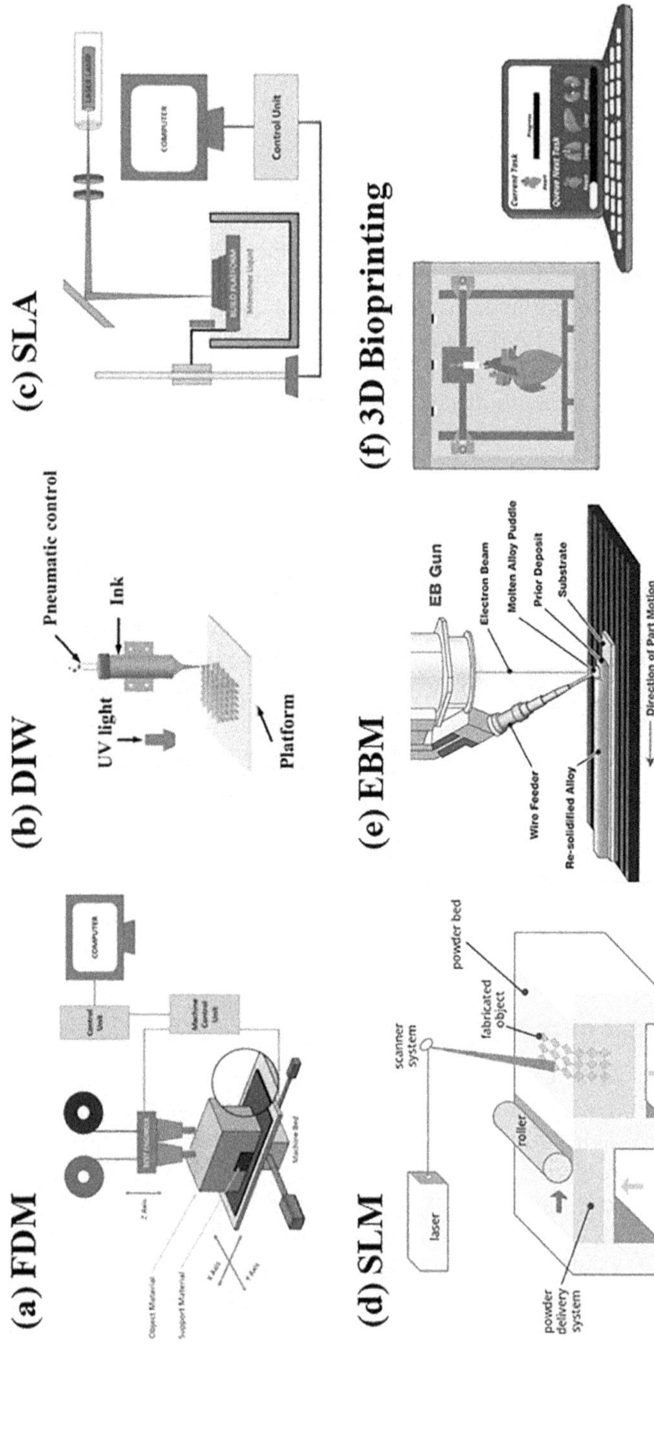

Figure 5.2 A schematic of important AM methods: (a) FDM, (b) DIW, (c) SLA, (d) SLM, (e) EBM, and (f) 3D bioprinting.

Table 5.1 Some important 3D AM methods for production of bioimplants

3D AM method	*Materials*	*Principal*	*Advantages*	*Disadvantages*	*Bioimplant Applications*	*Ref.*
FDM	Filaments made of thermoplastics, such as PLA, ABS, PA, and PC	Melted material is selectively deposited layer by layer along a predetermined path.	Economical; a variety of materials	Resolution with the lowest dimensions	Vertebrae, skull,	[8, 27] [28]
DIW	Sol-gel, hydrogel, ceramic inks, polymer, and HAp nanocomposites	Layer by layer, liquid-phase "ink" is deposited after being dispensed out under regulated pressure.	High density bulk; porous scaffold	Limited rheological ink selection; post-processing is required to eliminate polymer content for printing on ceramics and metal.	Vascularization, bone tissue, and cartilage	[29] [30] [31] [32]
SLA	Resin that reacts to light	Light processing is used to crosslink monomers and create layers of components	Great resolution, great speed, and a smooth surface	Expensive; fragile; requires post-processing to remove supporting component	Dental implants and bone implants	[8, 27] [33] [34]
SLM	Alloys of Mg, Ti, Al, Ti, and SS	Scanning and selectively fusing the metal powder particles with a laser to create a layer-by-layer model.	Lightweight construction, intricate geometry, and strong mechanical performance	Expensive; limited production size	Dental alloys, acetabular cups, spinal surgical templates, and locking plates	[8, 27] [33] [35] [36] [37]
EBM	Ni–Ti alloy, Ti–6Al–4V, and Co–Cr–Mo alloy	By using a high power electron beam to selectively melt the powder, components are constructed .	High operating temperatures, extremely high velocities in vacuum, and minimal residual stress.	Limited to conductive substances (alloys and metals).	Dental implants and orthopedic implants.	[38] [39] [40]

Acrylic cranioplasty implants customized for each patient were created by Tan et al. [28].

5.3.2 Direct ink writing

In the AM method known as "direct ink writing" (DIW), the material's melts or suspensions are extruded from the machine as filaments [30]. Hydrogels, suspensions of ceramic or metal powder in polymer solution, and thermoplastic polymer melts are only a few of the many sources of materials for DIW. Like FDM, the printing resolution depends on a number of factors, including the pressure, stage movement velocity, and printing nozzle diameter. Sintering or other post-treatment techniques are needed to eliminate the polymer composition in the printing inks for ceramic and metal components. The DIW technique has been used to create bioimplants for vascularization, bone tissue, and cartilage [29], [31], [32].

5.3.3 Stereolithography

One of the first AM techniques, SLA, was created in 1986 [44]. The SLA technique has been used to create dental implants and bone [33]. Ceramic powders can be mixed with photosensitive resin to create ceramic-based implants, and the polymers are then eliminated through sintering. The possible uses of SLA in maxillofacial prosthodontics, including, as obturators, surgical tents, and auricular and nasal prostheses, were compiled by Winder and Bibb [45]. Sanding, painting, and polishing are a few examples of post-treatments. SLA has the benefit of producing implants with a high resolution of 10 lm, but its drawbacks include high cost and scarce material resources [44].

5.3.4 Selective laser melting

The powder, which is free in the bed, is fused by the laser at a precise spot for each layer to create the intended structures during SLM procedures [37]. The SLM process often uses fiber lasers (1.09 lm) with a shorter wavelength or pure metal powders and laser beams (usually neodymium-doped yttrium aluminum garnet, 1.064 lm) with a higher absorptivity to metals. Its drawbacks include the fact that particle size affects printing accuracy, and that the inert gas printing environment stops particles from oxidizing. The creation of locking plates, acetabular cups, spinal surgery templates, and dental alloys are among the bioimplant applications of SLM [46], [35–37].

5.3.5 Electron beam melting

EBM is a powder-bed-based AM technique that was created in 1997 by Arcam AB Corporation [38]. It resembles the SLM procedure. But with

EBM, the heat source is an electron beam rather than a laser beam. Under vacuum, EBM can function at incredibly high speeds (up to 105 ms1) [38]. It has been reported that EBM fabricates Co–Cr–Mo, Ti–6Al–4V, and Ni–Ti alloys, for use in orthopedic and dental implants [1], [39], [40].

5.3.6 3D bioprinting

3D bioprinting techniques can be divided into three categories, depending on their working principles: inkjet-based, microextrusion-based, and laser-assisted bioprinting [1]. For bioprinting, the right bioink is essential; it should have the right mechanical strength, gelation process, biocompatibility, and other qualities. Replicating biological function through structure synthesis is the main issue in 3D bioprinting [47]. In order to potentially repair the mandible bone, calvarial bone, ear cartilage, and skeletal muscle, Kang et al. developed an integrated tissue–organ printer system [48]. A human heart was printed at different scales using a novel 3D bioprinting technique by Lee et al., that uses freeform reversible embedding of suspended hydrogels as a supporting printing medium [6]. Grigoryan and colleagues used SLA to create intravascular and multivascular structures using photopolymerizable hydrogels. Despite its lack of practical utility in clinics, 3D bioprinting technology has demonstrated a thriving foreground [7].

5.4 4D AM MATERIALS FOR BIOIMPLANTS

In 2014, a multi-material strand folded into the letter "MIT" served as the first example of 4D printing [49]. Numerous materials, such as metals, ceramics, and polymers, have been created thus far for 4D AM [1]. Light-driven 4D technology has garnered a lot of interest because of its benefits, which include quick reaction times, wireless control, precise focusing, and environmentally-friendly qualities [1]. A new generation of 4D-printed structures, such as light-thermal dual-responsive hydrogels, electrothermal and electrochemical actuation materials, magnetic-photo/thermal dual stimuli actuators, temperature-pH sensitive fluorescence bilayer actuators, and humidity–temperature–light triple-responsive hydrogels, have been made possible by the development of multi-responsive materials and technologies [50]. Figure 5.3 shows different bioimplant applications of additive manufacturing techniques.

5.5 CONCLUSIONS

Other binary and multiple-component systems can benefit from the current soft/rigid hybrid 4D AM idea, which is accomplished by 4D printing hybrid ceramic precursor/ceramic materials. More types of soft/rigid hybrid structures with functional gradient interfaces can be additively built with

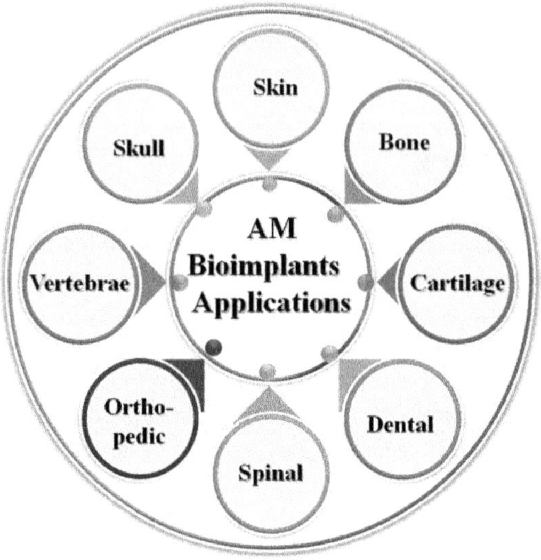

Figure 5.3 A depiction of various bioimplant applications of additive manufacturing.

the help of other technologies like local ceramization and multi-material printing. Combining 2D, 3D, and 4D AM materials could lead to further advancements in the creation of bioimplants for the human body's intricate and dynamic biological settings. Material combinations between printing host, printing support, and printing medium materials would be included in future studies on multi-material printing.

Acknowledgements: The author expresses gratitude to Jaiotec Labs (OPC) Pvt. Ltd., for providing the necessary facilities in completion of the current work.

REFERENCES

[1] G. Liu, He, Y., Liu, P., Chen, Z., Chen, X., Wan, L., Li, Y., & Lu, J. (2020). Development of bioimplants with 2D, 3D, and 4D additive manufacturing materials. *Engineering, 6*(11), 1232–1243.

[2] K. C. R. Kolan, M. C. Leu, G. E. Hilmas, R. F. Brown, and M. Velez, "Fabrication of 13-93 bioactive glass scaffolds for bone tissue engineering using indirect selective laser sintering," *Biofabrication*, vol. 3, no. 2, p. 025004, Jun. 2011.

[3] C. M. B. Ho, S. H. Ng, and Y.-J. Yoon, "A review on 3D printed bioimplants," *International Journal of Precision Engineering And Manufacturing*, vol. 16, no. 5, pp. 1035–1046, May 2015.

[4] M. Prakasam, J. Locs, K. Salma-Ancane, D. Loca, A. Largeteau, and L. Berzina-Cimdina, "Biodegradable materials and metallic implants—A review," *Journal of Functional Biomaterials*, vol. 8, no. 4, p. 44, Dec. 2017.
[5] M. Saini, Y. Singh, P. Arora, V. Arora, and K. Jain, "Implant biomaterials: A comprehensive review," *World Journal of Clinical Cases: WJCC*, vol. 3, no. 1, p. 52, Jan. 2015.
[6] A. Lee et al., "3D bioprinting of collagen to rebuild components of the human heart," *Science*, vol. 365, no. 6452, pp. 482–487, Aug. 2019.
[7] B. Grigoryan et al., "Multivascular networks and functional intravascular topologies within biocompatible hydrogels," *Science*, vol. 364, no. 6439, pp. 458–464, May 2019.
[8] T. D. Ngo, A. Kashani, G. Imbalzano, K. T. Q. Nguyen, and D. Hui, "Additive manufacturing (3D printing): A review of materials, methods, applications and challenges," *Composites Part B: Engineering*, vol. 143, pp. 172–196, Jun. 2018.
[9] M. R. Bogala, "Three-dimensional (3D) printing of hydroxyapatite-based scaffolds: A review," *Bioprinting*, vol. 28, p. e00244, Dec. 2022.
[10] A. Kurella and N. B. Dahotre, "Review paper: Surface modification for bioimplants: The role of laser surface engineering," *Journal of Biomaterials Applications*, vol. 20, no. 1, pp. 5–50, Jul. 2005.
[11] M. A. Surmeneva, T. M. Mukhametkaliyev, H. Khakbaz, R. A. Surmenev, and M. Bobby Kannan, "Ultrathin film coating of hydroxyapatite (HA) on a magnesium–calcium alloy using RF magnetron sputtering for bioimplant applications," *Materials Letters*, vol. 152, pp. 280–282, Aug. 2015.
[12] B. Subramanian, C. V. Muraleedharan, R. Ananthakumar, and M. Jayachandran, "Corrigendum to 'A comparative study of titanium nitride (TiN), titanium oxy nitride (TiON) and titanium aluminum nitride (TiAlN), as surface coatings for bioimplants' [Surf. Coat. Technol. 205 (2011) 5014–5020]," *Surface and Coatings Technology*, vol. 455, p. 129224, Feb. 2023.
[13] Y. Zhang et al., "Implant-derived magnesium induces local neuronal production of CGRP to improve bone-fracture healing in rats," *Natural Medicines*, vol. 22, no. 10, pp. 1160–1169, Oct. 2016.
[14] D. Martinez-Marquez, A. Mirnajafizadeh, C. P. Carty, and R. A. Stewart, "Application of quality by design for 3D printed bone prostheses and scaffolds," *PLOS ONE*, vol. 13, no. 4, p. e0195291, Apr. 2018.
[15] A. Haleem and M. Javaid, "Polyether ether ketone (PEEK) and its manufacturing of customised 3D printed dentistry parts using additive manufacturing," *Clinical Epidemiology and Global Health*, vol. 7, no. 4, pp. 654–660, Dec. 2019.
[16] C. Zhang, L. Wang, J. Kang, O. M. Fuentes, and D. Li, "Bionic design and verification of 3D printed PEEK costal cartilage prosthesis," *Journal of the Mechanical Behavior of Biomedical Materials*, vol. 103, p. 103561, Mar. 2020.

[17] V. V. Popov et al., "Design and 3D-printing of titanium bone implants: Brief review of approach and clinical cases," *Biomedical Engineering Letters*, vol. 8, no. 4, pp. 337–344, Nov. 2018.

[18] L. Hao, S. Dadbakhsh, O. Seaman, and M. Felstead, "Selective laser melting of a stainless steel and hydroxyapatite composite for load-bearing implant development," *Journal of Materials Processing Technology*, vol. 209, no. 17, pp. 5793–5801, Aug. 2009.

[19] H. Chai et al., "Antibacterial effect of 317L stainless steel contained copper in prevention of implant-related infection in vitro and in vivo," *Journal of Materials Science: Materials in Medicine*, vol. 22, no. 11, pp. 2525–2535, Nov. 2011.

[20] A. Purnama, H. Hermawan, J. Couet, and D. Mantovani, "Assessing the biocompatibility of degradable metallic materials: State-of-the-art and focus on the potential of genetic regulation," *Acta Biomaterialia*, vol. 6, no. 5, pp. 1800–1807, May 2010.

[21] N. S. Manam et al., "Study of corrosion in biocompatible metals for implants: A review," *Journal of Alloys and Compounds*, vol. 701, pp. 698–715, Apr. 2017.

[22] L. Li, M. Zhang, Y. Li, J. Zhao, L. Qin, and Y. Lai, "Corrosion and biocompatibility improvement of magnesium-based alloys as bone implant materials: A review," *Regenerative Biomaterials*, vol. 4, no. 2, pp. 129–137, Mar. 2017.

[23] E. Mostaed, M. Sikora-Jasinska, J. W. Drelich, and M. Vedani, "Zinc-based alloys for degradable vascular stent applications," *Acta Biomaterialia*, vol. 71, pp. 1–23, Apr. 2018.

[24] P. Bowen, J. Drelich, and J. Goldman, "Zinc exhibits physiological corrosion behavior for bioabsorbable stents," *Advanced Materials*, vol. 25, no. 18, pp. 2577–2582, May 2013.

[25] Z. Chen et al., "3D printing of ceramics: A review," *Journal of the European Ceramic Society*, vol. 39, no. 4, pp. 661–687, Apr. 2019.

[26] J. Schroers, G. Kumar, T. M. Hodges, S. Chan, and T. R. Kyriakides, "Bulk metallic glasses for biomedical applications," *JOM*, vol. 61, no. 9, pp. 21–29, Sep. 2009.

[27] V. J. Kharat et al., "Additive manufacturing (3D printing): A review of materials, methods, applications and challenges," *Materials Today: Proceedings*, Nov. 2023.

[28] E. T. W. Tan, J. M. Ling, and S. K. Dinesh, "The feasibility of producing patient-specific acrylic cranioplasty implants with a low-cost 3D printer," *Journal of Neurosurgery*, vol. 124, no. 5, pp. 1531–1537, May 2016.

[29] L. Chen et al., "3D printing of a lithium-calcium-silicate crystal bioscaffold with dual bioactivities for osteochondral interface reconstruction," *Biomaterials*, vol. 196, pp. 138–150, Mar. 2019.

[30] H. Ma, C. Feng, J. Chang, and C. Wu, "3D-printed bioceramic scaffolds: From bone tissue engineering to tumor therapy," *Acta Biomaterialia*, vol. 79, pp. 37–59, Oct. 2018.

[31] J. Winder and R. Bibb, "Medical rapid prototyping technologies: State of the art and current limitations for application in oral and maxillofacial

surgery," *Journal of Oral and Maxillofacial Surgery*, vol. 63, no. 7, pp. 1006–1015, Jul. 2005.

[32] W.-W. Song, J.-H. Heo, J.-H. Lee, Y.-M. Park, and Y.-D. Kim, "Osseointegration of magnesium-incorporated sand-blasted acid-etched implant in the dog mandible: Resonance frequency measurements and histomorphometric analysis," *Tissue Engineering and Regenerative Medicine*, vol. 13, no. 2, pp. 191–199, Apr. 2016.

[33] K. E. Smith et al., "Use of 3D printed bone plate in novel technique to surgically correct hallux valgus deformities," *Techniques in Orthopaedics*, vol. 31, no. 3, pp. 181–189, Sep. 2016.

[34] A. R. Studart, "Additive manufacturing of biologically-inspired materials," *Chemical Society Reviews*, vol. 45, no. 2, pp. 359–376, Jan. 2016.

[35] W. Zhang et al., "3D-printed scaffolds with synergistic effect of hollow-pipe structure and bioactive ions for vascularized bone regeneration," *Biomaterials*, vol. 135, pp. 85–95, Aug. 2017.

[36] M. Faveri, L. C. Figueiredo, and M. Feres, "Considerations about designing and reporting randomized clinical trials – Response to the letter to the editor from Preus et al," *Journal of Evidence Based Dental Practice*, vol. 15, no. 2, pp. 87–88, Jun. 2015.

[37] A. M. Khorasani, I. Gibson, M. Goldberg, and G. Littlefair, "A comprehensive study on surface quality in 5-axis milling of SLM Ti-6Al-4V spherical components," *International Journal of Advanced Manufacturing Technology*, vol. 94, no. 9, pp. 3765–3784, Feb. 2018.

[38] D. Wang et al., "Design and fabrication of a precision template for spine surgery using selective laser melting (SLM)," *Materials*, vol. 9, no. 7, p. 608, Jul. 2016.

[39] T. Koutsoukis, S. Zinelis, G. Eliades, K. Al-Wazzan, M. A. Rifaiy, and Y. S. Al Jabbari, "Selective laser melting technique of Co-Cr dental alloys: A review of structure and properties and comparative analysis with other available techniques," *Journal of Prosthodontics*, vol. 24, no. 4, pp. 303–312, Jun. 2015.

[40] C. Körner, "Additive manufacturing of metallic components by selective electron beam melting — A review," *International Materials Reviews*, vol. 61, no. 5, pp. 361–377, Jul. 2016.

[41] D. D. Xiang et al., "Anisotropic microstructure and mechanical properties of additively manufactured Co–Cr–Mo alloy using selective electron beam melting for orthopedic implants," *Materials Science and Engineering: A*, vol. 765, p. 138270, Sep. 2019.

[42] R. Ramakrishnaiah et al., "Preliminary fabrication and characterization of electron beam melted Ti–6Al–4V customized dental implant," *Saudi Journal of Biological Sciences*, vol. 24, no. 4, pp. 787–796, May 2017.

[43] K. V. Wong and A. Hernandez, "A review of additive manufacturing," *ISRN Mechanical Engineering*, vol. 2012, pp. 1–10, Aug. 2012.

[44] W. Zeng et al., "Fused deposition modelling of an auricle framework for microtia reconstruction based on CT images," *Rapid Prototyping Journal*, vol. 14, no. 5, pp. 280–284, Jan. 2008.

[45] P. M. Gronet, G. A. Waskewicz, and C. Richardson, "Preformed acrylic cranial implants using fused deposition modeling: A clinical report," *The Journal of Prosthetic Dentistry*, vol. 90, no. 5, pp. 429–433, Nov. 2003.

[46] F. P. W. Melchels, J. Feijen, and D. W. Grijpma, "A review on stereolithography and its applications in biomedical engineering," *Biomaterials*, vol. 31, no. 24, pp. 6121–6130, Aug. 2010.

[47] S. V. Murphy and A. Atala, "3D bioprinting of tissues and organs," *Nature Biotechnology*, vol. 32, no. 8, pp. 773–785, Aug. 2014.

[48] H.-W. Kang, S. J. Lee, I. K. Ko, C. Kengla, J. J. Yoo, and A. Atala, "A 3D bioprinting system to produce human-scale tissue constructs with structural integrity," *Nature Biotechnology*, vol. 34, no. 3, pp. 312–319, Mar. 2016.

[49] S. Tibbits, "4D printing: Multi-material shape change," *Architectural Design*, vol. 84, no. 1, pp. 116–121, Jan. 2014.

[50] Y. Dong et al., "Multi-stimuli-responsive programmable biomimetic actuator," *Nature Communications*, vol. 10, no. 1, p. 4087, Sep. 2019.

Chapter 6

Customized biomaterials architecture with additive manufacturing for tissue regeneration

Siddhartha Dan, Padmanava Mishra, Venkatesh Vakucherla, and Mahesh Kumar Sah

6.1 INTRODUCTION

Additive manufacturing (AM), commonly known as 3D printing, has recently become versatile and practical for advanced healthcare-related manufacturing. The core technology of AM, which was first developed in the last two decades, reached its refined version and standards that can meet practical applications in recent times (Zadpoor & Malda, 2017). A noted improvement is the capability of current AM techniques for precisely processing different biomedical materials. Furthermore, regulatory agencies had already cleared several AM methods and their associated products for clinical use; the FDA had even published draft guidance on additively manufactured devices (Ahlfeld et al., 2017). Concurrently, AM was also applied to produce living tissue constructs that could be used as regenerative implants and disease models and made landmark progress toward the development of "fabrication" (Groll et al., 2016). This domain-hastened growth [The rapid growth of this domain] underlines the advanced potential of AM in healthcare. Meanwhile, pharmacology, oncology, surgery, and rehabilitation were outstanding fields for research and clinical applications of additive manufacturing (Zadpoor & Malda, 2017). 3D printing is additive manufacturing or rapid prototyping, a technique to build a three-dimensional object using digital blueprints. The method was first developed by Charles Hull in the 1980s and has increased demand over time (Ventola, 2014). This technology offers a fast and efficient way to convert computer designs into actual models (Hoy, 2013). Sometimes, digital 3D models are created through Computer-aided design (CAD) software or through dimensions and images of an object that had been scanned and then processed using a computer. Healthcare and pharmaceuticals increasingly use 3D printing to formulate personalized medications, oral dosage forms, medical devices, and tissue-engineering products (Goyanes et al., 2016). Most 3D-printed objects result from stack-built layer-by-layer construction using thin slices of materials. Bioprinting made it possible in regenerative medicine to produce medical implants and scaffolds supporting cell growth (Cui et al., 2017). On

DOI: 10.1201/9781003581192-6

the otolaryngology front, application fields include preoperative planning for complex surgeries, surgeon education, and the production of individual anatomical models, implants, and tissue scaffolds. It also enhances surgical training and tackles difficult conditions (Kaye et al., 2016).

The selection of biomaterials and fabrication techniques are the basis for developing and applying scaffolds. Researchers have creatively sought to modify existing biomaterials and create new ones. Biomaterials that interact with biological systems can be broadly categorized based on attributes such as chemical and physical characteristics, biodegradability, origin, and generational advancements M. (Nair & Laurencin, 2006; Navarro et al., 2008). The choice of biomaterial generally depends on the specific requirements of the target tissue. Biodegradable biomaterials have recently gained much interest. From a chemical standpoint, biomaterials can be classified into ceramics, polymers, and composites. Ceramic biomaterials, mainly composed of inorganic metal compounds or calcium salts, are primarily used in orthopedic and dental applications. Because of their similarity to connective tissues, polymers are often used for soft tissue engineering. The composite biomaterials are composed of ceramics and polymers and have a significant application in orthopedic and dental tissue engineering (Jammalamadaka & Tappa, 2018).

Natural and synthetic polymers have been widely used in regenerative medicine (RM) and tissue engineering (TE). The natural origin of biomaterials like collagen, chitosan, hyaluronic acid, and alginate is preferred due to their biocompatibility, degradability, and availability. An essential characteristic of biomaterials is controlled degradation, which enables them to be easily adapted to biological systems. Biomaterials in the extracellular matrix (ECM) encourage excellent cellular growth and compatibility. Collagen is a frequently utilized natural biomaterial used in scaffolds that is versatile and not immunogenic across different species. Some commercially available collagen-based scaffolds include zyplast, zyderm, Collagen Meniscal Implant, and contigen. Another widely used natural material is chitosan, whose chemical structure is similar to hyaluronic acid, an ECM component (Jammalamadaka & Tappa, 2018). The degradation rate of chitosan can be controlled through acetylation. A more advanced approach involves the creation of scaffolds by making intact ECM obtained through the decellularization of tissues or organs. In this process, it is ensured that the ECM is retained, but all cellular components are extracted. Xenogeneic scaffolds have been applied even in clinical practices. Other natural biomaterials used in RM and tissue engineering (TE) include alginate, gelatin, agarose, and hyaluronic acid (Atala, 2009).

Bioprinting techniques primarily involve laser-assisted bioprinting (LaBP), droplet-based inkjet bioprinting, and extrusion bioprinting. Multihead deposition systems enable either simultaneous or sequential deposition of various materials. Besides, application-specific bioprinters have also been developed (Gungor-Ozkerim et al., 2018). These methods find their foundation in CAD/computer-aided manufacturing (CAM) systems upon which the 3D structures are constructed. A key feature of all these strategies is the bio-ink, which, after printing, is cross-linked or stabilized to maintain the shape of the engineered tissue. The selection of the appropriate bio-ink depends upon several parameters such as intended tissue, cell types, and the kind of bioprinter used. Despite the advancements in bioprinting techniques (Dababneh & Ozbolat, 2014; Khalil & Sun, 2009; Wang et al., 2015; Wüst et al., 2011). Advancement in this area still needs to be improved by the absence of bio-inks that meet the demands of bioprinting with cellular bioactivity. Ideally, the tailored mechanical, rheological, chemical, and biological properties should characterize the bio-inks (Lee et al., 2015). These include: (i) sufficient mechanical strength and flexibility for tissue constructs; (ii) tunable gelation and stabilization for structural precision; (iii) biocompatibility and biodegradability to mimic natural tissue environments; (iv) chemical adaptability to carry on specific tissue functions; and (v) scalability with minimal batch variation (Loo et al., 2015). As bio-ink formulations play a crucial role in the entire process of bioprinting, scientists have found novel natural and synthetic materials with unique properties Lee et al., 2016). However, it is urgently required to standardize these bio-ink formulations for greater use.

6.2 ADDITIVE MANUFACTURING TECHNOLOGIES AND BIOMATERIAL INTEGRATION

Three significant benefits are provided by 3D printing compared to the traditional manufacturing methods: unlimited design flexibility, the process is capable of producing complex geometric structures without bounds, and designers have a chance to provide detailed forms without charge. Thereby, doors for innovative designs are found. It makes it easier to produce manufacturing [make manufacturing easier] without requiring advanced operation skills to attain customized and personalized product designs. It permits the combination of different materials to create new items with unique characteristics, accelerates the development of products, provides better conditions for personalization, and enhances flexibility in production. Rather than a singular technology, 3D printing embodies the integration of several advanced disciplines, including digital modelling, electromechanical systems, material sciences, chemistry, and biomedical engineering. Some of the most frequently used methods include extrusion-based, inkjet-based, and laser-assisted bioprinting (Figure 6.1). While much more work remains before the complexity of biological tissue structures can be accurately mimicked, each of these techniques has peculiar strengths and weaknesses that together make up for one another's deficiencies (Groll et al., 2016). In other

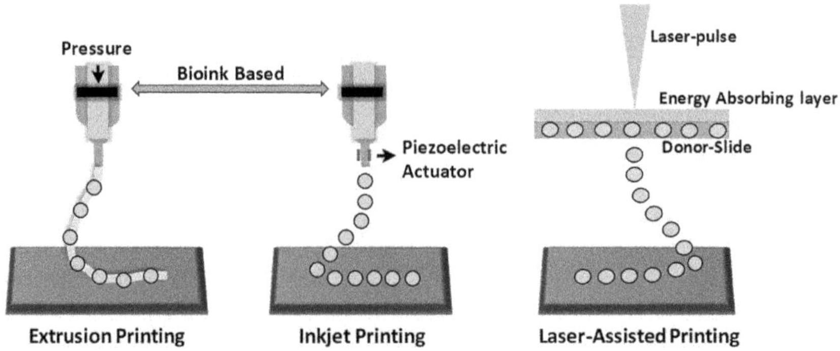

Figure 6.1 Exploring different types of printing technology.

words, it would depend on the complex biological issues and their resolution and cell structure in the applied bioprinting method.

Extrusion-based 3D printing is one of the most widely applied techniques, and its demand is exponentially increasing due to the practicality of this process (Baniasadi et al., 2021; Chen et al., 2021). The mechanism of extrusion bioprinting involves forcing bio-ink out of a nozzle to build tissue scaffolds and organs of any desired architecture (Daly et al., 2021). Inkjet printing, a pioneer in 3D printing, can also be used for cell printing to fabricate tissues or organs, giving rise to inkjet bioprinting as a subset of bioprinting (Moroni et al., 2018). Drop-on-demand inkjet printing, which ejects droplets only when an ejection signal is received, offers high accuracy and efficient ink usage, making it the preferred method in inkjet bioprinting (Li et al., 2020). The Laser-Assisted Bioprinter (LAB) could create tissues with near-physiological functions similar to autologous tissues. Stereolithography and selective laser sintering are variants of laser-assisted 3D printing technology. Unlike other methods, LAB does not suffer from nozzle clogging due to its open-type nozzle construction (Luo et al., 2018).

6.3 MATERIALS FOR 3D PRINTING IN TISSUE REGENERATION

Bioprinting is the process of printing biomaterials suspended in a liquid that can be frozen after being extruded to form a specific shape. The key to successful bioprinting lies in the biomaterial's ability to transition from sol to gel or undergo phase changes. Polymers and composites were widely used because they might be polymerized to make them "3D-printable." Important parameters related to bioprinting application include rheological properties, such as viscosity and non-Newtonian behavior, and crosslinking methods, which differ based on the bioprinting method: inkjet vs. extrusion.

For bioinks involving living cells, shear forces applied during printing must be considered to avoid damaging the cells. Fluids that were shear-thin and non-Newtonian should be used as their vicious behavior was low under shear forces, whilst shear-thickening or thixotropic fluids could cause nozzle clogs or variability in the distribution of particles. Polymers exhibiting the Barus effect, where they expand after ejection, should be minimized to avoid loss of print resolution (Jungst et al., 2016).

Bioinks, mostly hydrogels, can be cross-linked by physical, chemical, or enzymatic means. The cross-linking process induces a sol-gel transition that can impact the bioprinting process's printing rate, resolution, and accuracy. Hydrogels cross-linked by physical agents use non-covalent bonds, which usually result in weaker structures. These are mainly cross-linked by temperature, ionic interactions, or hydrogen bonding (Hospodiuk et al., 2017). On the other hand, chemically cross-linked hydrogels yield mechanically stable structures that can be used to create 3D-printed structures. Although many injectable hydrogels exist, their cross-linking kinetics must be optimized for successful 3D printing. In chemically crosslinked hydrogels, the process typically employs a photosensitive initiator that forms reactive species with exposure to ionizing radiation (Figure 6.2). Pre- and post-fabrication cross-linking has also been applied to increase mechanical stability of the printed objects (Jungst et al., 2016). Some of the commercially available bio inks include Gel4Cell®, CellInk®, BioInk®, OsteoInk®, Bio127®, and BioGel® (Hölzl et al., 2016).

Scaffolds for tissue engineering TE were fabricated using several 3D printing techniques and biomaterials with distinct chemical, mechanical, and biological properties. Tissue-engineered scaffolds in bone tissue engineering have drastically different properties than those used in connective

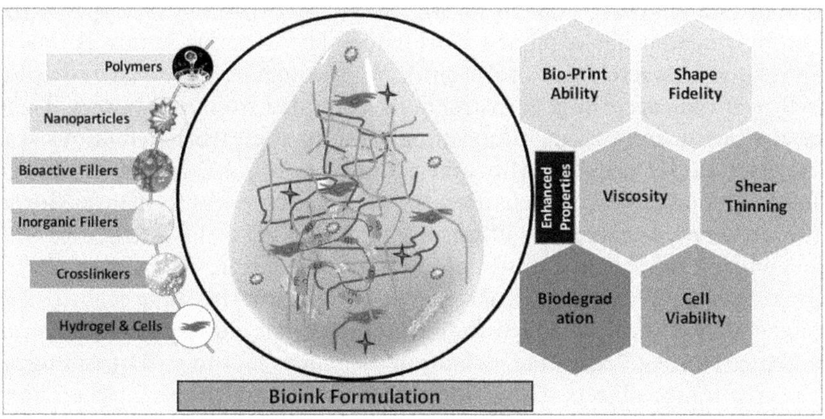

Figure 6.2 Bioink formulation and the requisite specifications for bone tissue regeneration.

tissue applications. The physical properties of the bone tissue scaffolds should be comparable to those of natural bones but vary according to the type of bone and location. The compressive strength of a cortical bone is about 100 MPa, whereas that of spongy bone is approximately 3.9 MPa (Misch et al., 1999). History compatibility and mechanical properties were also taken into account. Polymers and other biomaterials were incorporated into bone scaffolds to replace bone tissue's extracellular matrix (ECM) to support cell proliferation. This review focuses on the most commonly used biomaterials in 3D printing for bone tissue engineering, including bioceramics, bioglass (Afshar-Mohajer et al., 2015; Jang et al., 2017; Ye et al., 2014), natural biopolymers, synthetic degradable thermoplastics, and complex composites that incorporate cell-laden bioinks. A summarized overview of these processes, bioinks, and their applications is presented in Table 6.1.

6.4 4D PRINTING TECHNOLOGY

Skyranger Skylar Tibbits introduced in the TED conference at MIT in 2012 the idea of transformation happening over time in 3D printed products. He explained how something as simple as a 3D structure could become, over time, more complex (Tibbits, 2014). This discovery was a starting point for this new dimension in 3D printing, adding time alongside traditional dimensions- once famously known as 4D printing. In other words, 4D printing is 3D printing, with time being an additional variable, where materials evolve in time to form 4D printed structures. Following Tibbits' talk, several researchers and engineers in diverse fields quickly sparked interest in 4D printing. The first formal research on 4D printing was published a year after Tibbits' TED presentation in 2013. This research worked with the concept of printed active composites (PACs) and used the shape memory effect (SME) to transform a printed sheet into more complicated shapes (Momeni et al., 2019). Since then, the scope of 4D printing research has exploded worldwide. The dynamic nature is one of the unique characteristics of 4D printing, through the material reshaping itself over time according to instructions generated from a computer. There are various definitions of 4D printing. One of the earlier definitions was described as 3D printing with time (Ahmed et al., 2021; Tibbits, 2014). However, a more general definition is "4D printing refers to the transformation in shape, properties, and functionality of a 3D printed structure with time when it is subjected to stimuli such as temperature (Ding et al., 2017; Kotikian et al., 2018), light (Kuksenok & C. Balazs, 2016; Yang et al., 2017), water (Ahmed et al., 2021; Sydney Gladman et al., 2016), pH (Nadgorny et al., 2016), etc." Another definition elegantly captures 4D printing as "the creation of objects that change their shape after printing, where they self-assemble when exposed to stimuli such as heat, water, or air due to chemical reactions of the materials used." 4D printing is a combination

Table 6.1 A summarised table based on the provided details for the bioprinting processes, bio-inks, and applications

Sl. No.	*Bioink (Polymers)*	*Biomaterials*	*Printer Details*	*Nozzle Diameter and Speed*	*Layer Height and Structure*	*Application*	*Reference*
1	poly (3,4-ethylenedioxy-thiophene)	Lithium chloride (0%-40%)	Digital light processing 3D printer	-	Layer thickness = 100 μm	Monitoring human movements	(Mondal et al., 2024a)
2	Sodium Alginate	β-D-mannuronic acid and α-L guluronic acid	BIOVI 3D Bioprinter (REGEMAT 3D, Spain) (with 3 syringes)	27 G nozzle, speed: 5 mm/s	Scaffolds: 0.84 × 30 × 30 mm, 5 mm pore size	3D bioprinting scaffolds	(Gorroñogoitia et al., 2022)
3	PLMC (lactide: trimethylene carbonate 70: 30).	5% Fe_3O_4 composites	Extrusion-based printing 3D printer (BioX, CELLINK)	Nozzle temp:200°C,print speed: 4 mm/s	Two infill patterns (T and L), layer thickness = 1 mm	Vascular grafts, implants.	(Choudhury et al., 2024)
6	Poly(vinyl alcohol)	0.5%, 0.75%, 1%, and 2% of nanoceria	Cellink INKREDIBLE+ 3D Bioprinter	Nozzle diameter: 0.5 mm, pressure: 15-20 psi, speed: 4-6 mm/s		Peripheral nerve injury treatment	(Rizwana et al., 2024)
9	Gelatin type B, sodium alginate	Calcium chloride	Inkredible® bioprinter (CELLINK, Sweden)	Nozzle inner diameter (mm): 0.337 and 0.26	Dog bone geometries at 20 × 20 × 3 mm^3 and 30 × 10 × 5 mm^3 dimensions; Print speed: 2.5 mm/s	Wound dressing structure, effective burn healing	(Fayyazbakhsh et al., 2022)

(continued)

Table 6.1 (Cont.)

Sl. No.	*Bioink (Polymers)*	*Biomaterials*	*Printer Details*	*Nozzle Diameter and Speed*	*Layer Height and Structure*	*Application*	*Reference*
10	Alginate and Gelatin	Boron nitride nanotubes (0.05%-0.1%)	Cellink INKREDIBLE+ (Sweden)	Nozzle pressure: 75-105 kPa, speed: 2 mm/s	Layer height = 0.17 mm, pore size = 0.5 mm	Cell encapsulation	(Kakarla et al., 2022)
11	Sodium Alginate and Gelatin	calcium chloride	BioX bioprinter (Celllnk, Boston, MA, USA)	Speed: 15-30 mm/s, pressure: 10-30 kPa	Scaffolds (20 × 20 × 1 mm3); Layer height: 0.1-0.2 mm	Skeletal Muscle Tissue Engineering	(Sonaye et al., 2022)
12	Gelatin (GE), Polyvinyl Alcohol	Genipin (0.1%)	Biogens XI (3D Gens, Malaysia)	Inner diameter: 0.3 mm, speed: 4000 mm/s	Printed with 2.5 cm*2.5 cm length, 0.3 mm retraction length at 0.3 mm of retraction	Skin replacement, fluid absorption	(Masri et al., 2023)
13	Polyvinyl Alcohol (2.5%-10.5%)		AJ 300 (Optomec)	Nozzle: 200 µm, speed: 1 mm/s	Thickness = 5.7 µm, roughness = 1.8 µm	Micro-electro-mechanical-system (MEMS) device fabrication	(Monne et al., 2021)
14	Polyvinyl Alcohol and Gelatin	Carrageenan	BIO X6 bioprinter (CELLINK, USA)	Nozzle: 25G blunt, speed: 5 mm/s		Large human-sized heart valves	(Jafari et al., 2024)

of 3D printing, innovative materials, and accurate programming (Ahmed et al., 2021; Khoo et al., 2015; Momeni et al., 2017; Shin et al., 2017; Wu et al., 2018). Through 4D printing, different metamaterials are produced that change over time under the influence of environmental conditions. The present scientific research mainly deals with the shape-changing ability of 4D printed materials such as stretching, bending, twisting, and corrugation. These characteristics make 4D-printed materials suitable for applications in toys, robotics, lifters (Liu et al., 2018), microtubes (Ahmed et al., 2021), and lockers (Mao et al., 2015).

To assess the trend of 4D printing compared with other emerging technologies, the Gartner Hype Cycle (Ahmed et al., 2021) was further referred to. The Gartner Hype Cycle (Kuang et al., 2019) evaluates leading emerging technologies and plots the potential alignment with business trends and applications for the next 5-10 years. According to the cycle, 4D printing is now in the "trigger innovation" phase. The coming decade is expected to see a rise in expectations and development around 4D printing, as this technology is expected to gain mainstream focus for research during the coming decade.

Five key factors affect 4D printing and must be considered in the printing process. These include the AM process, material selection, the stimulus applied, the interaction mechanism, and the modelling approach (Ahmed et al., 2021). The first significant influencer in 4D printing was the AM process. In simple terms, AM is where designs are directly transformed into physical objects without needing extra tools apart from those used for physical conversion. Processes like SLA (Stereolithography), SLS (Selective Laser Sintering), FDM (Fused Deposition Modeling), 3DP (Three-Dimensional Printing), SLM (Selective Laser Melting), DIW (Direct Ink Writing), and EBM (Electron Beam Melting) are compatible with 4D printing, given that suitable materials are used. The other significant variable in those cases was the type of material used. To become functional, the material must exhibit sensitivity to certain stimuli applied during the process since it was printed layer after layer. Such sensitive materials can be termed programmable or intelligent materials, SMs, and are critical to the system. The natural properties of such materials decide what kind of external stimuli they would respond to, therefore allowing the material to transform. The third is the one about external stimulus applied in 4D printing, which are physical, chemical, or biological (Figure 6.3). The potential physical characteristics of external stimuli include light, humidity, magnetic and electric fields, temperature variation, and ultraviolet (UV) radiation. Chemical stimuli may be through alterations in pH or the presence of an oxidant or a reductant, whereas biological stimuli may come from incorporating enzymes or glucose. Such stimuli induce physical or chemical responses, stress relaxation, molecular rearrangements, or phase transitions that create structural deformations. The mechanism of interaction and mathematical modelling are the fourth and fifth factors. Not every material can undergo the transformation that a

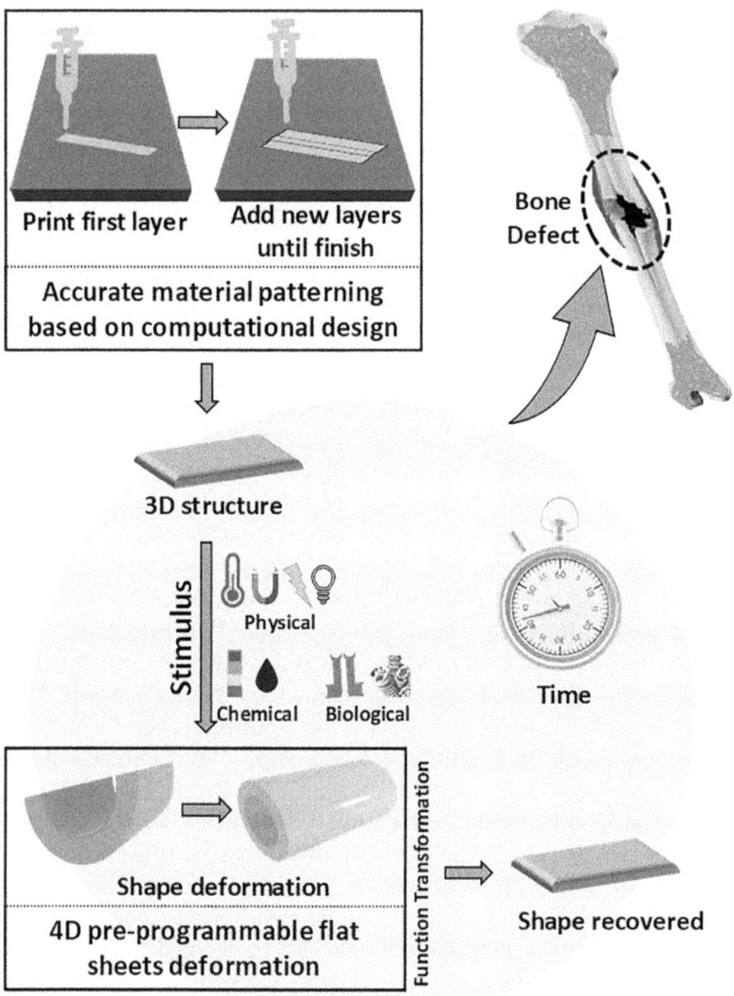

Figure 6.3 4D-printed sheets transform into functional 3D structures under stimuli for bone regeneration.

specific stimulus needs. Therefore, interaction mechanisms- such as mechanical forces or structural manipulation- are required to aid and guide these shape-changing processes. Mathematical modelling also determines how long the stimulus would act on the innovative material. In light of the above, 4D printing can be summarized as "applying a stimulus to an smart material through a suitable interaction mechanism and mathematical modelling during an AM process, resulting in a 4D-printed structure" (Ahmed et al., 2021).

It is argued that the enhancement in 3D printing led to placing materials with much more precision and flexibility. This development largely contributed to the growth of 4D printing (Vaezi et al., 2013). Intelligent materials are typically used in 4D printing, which can change properties based on external stimuli over time (Leist & Zhou, 2016). The behavior of self-assembly, self-healing, shape memory, and self-adjustment has been observed in these materials (Ahmed et al., 2021). Besides changing their shapes, 4D printing could also cause color changes depending on the exposure to UV and visible light. This chapter will consider the types of 4D printing responses to the stimuli they react to. As the years have passed since the conception of 4D printing, its potential applications in different research and technological sectors have been discussed. This technology has dramatically reduced the volume of material within printed structures and has enabled novel possibilities for transformation in printed devices (Campbell et al., 2014). Complex structures can be printed directly with 3D printers, or initial simple 3D structures can be printed and assembled into more complex forms (Zhou et al., 2015). Unlike traditional 3D printing, which uses static materials for various applications, the 4D printing technique offers the flexibility of material and process since it will utilize dynamic features. The versatility of this concept has made researchers focus more on the 4D-printed structures. All these things give such structures improved capabilities for being applicable. They can create surgical devices that self-assemble at the location required within the body (Zhou et al., 2015). The unique features of 4D-printed structures, such as the ability to assemble independently, adapt to environmental conditions, and undergo self-healing, contribute to exploring it for various applications.

6.5 APPLICATIONS OF CUSTOMIZED BIOMATERIALS AND CHALLENGES IN ADDITIVE MANUFACTURING

3D bioprinting develops rapidly and shows good prospects in the healthcare industry because of the growing need for care for an ageing population, reduced dependence on animal testing, and filling gaps in organ donor supply. It will prove crucial in cancer research, drug resistance, and diseases that cause infections. Generally, 3D bioprinting will also enhance the process of drug testing by eliminating dependency on animal models. With all these promises, it still comes with challenges like proper cell growth, tissue arrays, and, most importantly, biocompatibility in its chosen material. In addition, there are persisting issues with the affordability and compatibility of the bio-inks, satisfactory vascular network formation, and organoid synthesis. However, 3D bioprinting displays excellent promise in personalized medicine, surgical planning, or even just making organs, which could revolutionize health care by allowing tissues to be repaired and regenerated. Advances in drug printing also indicate its potential use for mass production of drugs. Table 6.2 provides a comparative analysis of various polymer composites and their applications in bone tissue engineering. Ethical concerns, material limitations, and the regulatory environment will be addressed as the technology develops (Bejoy et al., 2021).

The revolution in 4D printing began with the work of Tibbits and others in 2014, who demonstrated self-evolving structures derived from 3D-printed geometries interacting with the environment and proposing the concept of multi-material assemblies (Raviv et al., 2014; Tibbits, 2014). Lewis's group pushed this further ahead in 2016 with the work on biomimetic anisotropic hydrogel composites motivated by plant cell walls; these composites would be capable of transforming into complex shapes upon water exposure, enabled by a theoretical framework for the precise control of transformations (Sydney Gladman et al., 2016). 4D printing eliminates several limitations of traditional 3D bioprinting, especially in the context of the difficult task of fabricating small tubular tissue structures in nature like blood vessels and trachea, as they suffer from misalignment and resolution issues. There are innovations like self-folding cell-laden hydrogel sheets for creating high-resolution constructs for tubular geometries applicable in tissue repair drug testing and generating related natural tissue geometries (Figure 6.4) (Miller et al., 2012; Pi et al., 2018; Zhang et al., 2020; Zhang et al., 2014). While still in its infancy, 4D bioprinting holds a strong promise toward in vivo applications, from self-folding nerve conduits for peripheral nerve repair to targeted drug release and overcoming existing constraints of bioprinting. These strategies rely on post-printing transformations to enhance the versatility, complexity, and functionality of printed constructs (Joshi et al., 2023; Mandal & Chatterjee, 2023).

6.6 CONCLUSION AND FUTURE PERSPECTIVES

The impact of additive manufacturing on tissue engineering has been ground breaking: it enabled the design and fabrication of highly customized biomaterials tailored for specific tissue regeneration needs. In other words, 3D and 4D printing technologies form a crucial platform with significant promise for creating implantable biomaterials that are biocompatible, mechanically strong, and bioactive enough to sustain the native microenvironment. While 4D printing can provide dynamic materials that respond to stimuli after implantation, material choice, printability, and precision can limit the more profound potential of AM for tissue engineering applications. Exploring multi-material printing and hybrid fabrication methods stands to help mitigate these challenges, further opening up possibilities in personal and functional implants. As new technology matures, advances will be taken from bench to bedside and closer to real-world clinical applications, eventually transforming tissue regeneration practice and personalized healthcare solutions.

Table 6.2 Comparison of various polymer composites and their applications in bone tissue engineering

Sl. No.	*Polymer and Biomaterials*	*Study Type*	*Application*	*Reference*
1.	Polylactic Acid/Graphene Oxide	MG-63 osteosarcoma cells and MC3T3-E1 preosteoblast cells	Bone tissue engineering	(Belaid et al., 2020)
2.	Keratin	L929 murine fibroblasts	Clinically relevant applications	(S. Wang et al., 2015)
3.	Hydroxyapatite/Gelatin type-A/ Graphene Oxide	Rat adipose-derived stem cells	Cancellous bone	(H. Lee et al., 2022)
4.	Polylactic acid/hydroxyapatite and Polylactic acid/bioglass	Rat dental pulp stem cells	Bone regeneration	(Alksne et al., 2020)
5.	Polycaprolactone/Graphene Oxide	Rabbit tibia defect model	Bone regeneration	(Alazab et al., 2023)
6.	Hyaluronic acid with glycidyl methacrylate	Adult male C57BL/6 mice	Recovery of nerve tissue after traumatic brain injury	(Mishchenko et al., 2022)
7.	Cellulose acetate/Graphene Oxide/ Hydroxyapatite	Human Dental Pulp Stem Cells	Regenerative medicine and tissue engineering	(dos Santos Menezes et al., 2024)
8.	Gelatin–Hydroxyapatite /Graphene Oxide	Buccal Fat Pad-Derived Stem Cells	Bone tissue engineering	(Mahdavi et al., 2020)
9.	Polylactic acid/hydroxyapatite	Human mesenchymal stem cells	Bone tissue engineering	(Bernardo et al., 2022)
10.	Gelatin-Hyaluronic Acid-Genipin	Mouse osteoblast MC3T3 cells	Tissue engineering, regenerative medicine	(Khatun et al., 2023)
11.	Chitosan/Acetic acid/D-(+) Raffinose pentahydrate	Normal dermal human fibroblast cells (Nhdf cells) and aneuploid immortal keratinocyte cells (HaCaT cells)	Wound healing	(Intini et al., 2018)
12.	Xanthan gum/Guar gum	Bone-marrow-derived mesenchymal stem cells – normal human	Wound healing	(Virzì et al., 2024)
13.	Collagen and Tannic Acid	Neonatal human dermal fibroblasts	Cell-laden pure collagen scaffold	(Palladino et al., 2024)

(continued)

Table 6.2 (Cont.)

Sl. No.	*Polymer and Biomaterials*	*Study Type*	*Application*	*Reference*
14.	Bioactive glass S53P4/sodium alginate	Mouse osteoblastic cell line (MC3T3-E1)	Treatment of bone infections	(Oliveira et al., 2022)
15.	Hydroxyapatite/TPU/PLA nanocomposites	Mouse embryo fibroblast cells (L929)	Bone, cartilage, and tendon engineering	(Faghihi-Rezaei et al., 2022)
16.	PLLA/Graphene Oxide-Hydroxyapatite	MG63 cells	Bone tissue engineering.	(Shuai et al., 2022)
17.	Type I Bovine Collagen/N-(3-Dimethylaminopropyl)-N′-ethylcarbodiimide	hOP cells	Customized, patient-specific tissue regenerative applications	(Nayak et al., 2023)
18.	Graphene Oxide/Poly-L-Lactic Acid	Goat mesenchymal cells and murine 3T3 fibroblast cells	Bone tissue engineering and implants	(da Silva et al., 2023)
19.	Chitosan/Alginate/ Silver Sulfadiazine	Fibroblast cells	Wound Healing	(Bergonzi et al., 2023)
20.	Polyetheretherketone	human osteosarcoma cell line (SAOS-2)	Cranio-maxillofacial surgeries	(Oliveira et al., 2022)
21.	Keratin-based bioink	Adult normal human dermal fibroblasts	Severe burn wounds	(J. Navarro et al., 2020)
22.	Polylactic acid/Keratin and Chitosan	Human gingival fibroblasts	Bone regeneration	(Rojas-Martínez et al., 2020)
23.	Polyetheretherketone/ Hydroxyapatite	-na-	Orthopaedic applications	(Rodzeń et al., 2021)
24.	Cellulose acetate/ Graphene oxide / Hydroxyapatite	Human Dental Pulp Stem Cells	Tissue engineering & regenerative therapies	(Menezes et al., 2024)
25.	Polylactide/Hydroxyapatite Nonwovens/ Chitosan/ Graphene	Simulated body fluid	Bone regeneration	(Kosowska et al., 2020)
26.	Conductive extracellular matrix/ chitosan methacrylate/ graphene oxide-pegylated	Umbilical cord blood cells	Nutrient exchange & supporting cell migration	(Jaramillo et al., 2024)
27.	Novel Zwitterionic Hydrogel Incorporated with Graphene Oxide	Rat bone marrow mesenchymal stem cells (rBMSCs)	Bone formation	(Jaramillo et al., 2024)
28.	Hydroxyapatite/Polyvinyl alcohol	-na-	Soft tissue scaffold	(Qu et al., 2023)

29.	Magnetic nanocomposite /polyvinyl alcohol-chitosan/ hydroxyapatite and clay modified with graphene oxide	Rat bone marrow mesenchymal stem cells	Bone tissue applications	(Babakhani et al., 2024)
30.	Ti–6Al–4V (90% titanium, 6% aluminium and 4% vanadium) with Graphene oxide	MC3T3-E1 murine preosteoblast cell line, derived from C57BL/6 mouse calvaria	Protein adsorption properties	(H. J. Jang et al., 2024)
31.	Strontium-hydroxyapatite/ graphene oxide/ chitosan	Sprague Dawley rat cranial defect	Promote differentiation of osteoblasts	(T. Wu et al., 2020)
32.	Poly(3,4-ethylenedioxythiophene) polystyrene sulfonate/ Acrylamide/ Pluronic F-127 dimethacrylate/LiCl	L929 mouse fibroblasts	Bone regeneration	(Mondal et al., 2024b)
33.	liquid crystal elastomer ink, RM257 polymer	-na-	Bone regeneration	(Jiang et al., 2024)
34.	Polylactide-co-trimethylene carbonate/ Fe_3O_4	NIH-3T3 fibroblast cells, then Wistar rats	Bone Implants	(Choudhury et al., 2024)
35.	Methacrylated carboxymethyl cellulose, photoinitiator (Lithium phenyl-2,4,6-trimethyl benzoylphosphinate and methyl cellulose	L929 mouse fibroblasts	Bone regeneration	(Mondal et al., 2023)
36.	Chitosan	NIH 3T3 cells	shape morphing capabilities.	(Malappuram et al., 2024)

n.a: data not available

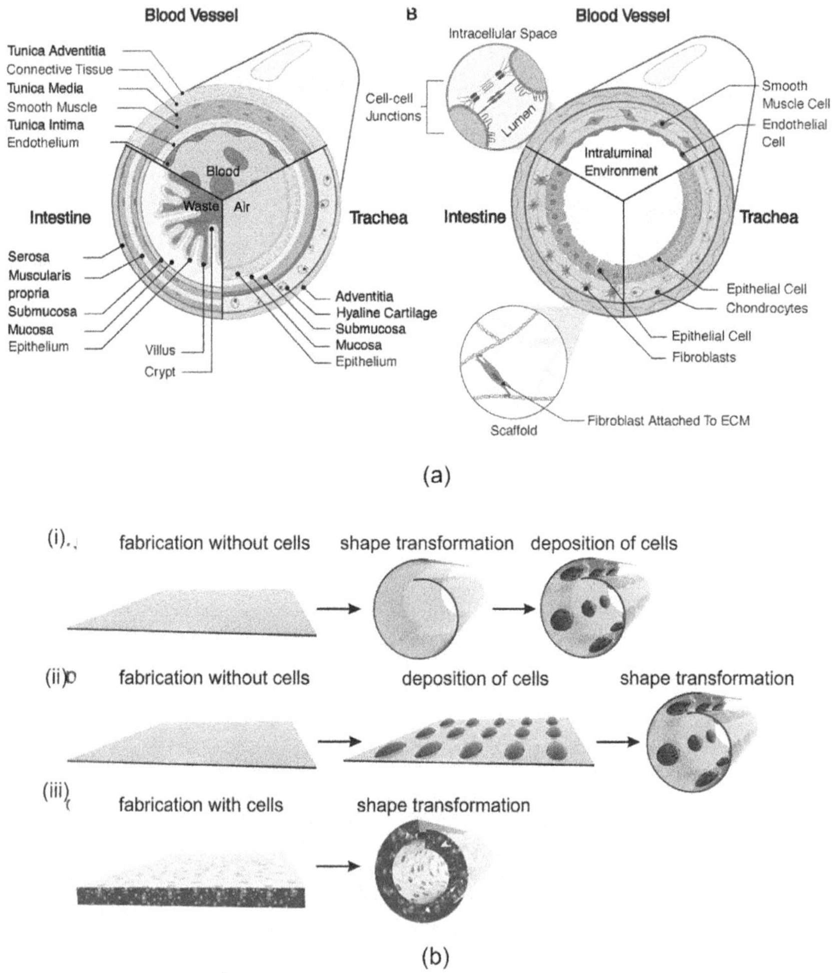

Figure 6.4 **(a)** The architecture and cellular arrangement within tubular tissue systems (Boys et al., 2020), **(b)** Application of 4D bioprinting for fabricating curved structures (Ionov, 2018). Reused with permission from *Elsevier* (Mandal & Chatterjee, 2023).

REFERENCES

Afshar-Mohajer, N., Wu, C.-Y., Ladun, T., Rajon, D. A., & Huang, Y. (2015). Characterization of particulate matters and total VOC emissions from a binder jetting 3D printer. *Building and Environment*, *P2*(93), 293–301. https://doi.org/10.1016/j.buildenv.2015.07.013

Ahlfeld, T., Akkineni, A. R., Förster, Y., Köhler, T., Knaack, S., Gelinsky, M., & Lode, A. (2017). Design and fabrication of complex scaffolds for bone defect healing: Combined 3D plotting of a calcium phosphate cement and a growth factor-loaded hydrogel. *Annals of Biomedical Engineering*, *45*(1), 224–236. https://doi.org/10.1007/s10439-016-1685-4

Ahmed, A., Arya, S., Gupta, V., Furukawa, H., & Khosla, A. (2021). 4D printing: Fundamentals, materials, applications and challenges. *Polymer*, *228*, 123926. https://doi.org/10.1016/j.polymer.2021.123926

Alazab, M. H., Abouelgeit, S. A., & Aboushelib, M. N. (2023). Histomorphometric evaluation of 3D printed graphene oxide-enriched poly(ε-caprolactone) scaffolds for bone regeneration. *Heliyon*, *9*(5), e15844. https://doi.org/10.1016/j.heliyon.2023.e15844

Alksne, M., Kalvaityte, M., Simoliunas, E., Rinkunaite, I., Gendviliene, I., Locs, J., Rutkunas, V., & Bukelskiene, V. (2020). *In vitro* comparison of 3D printed polylactic acid/hydroxyapatite and polylactic acid/bioglass composite scaffolds: Insights into materials for bone regeneration. *Journal of the Mechanical Behavior of Biomedical Materials*, *104*, 103641. https://doi.org/10.1016/j.jmbbm.2020.103641

Atala, A. (2009). *Foundations of Regenerative Medicine: Clinical and Therapeutic Applications*. Academic Press.

Babakhani, A., Peighambardoust, S. J., & Olad, A. (2024). Fabrication of magnetic nanocomposite scaffolds based on polyvinyl alcohol-chitosan containing hydroxyapatite and clay modified with graphene oxide: Evaluation of their properties for bone tissue engineering applications. *Journal of the Mechanical Behavior of Biomedical Materials*, *150*, 106263. https://doi.org/10.1016/j.jmbbm.2023.106263

Baniasadi, H., Madani, Z., Ajdary, R., Rojas, O. J., & Seppälä, J. (2021). Ascorbic acid-loaded polyvinyl alcohol/cellulose nanofibril hydrogels as precursors for 3D printed materials. *Materials Science and Engineering: C*, *130*, 112424. https://doi.org/10.1016/j.msec.2021.112424

Bejoy, Aathma Merin, Makkithaya, Kausalya Neelavara, Hunakunti, Bhagesh Basavraj, Hegde, Anarghya, Krishnamurthy, Keerthana, Sarkar, Aparajita, Lobo, Carol Felcita, Keshav, D. V. S., Dharshini, G., Dhivya Dharshini, S., Mascarenhas, Selinda, Chakrabarti, Shweta, Kalepu, Sree Raja Rajeswari Devi, Paul, Bobby, & Mazumder, Nirmal. (2021). *An insight on advances and applications of 3D bioprinting: A review*. *Bioprinting*, *24*, e00176. https://doi.org/10.1016/j.bprint.2021.e00176.

Belaid, H., Nagarajan, S., Teyssier, C., Barou, C., Barés, J., Balme, S., Garay, H., Huon, V., Cornu, D., Cavaillès, V., & Bechelany, M. (2020). Development of new biocompatible 3D printed graphene oxide-based scaffolds. *Materials Science and Engineering: C*, *110*, 110595. https://doi.org/10.1016/j.msec.2019.110595

Bergonzi, C., Bianchera, A., Remaggi, G., Ossiprandi, M. C., Bettini, R., & Elviri, L. (2023). 3D printed chitosan/alginate hydrogels for the controlled release of silver sulfadiazine in wound healing applications: Design, characterization and antimicrobial activity. *Micromachines*, *14*(1), 137. Article 1. https://doi.org/10.3390/mi14010137

Bernardo, M. P., da Silva, B. C. R., Hamouda, A. E. I., de Toledo, M. A. S., Schalla, C., Rütten, S., Goetzke, R., Mattoso, L. H. C., Zenke, M., & Sechi, A. (2022). PLA/Hydroxyapatite scaffolds exhibit in vitro immunological inertness and promote robust osteogenic differentiation of human mesenchymal stem cells without osteogenic stimuli. *Scientific Reports*, *12*(1), 2333. https://doi.org/10.1038/s41598-022-05207-w

Boys, A. J., Barron, S. L., Tilev, D., & Owens, R. M. (2020). Building scaffolds for tubular tissue engineering. *Frontiers in Bioengineering and Biotechnology*, *8*, 589960. https://doi.org/10.3389/fbioe.2020.589960

Campbell, T. A., Tibbits, S., & Garrett, B. (2014). The programmable world. *Scientific American*, *311*(5), 60–65.

Chen, X., Yue, Z., Winberg, P. C., Lou, Y.-R., Beirne, S., & Wallace, G. G. (2021). 3D bioprinting dermal-like structures using species-specific ulvan. *Biomaterials Science*, *9*(7), 2424–2438. https://doi.org/10.1039/D0BM01784A

Choudhury, S., Joshi, A., Baghel, V. S., Ananthasuresh, G. K., Asthana, S., Homer-Vanniasinkam, S., & Chatterjee, K. (2024). Design-encoded dual shape-morphing and shape-memory in 4D printed polymer parts toward cellularized vascular grafts. *Journal of Materials Chemistry B*, *12*(23), 5678–5689. https://doi.org/10.1039/D4TB00437J

Cui, H., Nowicki, M., Fisher, J. P., & Zhang, L. G. (2017). 3D bioprinting for organ regeneration. *Advanced Healthcare Materials*, *6*(1), 1601118. https://doi.org/10.1002/adhm.201601118

da Silva, T. S., Horvath-Pereira, B. de O., da Silva-Júnior, L. N., Tenório Fireman, J. V. B., Mattar, M., Félix, M., Buchaim, R. L., Carreira, A. C. O., Miglino, M. A., & Soares, M. M. (2023). Three-dimensional printing of graphene oxide/poly-L-lactic acid scaffolds using Fischer–Koch modeling. *Polymers*, 15(21), 4213, Article 21. https://doi.org/10.3390/polym15214213

Dababneh, A. B., & Ozbolat, I. T. (2014). Bioprinting technology: A current state-of-the-art review. *Journal of Manufacturing Science and Engineering*, 136, 061016.

Daly, A. C., Prendergast, M. E., Hughes, A. J., & Burdick, J. A. (2021). Bioprinting for the biologist. *Cell*, *184*(1), 18–32. https://doi.org/10.1016/j.cell.2020.12.002

Ding, Z., Yuan, C., Peng, X., Wang, T., Qi, H. J., & Dunn, M. L. (2017). Direct 4D printing via active composite materials. *Science Advances*, *3*(4), e1602890. https://doi.org/10.1126/sciadv.1602890

dos Santos Menezes, L., Navarro da Rocha, D., Nonato, R. C., Costa, A. R., Morales, A. R., Correr-Sobrinho, L., Correr, A. B., & Neves, J. G. (2024). Cellulose acetate scaffold coated with a hydroxyapatite/graphene oxide nanocomposite for application in tissue engineering. *Proceedings of the Institution of Mechanical Engineers, Part H: Journal of Engineering in Medicine*, *238*(7), 793–802. https://doi.org/10.1177/09544119241256715

Faghihi-Rezaei, V., Khonakdar, H. A., Goodarzi, V., Darbemamieh, G., & Otadi, M. (2022). Hydroxyapatite/TPU/PLA nanocomposites: Morphological, dynamic-mechanical, and thermal study. *Green Processing and Synthesis*, *11*(1), 996–1012. https://doi.org/10.1515/gps-2022-0087

Fayyazbakhsh, F., Khayat, M. J., & Leu, M. C. (2022). 3D-printed gelatin-alginate hydrogel dressings for burn wound healing: A comprehensive study. *International Journal of Bioprinting*, *8*(4), 618, Article 4. https://doi.org/10.18063/ijb.v8i4.618

Gorroñogoitia, I., Urtaza, U., Zubiarrain-Laserna, A., Alonso-Varona, A., & Zaldua, A. M. (2022). A study of the printability of alginate-based bioinks by

3D bioprinting for articular cartilage tissue engineering. *Polymers*, *14*(2), 354, Article 2. https://doi.org/10.3390/polym14020354

Goyanes, A., Det-Amornrat, U., Wang, J., Basit, A. W., & Gaisford, S. (2016). 3D scanning and 3D printing as innovative technologies for fabricating personalized topical drug delivery systems. *Journal of Controlled Release*, *234*, 41–48. https://doi.org/10.1016/j.jconrel.2016.05.034

Groll, J., Boland, T., Blunk, T., Burdick, J. A., Cho, D.-W., Dalton, P. D., Derby, B., Forgacs, G., Li, Q., Mironov, V. A., Moroni, L., Nakamura, M., Shu, W., Takeuchi, S., Vozzi, G., Woodfield, T. B. F., Xu, T., Yoo, J. J., & Malda, J. (2016). Biofabrication: Reappraising the definition of an evolving field. *Biofabrication*, *8*(1), 013001. https://doi.org/10.1088/1758-5090/8/1/013001

Gungor-Ozkerim, P. S., Inci, I., Zhang, Y. S., Khademhosseini, A., & Dokmeci, M. R. (2018). Bioinks for 3D bioprinting: An overview. *Biomaterials Science*, *6*(5), 915. https://doi.org/10.1039/c7bm00765e

Hölzl, K., Lin, S., Tytgat, L., Vlierberghe, S. V., Gu, L., & Ovsianikov, A. (2016). Bioink properties before, during and after 3D bioprinting. *Biofabrication*, *8*(3), 032002. https://doi.org/10.1088/1758-5090/8/3/032002

Hospodiuk, M., Dey, M., Sosnoski, D., & Ozbolat, I. T. (2017). The bioink: A comprehensive review on bioprintable materials. *Biotechnology Advances*, *35*(2), 217–239. https://doi.org/10.1016/j.biotechadv.2016.12.006

Hoy, M. B. (2013). 3D printing: Making things at the library. *Medical Reference Services Quarterly*, *32*(1), 93–99. https://doi.org/10.1080/02763869.2013.749139

Intini, C., Elviri, L., Cabral, J., Mros, S., Bergonzi, C., Bianchera, A., Flammini, L., Govoni, P., Barocelli, E., Bettini, R., & McConnell, M. (2018). 3D-printed chitosan-based scaffolds: An *in vitro* study of human skin cell growth and an *in-vivo* wound healing evaluation in experimental diabetes in rats. *Carbohydrate Polymers*, *199*, 593–602. https://doi.org/10.1016/j.carbpol.2018.07.057

Ionov, L. (2018). 4D biofabrication: Materials, methods, and applications. *Advanced Healthcare Materials*, 7(17), 1800412. https://doi.org/10.1002/adhm.201800412

Jafari, A., Vahid Niknezhad, S., Kaviani, M., Saleh, W., Wong, N., Van Vliet, P. P., Moraes, C., Ajji, A., Kadem, L., Azarpira, N., Andelfinger, G., & Savoji, H. (2024). Formulation and evaluation of PVA/gelatin/carrageenan inks for 3D printing and development of tissue-engineered heart valves. *Advanced Functional Materials, 34*(7), 2305188. https://doi.org/10.1002/adfm.202305188

Jammalamadaka, U., & Tappa, K. (2018). Recent advances in biomaterials for 3D printing and tissue engineering. *Journal of Functional Biomaterials*, *9*(1), 22, Article 1. https://doi.org/10.3390/jfb9010022

Jang, H. J., Kang, M. S., Jang, J., Lim, D., Choi, S.-W., Jung, T.-G., Chun, H.-J., Kim, B., & Han, D.-W. (2024). Harnessing 3D printed highly porous Ti–6Al–4V scaffolds coated with graphene oxide to promote osteogenesis. *Biomaterials Science*, *12*(21), 5491–5503. https://doi.org/10.1039/D4BM00970C

Jang, J., Park, H.-J., Kim, S.-W., Kim, H., Park, J. Y., Na, S. J., Kim, H. J., Park, M. N., Choi, S. H., Park, S. H., Kim, S. W., Kwon, S.-M., Kim, P.-J., & Cho, D.-W. (2017). 3D printed complex tissue construct using stem cell-laden decellularized extracellular matrix bioinks for cardiac repair. *Biomaterials*, *112*, 264–274. https://doi.org/10.1016/j.biomaterials.2016.10.026

Jaramillo, V., Arévalo, D. F., González-Hernández, M., Cortés, M. T., Perdomo-Arciniegas, A. M., Cruz, J. C., & Muñoz-Camargo, C. (2024). Conductive extracellular matrix derived/chitosan methacrylate/ graphene oxide-pegylated hybrid hydrogel for cell expansion. *Frontiers in Bioengineering and Biotechnology*, 12, 1398052. https://doi.org/10.3389/fbioe.2024.1398052

Jiang, H., Chung, C., Dunn, M. L., & Yu, K. (2024). 4D printing of liquid crystal elastomer composites with continuous fiber reinforcement. *Nature Communications*, *15*(1), 8491. https://doi.org/10.1038/s41467-024-52716-5

Joshi, A., Choudhury, S., Baghel, V. S., Ghosh, S., Gupta, S., Lahiri, D., Ananthasuresh, G. K., & Chatterjee, K. (2023). 4D printed programmable shape-morphing hydrogels as intraoperative self-folding nerve conduits for sutureless neurorrhaphy. *Advanced Healthcare Materials*, *12*(24), 2300701. https://doi.org/10.1002/adhm.202300701

Jungst, T., Smolan, W., Schacht, K., Scheibel, T., & Groll, J. (2016). Strategies and molecular design criteria for 3D printable hydrogels. *Chemical Reviews*, *116*(3), 1496–1539. https://doi.org/10.1021/acs.chemrev.5b00303

Kakarla, A. B., Kong, I., Turek, I., Kong, C., & Irving, H. (2022). Printable gelatin, alginate and boron nitride nanotubes hydrogel-based ink for 3D bioprinting and tissue engineering applications. *Materials & Design*, *213*, 110362. https://doi.org/10.1016/j.matdes.2021.110362

Kaye, R., Goldstein, T., Zeltsman, D., Grande, D. A., & Smith, L. P. (2016). Three dimensional printing: A review on the utility within medicine and otolaryngology. *International Journal of Pediatric Otorhinolaryngology*, *89*, 145–148. https://doi.org/10.1016/j.ijporl.2016.08.007

Khalil, S., & Sun, W. (2009). Bioprinting endothelial cells with alginate for 3D tissue constructs. *Journal of Biomechanical Engineering*, 12, 1398052. https://doi.org/10.1115/1.3128729

Khatun, M. R., Bhattacharyya, A., Gunbayar, M., Jung, M., & Noh, I. (2023). Study on bioresponsive gelatin-hyaluronic acid-genipin hydrogel for high cell-density 3D bioprinting. *Gels*, *9*(8), 601. Article 8. https://doi.org/10.3390/gels9080601

Khoo, Z. X., Teoh, J. E. M., Liu, Y., Chua, C. K., Yang, S., An, J., Leong, K. F., & Yeong, W. Y. (2015). 3D printing of smart materials: A review on recent progresses in 4D printing. *Virtual and Physical Prototyping*, *10*(3), 103–122. https://doi.org/10.1080/17452759.2015.1097054

Kosowska, K., Domalik-Pyzik, P., Krok-Borkowicz, M., & Chłopek, J. (2020). Polylactide/hydroxyapatite nonwovens incorporated into chitosan/graphene materials hydrogels to form novel hierarchical scaffolds. *International Journal of Molecular Sciences*, *21*(7), Article 7. https://doi.org/10.3390/ijms21072330

Kotikian, A., Truby, R. L., Boley, J. W., White, T. J., & Lewis, J. A. (2018). 3D printing of liquid crystal elastomeric actuators with spatially programed nematic order. *Advanced Materials*, *21*(7), 2330 https://doi.org/10.1002/adma.201706164

Kuang, X., Roach, D. J., Wu, J., Hamel, C. M., Ding, Z., Wang, T., Dunn, M. L., & Qi, H. J. (2019). Advances in 4D printing: Materials and applications.

Advanced Functional Materials, *29*(2), 1805290. https://doi.org/10.1002/adfm.201805290
Kuksenok, O., & C. Balazs, A. (2016). Stimuli-responsive behavior of composites integrating thermo-responsive gels with photo-responsive fibers. *Materials Horizons*, *3*(1), 53–62. https://doi.org/10.1039/C5MH00212E
Lee, D.-Y., Lee, H., Kim, Y., Yoo, S. Y., Chung, W.-J., & Kim, G. (2016). Phage as versatile nanoink for printing 3-D cell-laden scaffolds. *Acta Biomaterialia*, *29*, 112–124. https://doi.org/10.1016/j.actbio.2015.10.004
Lee, H., Yoo, J. M., Ponnusamy, N. K., & Nam, S. Y. (2022). 3D-printed hydroxyapatite/gelatin bone scaffolds reinforced with graphene oxide: Optimized fabrication and mechanical characterization. *Ceramics International*, *48*(7), 10155–10163. https://doi.org/10.1016/j.ceramint.2021.12.227
Lee, H. J., Kim, Y. B., Ahn, S. H., Lee, J.-S., Jang, C. H., Yoon, H., Chun, W., & Kim, G. H. (2015). A new approach for fabricating collagen/ECM-based bioinks using preosteoblasts and human adipose stem cells. *Advanced Healthcare Materials*, *4*(9), 1359–1368. https://doi.org/10.1002/adhm.201500193
Leist, S. K., & Zhou, J. (2016). Current status of 4D printing technology and the potential of light-reactive smart materials as 4D printable materials. *Virtual and Physical Prototyping*. www.tandfonline.com/doi/abs/10.1080/17452759.2016.1198630
Li, X., Liu, B., Pei, B., Chen, J., Zhou, D., Peng, J., Zhang, X., Jia, W., & Xu, T. (2020). Inkjet bioprinting of biomaterials. *Chemical Reviews*, *120*(19), 10793–10833. https://doi.org/10.1021/acs.chemrev.0c00008
Liu, Y., Zhang, W., Zhang, F., Lan, X., Leng, J., Liu, S., Jia, X., Cotton, C., Sun, B., Gu, B., & Chou, T.-W. (2018). Shape memory behavior and recovery force of 4D printed laminated Miura-origami structures subjected to compressive loading. *Composites Part B: Engineering*, *153*, 233–242. https://doi.org/10.1016/j.compositesb.2018.07.053
Loo, Y., Lakshmanan, A., Ni, M., Toh, L. L., Wang, S., & Hauser, C. A. E. (2015). Peptide bioink: Self-assembling nanofibrous scaffolds for three-dimensional organotypic cultures. *Nano Letters*, *15*(10), 6919–6925. https://doi.org/10.1021/acs.nanolett.5b02859
Luo, Y., Lin, X., & Huang, P. (2018). 3D bioprinting of artificial tissues: Construction of biomimetic microstructures. *Macromolecular Bioscience*, *18*(6), 1800034. https://doi.org/10.1002/mabi.201800034
Mahdavi, R., Belgheisi, G., Haghbin-Nazarpak, M., Omidi, M., Khojasteh, A., & Solati-Hashjin, M. (2020). Bone tissue engineering gelatin–Hydroxyapatite/graphene oxide scaffolds with the ability to release vitamin D: Fabrication, characterization, and in vitro study. *Journal of Materials Science: Materials in Medicine*, *31*(11), 97. https://doi.org/10.1007/s10856-020-06430-5
Malappuram, K. M., Chatterjee, A., Chakraborty, S., Debnath, S., Chatterjee, K., & Nain, A. (2024). Shape programmable chitosan films as soft microrobots toward the development of chemo-mechanical sensors. *ChemRxiv*. https://doi.org/10.26434/chemrxiv-2024-6xlj9
Mandal, A., & Chatterjee, K. (2023). Emerging trends in humidity-responsive 4D bioprinting. *Chemical Engineering Journal*, *455*, 140550. https://doi.org/10.1016/j.cej.2022.140550

Mao, Y., Yu, K., Isakov, M. S., Wu, J., Dunn, M. L., & Jerry Qi, H. (2015). Sequential self-folding structures by 3D printed digital shape memory polymers. *Scientific Reports*, *5*(1), 13616. https://doi.org/10.1038/srep13616

Masri, S., Maarof, M., Aziz, I. A., Idrus, R., & Fauzi, M. B. (2023). Performance of hybrid gelatin-PVA bioinks integrated with genipin through extrusionbased 3D bioprinting: An in vitro evaluation using human dermal fibroblasts. *International Journal of Bioprinting*, *9*(3), 677. Article 3. https://doi.org/10.18063/ijb.677

Menezes, L. dos S., Navarro da Rocha, D., Carajelescov Nonato, R., Costa, A. R., Morales, A. R., Correr-Sobrinho, L., Correr, A. B., & Neves, J. G. (2024). Cellulose acetate scaffold containing hydroxyapatite/graphene oxide nanocomposite by electrospinning for advanced regenerative therapies. *Journal of Bioactive and Compatible Polymers, 39*(2), 91–103. https://doi.org/10.1177/08839115241233345

Miller, J. S., Stevens, K. R., Yang, M. T., Baker, B. M., Nguyen, D.-H. T., Cohen, D. M., Toro, E., Chen, A. A., Galie, P. A., Yu, X., Chaturvedi, R., Bhatia, S. N., & Chen, C. S. (2012). Rapid casting of patterned vascular networks for perfusable engineered three-dimensional tissues. *Nature Materials*, *11*(9), 768–774. https://doi.org/10.1038/nmat3357

Misch, C. E., Qu, Z., & Bidez, M. W. (1999). Mechanical properties of trabecular bone in the human mandible: Implications for dental implant treatment planning and surgical placement. *Journal of Oral and Maxillofacial Surgery*, *57*(6), 700–706. https://doi.org/10.1016/S0278-2391(99)90437-8

Mishchenko, T. A., Klimenko, M. O., Kuznetsova, A. I., Yarkov, R. S., Savelyev, A. G., Sochilina, A. V., Mariyanats, A. O., Popov, V. K., Khaydukov, E. V., Zvyagin, A. V., & Vedunova, M. V. (2022). 3D-printed hyaluronic acid hydrogel scaffolds impregnated with neurotrophic factors (BDNF, GDNF) for post-traumatic brain tissue reconstruction. *Frontiers in Bioengineering and Biotechnology*, *10*, 895406. https://doi.org/10.3389/fbioe.2022.895406

Momeni, F., Liu, X., & Ni, J. (2017). A review of 4D printing. *Materials & Design*, *122*, 42–79. https://doi.org/10.1016/j.matdes.2017.02.068

Momeni, F., Sabzpoushan, S., Valizadeh, R., Morad, M. R., Liu, X., & Ni, J. (2019). Plant leaf-mimetic smart wind turbine blades by 4D printing. *Renewable Energy*, *130*, 329–351. https://doi.org/10.1016/j.renene.2018.05.095

Mondal, P., Mandal, A., & Chatterjee, K. (2023). Bi-Directional shape morphing in 4D-Bioprinted hydrogels on a single stimulation. *Advanced Materials Technologies*, *8*(19), 2300894. https://doi.org/10.1002/admt.202300894

Mondal, P., Mandal, A., & Chatterjee, K. (2024a). "All-in-one" ink for light-based 4D printing of conducting, tough, anti-freezing, and cytocompatible hydrogels. *Chemical Engineering Journal*, *496*, 153883. https://doi.org/10.1016/j.cej.2024.153883

Mondal, P., Mandal, A., & Chatterjee, K. (2024b). "All-in-one" ink for light-based 4D printing of conducting, tough, anti-freezing, and cytocompatible hydrogels. *Chemical Engineering Journal*, *496*, 153883. https://doi.org/10.1016/j.cej.2024.153883

Monne, M. A., Howlader, C. Q., Mishra, B., & Chen, M. Y. (2021). Synthesis of printable polyvinyl alcohol for aerosol jet and inkjet printing technology. *Micromachines*, *12*(2),220. Article 2. https://doi.org/10.3390/mi12020220

Moroni, L., Boland, T., Burdick, J. A., De Maria, C., Derby, B., Forgacs, G., Groll, J., Li, Q., Malda, J., Mironov, V. A., Mota, C., Nakamura, M., Shu, W., Takeuchi, S., Woodfield, T. B. F., Xu, T., Yoo, J. J., & Vozzi, G. (2018). Biofabrication: A guide to technology and terminology. *Trends in Biotechnology*, *36*(4), 384–402. https://doi.org/10.1016/j.tibtech.2017.10.015

Nadgorny, M., Xiao, Z., Chen, C., & Connal, L. A. (2016). Three-dimensional printing of pH-responsive and functional polymers on an affordable desktop printer. *ACS Applied Materials & Interfaces*, *8*(42), 28946–28954. https://doi.org/10.1021/acsami.6b07388

Nair, L. S., & Laurencin, C. T. (2006). Polymers as biomaterials for tissue engineering and controlled drug delivery. In K. Lee & D. Kaplan (Eds.), *Tissue Engineering I* (pp. 47–90). Springer. https://doi.org/10.1007/b137240

Navarro, J., Clohessy, R. M., Holder, R. C., Gabard, A. R., Herendeen, G. J., Christy, R. J., Burnett, L. R., & Fisher, J. P. (2020). *In Vivo* evaluation of three-dimensional printed, keratin-based hydrogels in a porcine thermal burn model. *Tissue Engineering Part A*, *26*(5–6), 265–278. https://doi.org/10.1089/ten.tea.2019.0181

Navarro, M., Michiardi, A., Castaño, O., & Planell, J. A. (2008). Biomaterials in orthopaedics. *Journal of the Royal Society Interface*, *5*(27), 1137–1158. https://doi.org/10.1098/rsif.2008.0151

Nayak, V. V., Tovar, N., Khan, D., Pereira, A. C., Mijares, D. Q., Weck, M., Durand, A., Smay, J. E., Torroni, A., Coelho, P. G., & Witek, L. (2023). 3D printing type 1 bovine collagen scaffolds for tissue engineering applications—Physicochemical characterization and in vitro evaluation. *Gels*, *9*(8), 637. Article 8. https://doi.org/10.3390/gels9080637

Oliveira, R. L. M. S., Alves, A. P. N., Barbosa, L., Silva, A. P., de Cena, G. L., Conceição, K., Tada, D. B., & Trichês, E. de S. (2022). 3D printing of bioactive glass S53P4/sodium alginate sintering-free scaffolds. *Bioprinting, 27*, e00226. https://doi.org/10.1016/j.bprint.2022.e00226

Palladino, S., Copes, F., Chevallier, P., Candiani, G., & Mantovani, D. (2024). Enabling 3D bioprinting of cell-laden pure collagen scaffolds via tannic acid supporting bath. *Frontiers in Bioengineering and Biotechnology*, 12, 1434435, https://doi.org/10.3389/fbioe.2024.1434435

Pi, Q., Maharjan, S., Yan, X., Liu, X., Singh, B., van Genderen, A. M., Robledo-Padilla, F., Parra-Saldivar, R., Hu, N., Jia, W., Xu, C., Kang, J., Hassan, S., Cheng, H., Hou, X., Khademhosseini, A., & Zhang, Y. S. (2018). Digitally tunable microfluidic bioprinting of multilayered cannular tissues. *Advanced Materials*, *30*(43), 1706913. https://doi.org/10.1002/adma.201706913

Qu, R., Song, X., Wang, Y., Zhao, Y., & Fu, X. (2023). Hydroxyapatite cross-linked in situ polyvinyl alcohol hydrogel for bionic calcified cartilage layer. *Colloids and Surfaces B: Biointerfaces*, *230*, 113510. https://doi.org/10.1016/j.colsurfb.2023.113510

Raviv, D., Zhao, W., McKnelly, C., Papadopoulou, A., Kadambi, A., Shi, B., Hirsch, S., Dikovsky, D., Zyracki, M., Olguin, C., Raskar, R., & Tibbits, S. (2014). Active printed materials for complex self-evolving deformations. *Scientific Reports*, *4*(1), 7422. https://doi.org/10.1038/srep07422

Rizwana, N., Maslekar, N., Chatterjee, K., Yao, Y., Agarwal, V., & Nune, M. (2024). Dual crosslinked antioxidant mixture of poly(vinyl alcohol) and cerium oxide nanoparticles as a bioink for 3D bioprinting. *ACS Applied Nano Materials*, 7(16), 18177–18188. https://doi.org/10.1021/acsanm.3c02962

Rodzeń, K., Sharma, P. K., McIlhagger, A., Mokhtari, M., Dave, F., Tormey, D., Sherlock, R., Meenan, B. J., & Boyd, A. (2021). The direct 3D printing of functional PEEK/hydroxyapatite composites via a fused filament fabrication approach. *Polymers*, *13*(4),545, Article 4. https://doi.org/10.3390/polym13040545

Rojas-Martínez, L. E., Flores-Hernandez, C. G., López-Marín, L. M., Martinez-Hernandez, A. L., Thorat, S. B., Reyes Vasquez, C. D., Del Rio-Castillo, A. E., & Velasco-Santos, C. (2020). 3D printing of PLA composites scaffolds reinforced with keratin and chitosan: Effect of geometry and structure. *European Polymer Journal*, *141*, 110088. https://doi.org/10.1016/j.eurpolymj.2020.110088

Shin, D.-G., Kim, T.-H., & Kim, D.-E. (2017). Review of 4D printing materials and their properties. *International Journal of Precision Engineering and Manufacturing-Green Technology*, *4*(3), 349–357. https://doi.org/10.1007/s40684-017-0040-z

Shuai, C., Peng, B., Feng, P., Yu, L., Lai, R., & Min, A. (2022). In situ synthesis of hydroxyapatite nanorods on graphene oxide nanosheets and their reinforcement in biopolymer scaffold. *Journal of Advanced Research*, *35*, 13–24. https://doi.org/10.1016/j.jare.2021.03.009

Sonaye, S. Y., Ertugral, E. G., Kothapalli, C. R., & Sikder, P. (2022). Extrusion 3D (bio)printing of alginate-gelatin-based composite scaffolds for skeletal muscle tissue engineering. *Materials*, *15*(22),7945, Article 22. https://doi.org/10.3390/ma15227945

Sydney Gladman, A., Matsumoto, E. A., Nuzzo, R. G., Mahadevan, L., & Lewis, J. A. (2016). Biomimetic 4D printing. *Nature Materials*, *15*(4), 413–418. https://doi.org/10.1038/nmat4544

Tibbits, S. (2014). 4D printing: Multi-material shape change. *Architectural Design*, *84*(1), 116–121. https://doi.org/10.1002/ad.1710

Vaezi, M., Chianrabutra, S., Mellor, B., & Yang, S. (2013). Multiple material additive manufacturing – Part 1: A review. *Virtual and Physical Prototyping*, *8*(1), 19–50. https://doi.org/10.1080/17452759.2013.778175

Ventola, C. L. (2014). Medical applications for 3D printing: Current and projected uses. *Pharmacy and Therapeutics*, *39*(10), 704.

Virzì, N. F., Diaz-Rodriguez, P., Concheiro, A., Pittalà, V., & Alvarez-Lorenzo, C. (2024). Xanthan gum/Guar gum-based 3D-printed scaffolds for wound healing: Production, characterization, and biocompatibility screening. *Carbohydrate Polymer Technologies and Applications*, 7, 100523. https://doi.org/10.1016/j.carpta.2024.100523

Wang, S., Wang, Z., Foo, S. E. M., Tan, N. S., Yuan, Y., Lin, W., Zhang, Z., & Ng, K. W. (2015). Culturing fibroblasts in 3D human hair keratin hydrogels. *ACS Applied Materials & Interfaces*, 7(9), 5187–5198. https://doi.org/10.1021/acsami.5b00854

Wang, Z., Abdulla, R., Parker, B., Samanipour, R., Ghosh, S., & Kim, K. (2015). A simple and high-resolution stereolithography-based 3D bioprinting system using visible light crosslinkable bioinks. *Biofabrication*, 7(4), 045009. https://doi.org/10.1088/1758-5090/7/4/045009

Wu, J.-J., Huang, L.-M., Zhao, Q., & Xie, T. (2018). 4D printing: History and recent progress. *Chinese Journal of Polymer Science*, *36*(5), 563–575. https://doi.org/10.1007/s10118-018-2089-8

Wu, T., Li, B., Wang, W., Chen, L., Li, Z., Wang, M., Zha, Z., Lin, Z., Xia, H., & Zhang, T. (2020). Strontium-substituted hydroxyapatite grown on graphene oxide nanosheet-reinforced chitosan scaffold to promote bone regeneration. *Biomaterials Science*, *8*(16), 4603–4615. https://doi.org/10.1039/D0BM00523A

Wüst, S., Müller, R., & Hofmann, S. (2011). Controlled positioning of cells in biomaterials—Approaches towards 3D tissue printing. *Journal of Functional Biomaterials*, *2*(3), 119, Article 3. https://doi.org/10.3390/jfb2030119

Yang, H., Leow, W. R., Wang, T., Wang, J., Yu, J., He, K., Qi, D., Wan, C., & Chen, X. (2017). 3D printed photoresponsive devices based on shape memory composites. *Advanced Materials*, *29*(33), 1701627. https://doi.org/10.1002/adma.201701627

Ye, K., Felimban, R., Traianedes, K., Moulton, S. E., Wallace, G. G., Chung, J., Quigley, A., Choong, P. F. M., & Myers, D. E. (2014). Chondrogenesis of infrapatellar fat pad derived adipose stem cells in 3D printed chitosan scaffold. *PLOS ONE*, *9*(6), e99410. https://doi.org/10.1371/journal.pone.0099410

Zadpoor, A. A., & Malda, J. (2017). Additive manufacturing of biomaterials, tissues, and organs. *Annals of Biomedical Engineering*, *45*(1), 1–11. https://doi.org/10.1007/s10439-016-1719-y

Zhang, L., Xiang, Y., Zhang, H., Cheng, L., Mao, X., An, N., Zhang, L., Zhou, J., Deng, L., Zhang, Y., Sun, X., Santos, H. A., & Cui, W. (2020). A biomimetic 3D-self-forming approach for microvascular scaffolds. *Advanced Science*, *7*(9), 1903553. https://doi.org/10.1002/advs.201903553

Zhang, Y., Yu, Y., Akkouch, A., Dababneh, A., Dolati, F., & Ozbolat, I. T. (2014). In vitro study of directly bioprinted perfusable vasculature conduits. *Biomaterials Science*, *3*(1), 134–143. https://doi.org/10.1039/C4BM00234B

Zhou, Y., Huang, W. M., Kang, S. F., Wu, X. L., Lu, H. B., Fu, J., & Cui, H. (2015). From 3D to 4D printing: Approaches and typical applications. *Journal of Mechanical Science and Technology*, *29*(10), 4281–4288. https://doi.org/10.1007/s12206-015-0925-0

Chapter 7

Additive electrochemical micro-manufacturing technology for biomedical application

Sourabh Tandon, Divyansh Singh Patel, and Ruchin Kacker

7.1 INTRODUCTION TO ADDITIVE MANUFACTURING

Additive Manufacturing (AM), commonly known as 3D printing, is a technology used to create complex three-dimensional parts directly from a computer-aided design (CAD) model. Compared to traditional manufacturing methods, AM requires less time to fabricate objects and offers unique advantages in sectors such as biomedical, aerospace, and automotive industries.

Several techniques are employed in 3D printing, including VAT photopolymerization, material jetting, material extrusion, sheet lamination, powder bed fusion, and direct energy deposition, as illustrated in Figure 7.1. Recently, the demand for micro-sized components has grown significantly, particularly in the biomedical field, where AM has been successfully used to fabricate tools like tissue saws and tissue approximation clips.

In this chapter, the authors will provide a detailed discussion on micro-manufacturing technology, the history of Electrochemical Additive Manufacturing (ECAM), its working principles and classifications, process parameters, and associated challenges.

7.1.1 Micro manufacturing

Today, a vast range of microproducts exists, with key categories including microelectromechanical systems (MEMS) and micro-opto-electromechanical systems (MOEMS), which are defined by their functional applications and operational principles. Additive manufacturing (AM) of metal microstructure arrays has become essential for producing miniaturized components, widely used as core carriers in aerospace, microelectronics packaging, microsensors, and biomedical applications (Wang et al., 2024; Li et al., 2022).

Over the years, numerous metal microfabrication techniques have been developed, including mechanical micromachining methods such as micro-milling, micro-turning, and micro-drilling (Balazs et al., 2021; Hasan

DOI: 10.1201/9781003581192-7

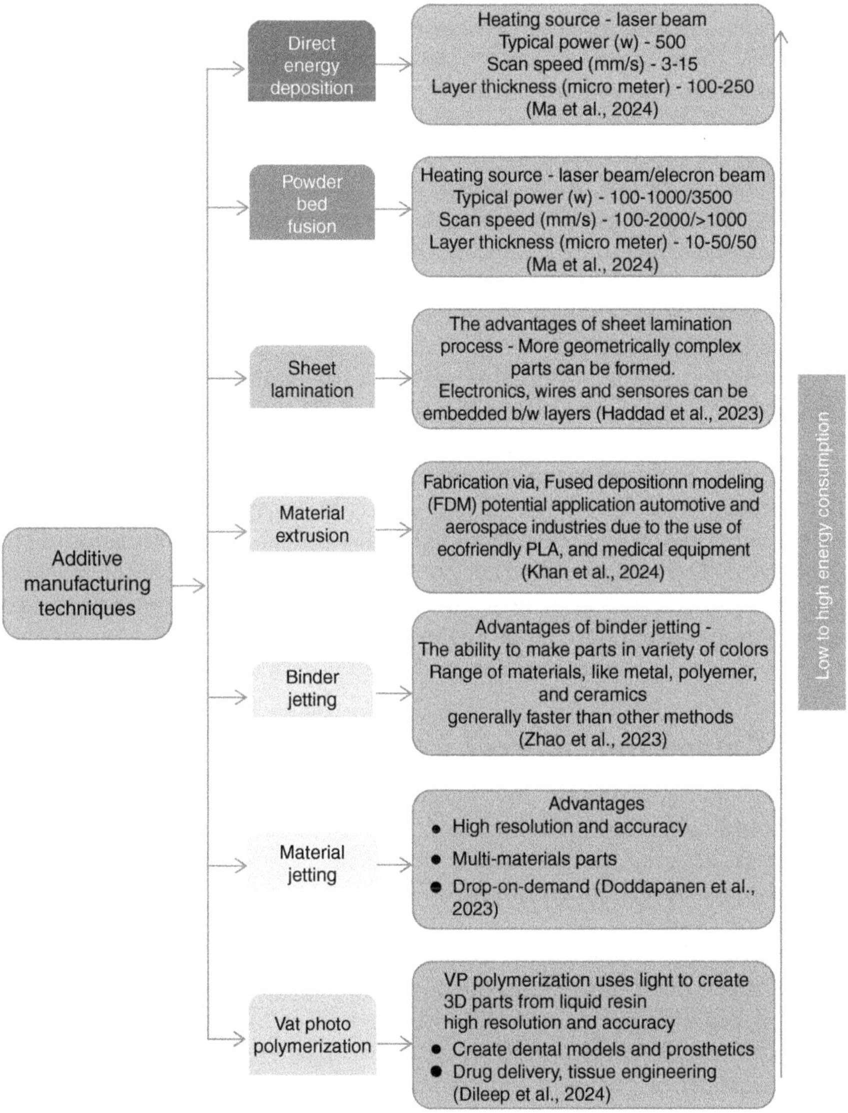

Figure 7.1 Additive manufacturing classification.

et al., 2017); high-energy beam micromachining using laser beams, electron beams, and ion beams (Raj et al., 2019); electrical discharge micromachining (micro-EDM); micro-electrochemical machining (micro-ECM) (Saxena et al., 2018); and electrochemical deposition (ECD) (Qin et al., 2024).

7.1.2 Micro-AM techniques

Numerous microfabrication processes have been developed over time. However, these techniques often face limitations when applied to new microproducts that require the use of diverse materials and complex three-dimensional (3D) microstructures with high aspect ratios.

Among the most commonly used micro-AM techniques are those driven by high-energy beams, such as electron or laser beam selective melting and sintering. However, micro components fabricated using these methods often face challenges, including significant thermal and stress-induced distortions, as well as the formation of cracks and voids. These issues arise due to the drastic temperature changes experienced by micro geometries over a short time frame (Li et al., 2022; Wang et al., 2017).

Over the last decade, AM technologies have been extensively used to produce intricate 3D components. The fabrication of 3D microparts and structures has also become feasible through specific AM technologies, aided by essential modifications and improvements to meet the requirements of microfabrication. For instance, stereolithography (SL) is a layer-by-layer 3D printing technique that creates objects by curing liquid materials through photoirradiation. This light-based 3D printing method has proven effective in manufacturing biomedical microdevices, such as tissue scaffolds, due to its high resolution and precise construction capabilities. These advantages stem from its ability to control various aspects of photon application (Muldoon et al., 2022).

7.1.3 Comparison between micro-AECM and micro-AM

Selecting the appropriate 3D micro-AM process requires a thorough understanding of the capabilities and limitations of each technique. A key distinction between micro Additive Electrochemical Manufacturing (micro-AECM) and thermally-driven micro-AM techniques lies in the use of laser or electron beams.

Thermally-driven micro-AM techniques often fall short in producing high-quality metal micro-geometries due to issues such as thermal distortion and material degradation. As a result, non-thermal or low-temperature micro-AM techniques, like micro-AECM, are increasingly preferred for applications requiring superior precision and quality, as illustrated in Figure 7.2.

7.1.4 Challenges of micro-AM

Major challenges for 3D micro-AM are process modeling, development of new The major challenges faced by 3D micro-AM processes include process modeling, the development of new mechanisms and optimization strategies, integration issues for microdevice applications, and the evaluation of the functional performance of 3D microstructures (Vaezi et al., 2013). Despite these challenges, advancements in 3D micro-AM are expected to

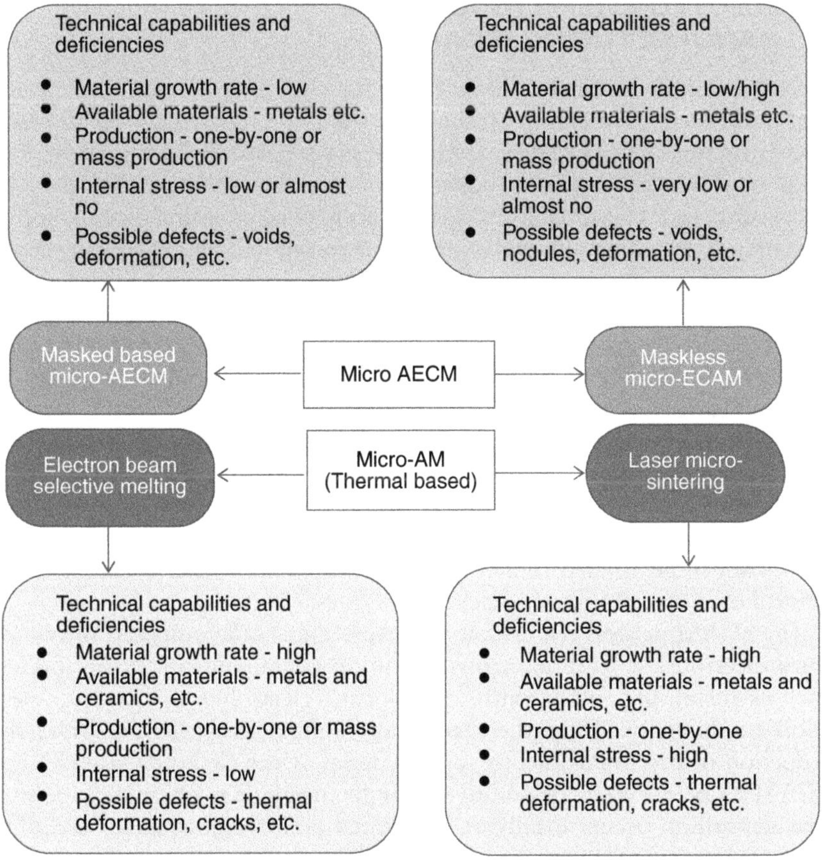

Figure 7.2 Comparison between micro-AECM and micro-AM (thermal based).

drive significant progress in micro- and nanosystems, enabling innovations in areas such as microfluidics, optics, biological systems, and electronics.

One critical application of micro-AM is the fabrication of blood vessels, which requires ultra-precise printing capabilities to match the intricate dimensions of various blood vessel types. Techniques such as extrusion, inkjet printing, laser-assisted methods, and VAT polymerization have shown promise, as they can produce structures as small as 10 μm—the approximate inner diameter of capillaries, the smallest blood vessels.

The ability to accurately 3D print blood vessels offers significant advantages in the medical field, as manually manufacturing such small and complex structures is extremely challenging. By utilizing highly precise methods, micro-AM can create biologically realistic blood vessels at scales that closely resemble natural anatomy. However, challenges remain, particularly in developing suitable bio-inks and managing the delicate process of shaping cells into desired structures (Cao et al., 2021; Diba et al., 2021).

7.2 ELECTRO-CHEMICAL ADDITIVE MANUFACTURING (ECAM)

Electrochemical Additive Manufacturing (ECAM) is an advanced, non-traditional fabrication technique used to construct metal-based microstructures layer by layer. Traditional mask-based ECAM has primarily been used for large-scale production of two-dimensional (2D) metallic microstructures. However, ECAM is rapidly gaining attention globally for its advantages, including minimal material waste, reduced manufacturing costs, and the ability to produce complex microstructures. As a true additive manufacturing (AM) technology, ECAM offers superior surface quality and high geometric precision, making it increasingly popular for diverse applications.

Recent developments in ECAM methods have expanded its range of use, and several of these methods are already implemented in the market. ECAM stands out as a versatile technique capable of creating intricate 3D micro- and nano-scale metal geometries (Ayalew et al., 2023). One of the key benefits of electrochemistry in 3D printing is its ability to convert liquid inks into solid materials through electrodeposition. The process is straightforward, can be applied to a wide range of materials, and offers excellent control over morphology and deposition rates.

The ECAM process requires an electrochemical cell composed of two or three electrodes and an electrolyte solution containing precursor species, such as metal ions, along with a supporting electrolyte to maintain electrical conductivity. When the appropriate voltage is applied, it drives the reduction of precursor ions to solid material at the electrode surface. For ECAM to be adapted for additive manufacturing, it is essential to ensure that deposition occurs locally at designated points, allowing for layer-by-layer construction (Hengsteler et al., 2023).

In recent decades, ECAM techniques for micro- and nano-scale additive manufacturing have received significant attention in both academic and industrial sectors. A variety of ECAM methods have been developed, including localized electrochemical deposition, meniscus-confined 3D electrodeposition, electrochemical fabrication, jet electrochemical deposition, mask electroplating, and electrochemical printing.

7.2.1 History of ECAM

7.2.1 History of electrochemical additive manufacturing (ECAM)

Electrochemical Additive Manufacturing (ECAM) is a relatively new and evolving microfabrication technique, but its development is part of the broader history of additive manufacturing (AM). The journey of AM began with innovations that paved the way for advanced techniques like ECAM.

7.2.1.1 *Early Milestones in Additive Manufacturing*

The concept of additive manufacturing was introduced in 1980, when Dr. Hideo Kodama of the Nagoya Municipal Industrial Research Institute filed the first AM patent. Kodama's process involved the use of photopolymers and light exposure to create three-dimensional prototypes. This idea laid the foundation for future innovations in AM.

In 1983, **stereolithography (SLA)** was invented, becoming the first practical AM technique. This method used a laser to cure liquid photopolymers layer by layer, forming solid structures (Afridi et al., 2024). Following this, in 1986, Dr. Joseph Beaman developed **Selective Laser Sintering (SLS)**, which employed lasers to selectively fuse powdered materials. The first commercial SLS machine was introduced in 1990.

Advancements in AM for Medical Applications

Over time, AM technologies like Selective Laser Melting (SLM) have advanced significantly, particularly in the field of biomedicine. SLM is now widely used to produce complex, near-dense biometallic implants for applications such as tissue repair, dentistry, surgical tools, and orthopedics. The precision of SLM allows it to print materials ranging from metals and polymers to combinations of metal-ceramic components, enabling the creation of implants based on anatomical structures (Aufa et al., 2024).

By the late 20th century, **bio-printing** emerged as a specialized form of AM. The development of the first bio-printers enabled the fabrication of biological constructs —opening new possibilities in medical science.

Emergence of ECAM

Building on these advancements, ECAM has developed as a distinct AM technology capable of fabricating complex 3D nano- and micro-sized metallic geometries. Unlike thermally driven AM methods like SLS and SLM, ECAM utilizes electrochemical principles to achieve layer-by-layer deposition, ensuring low material waste, smooth surfaces, and high geometric precision. While still in its early stages of development, ECAM's versatility and potential for customization have garnered significant interest in academia and industry.

As the field continues to evolve, ECAM is poised to expand its applications across various industries, including electronics, aerospace, and biomedicine.

Electrochemical Additive Manufacturing (ECAM) is an advanced microfabrication technology that offers the ability to produce structures with nearly unlimited geometrical complexity. This technique holds immense potential for applications in fields such as microelectronics, sensing, robotics, and energy storage (Khalid et al., 2024).

Evolution of EFAB Technology

One significant development in the realm of ECAM is **EFAB (Electrochemical Fabrication) technology**, which was invented in the mid-1990s at the University of Southern California with funding from DARPA. EFAB was commercialized by Microfabrica, Inc. (formerly MEMGen Corporation), a venture-funded company based in Van Nuys, California. The technology was first publicly introduced at the Solid Freeform Fabrication Symposium in 1998.

EFAB technology enables the production of intricate metal devices ranging from millimeters to centimeters in size, with features as small as a few microns. Its hallmark lies in its **wafer-scale fabrication**, producing devices in batches of hundreds to thousands, using a combination of **additive and subtractive processes**. During the EFAB process, metal is deposited through electroplating, creating fully dense materials with exceptional mechanical properties and biocompatibility (Cohen et al., 2010).

Applications of EFAB in the Medical Device Industry

In the medical field, EFAB has enabled the production of devices for minimally invasive surgeries, microinvasive therapies, and other precision applications. Specific examples include:

- **Microtissue debriders**
- **Monolithically fabricated articulated biopsy forceps**
- **Tools for minimally invasive surgical interventions**

The adaptability and precision of EFAB technology make it particularly suitable for producing devices that require intricate designs and biocompatible materials—further underscoring its potential for widespread adoption in medical, electronic, and industrial applications.

7.2.2 Principle

The principle underlying **Electrochemical Additive Manufacturing** (**ECAM**) is the localized **electrodeposition** of material between an anode and a cathode, both submerged in a metal plating bath. Unlike conventional techniques such as electroplating or electroforming, which apply material over a large area, ECAM precisely deposits material in a controlled, localized manner as shown in Figure 7.3.

In this process, the tool with a localized geometry acts as the **anode**, while the flat substrate serves as the **cathode**. An externally applied voltage bias facilitates the migration of metal ions from the electrolyte solution toward the substrate near the tool. At the cathode surface, these ions undergo a

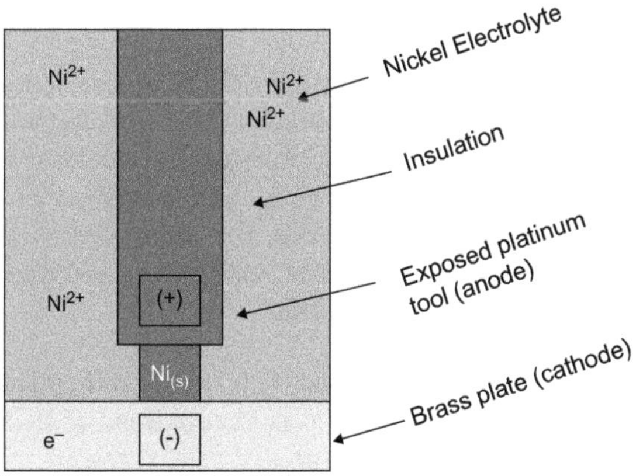

Figure 7.3 Working principle of ECAM.

reduction in charge, leading to the formation of a solid metal deposit on the substrate. This localized material addition enables the fabrication of intricate geometries with high precision (Mbugua et al., 2020).

7.3 CLASSIFICATIONS

Additive Manufacturing (AM) technologies, particularly those based on layer-by-layer fabrication, have emerged as effective methods for producing intricate 3D microproducts. Over the past decade, AM processes have been extensively utilized for creating complex 3D components, including microparts and microstructures. Achieving true microfabrication often requires tailoring existing AM technologies through essential modifications and improvements.

Some scalable AM technologies adapted for microscale applications include:

- **Stereolithography** (SL), referred to as **micro-SL** (MSL) in microscale applications,
- **Selective Laser Sintering** (SLS), termed **microlaser sintering** (MLS) at microscale,
- **3D Printing** (3DP),
- **Inkjet Printing**,
- **Fused Deposition Modeling** (FDM), and
- **Laminated Object Manufacturing** (LOM).

These technologies enable precise fabrication of microstructures with advanced design flexibility and are illustrated in Figure 7.1 (Vaezi et al., 2013).

Electrochemical Additive Manufacturing (ECAM) Classifications
In the realm of Electrochemical Deposition (ECD), two electrodes—an anode and a cathode—are connected to the positive and negative terminals of a power supply, respectively. The properties and behaviors of the deposited material can be fine-tuned by regulating the electrolyte composition and operating conditions. Depending on the application, **electrodeposition** can be categorized into two primary methods:

1. **Mask-Based Electrodeposition:** This method involves the use of a patterned mask, referred to as **through-mask ECD,** to deposit material selectively on specific areas of the substrate.
2. **Maskless Electrodeposition:** Here, the cathode is blank, allowing for deposition without a mask, offering greater flexibility for complex geometries.

Similarly, **Micro-AECM (Advanced Electrochemical Additive Manufacturing)** processes are categorized based on the use of a mask:

- **Mask-Based Micro-AECM:** Utilizes a patterned mask to confine deposition to precise regions.
- **Maskless Micro-ECAM:** Achieves deposition directly without the need for masking, suitable for creating intricate freeform structures (Li et al., 2022).

7.3.1 Through mask-based additive manufacturing

Through mask-based additive manufacturing (AM) involves the use of an electrically insulating photoresist mask to define and confine the areas for material deposition. This approach relies on a patterned through-mask to expose specific regions on the substrate where metal deposition is required. The unmasked areas serve as molds, guiding the electrochemical deposition of metal material into the predefined shapes. Figure 7.4 shows the schematic diagram of through mask ECAM and the working principle is illustrated in Figure 7.5.

This technique can be considered a metal duplication process, where the deposited metal structures reverse-replicate the geometry of the patterned through-mask. The photoresist mask ensures high precision and consistency in shaping the deposited features, making this method particularly suitable for fabricating intricate metal components and microstructures with high dimensional accuracy.

The following are some of the experiments conducted in our laboratory, along with the results obtained from Masked ECAM performed on copper, brass, and other materials.

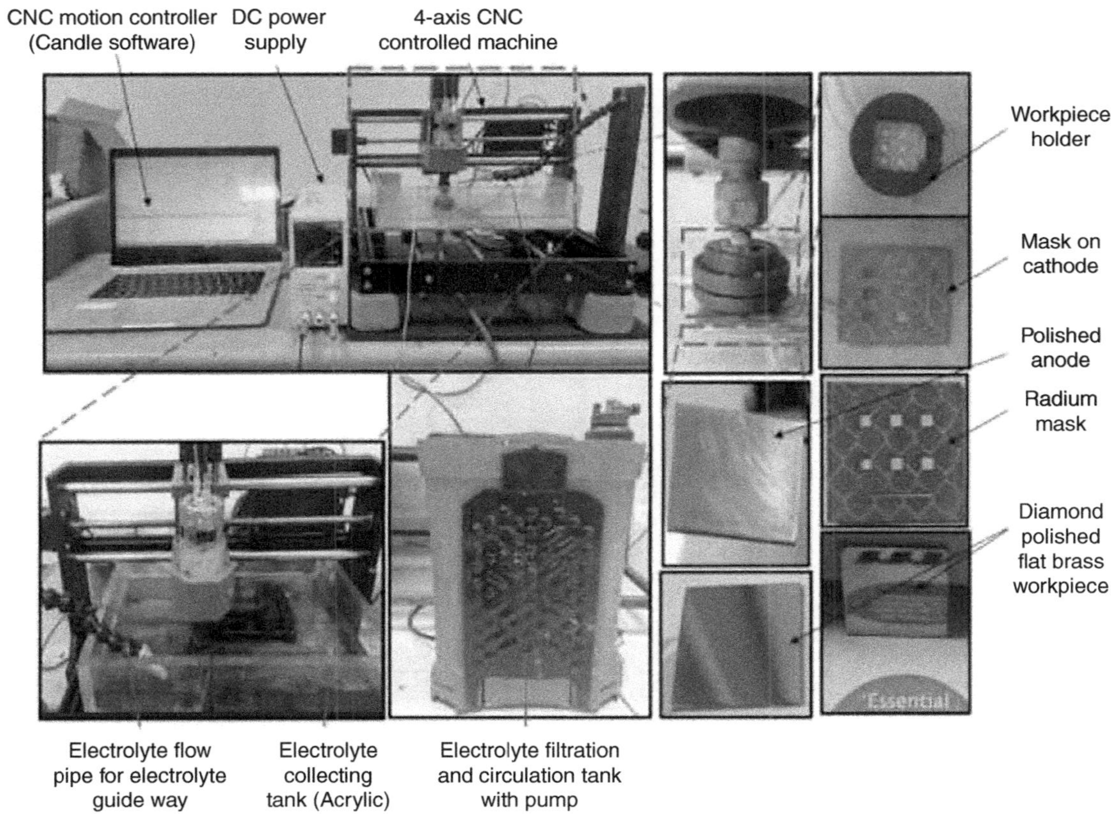

Figure 7.4 Schematic diagram of through mask ECAM.

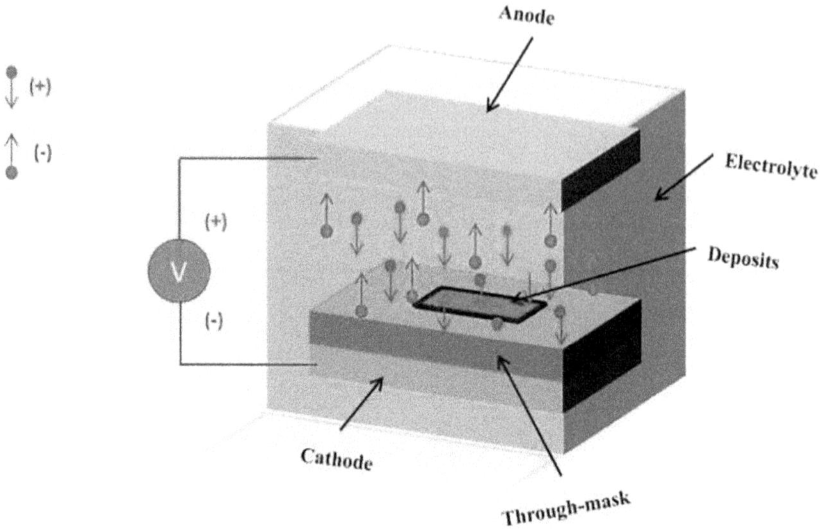

Figure 7.5 Through mask ECAM principle.

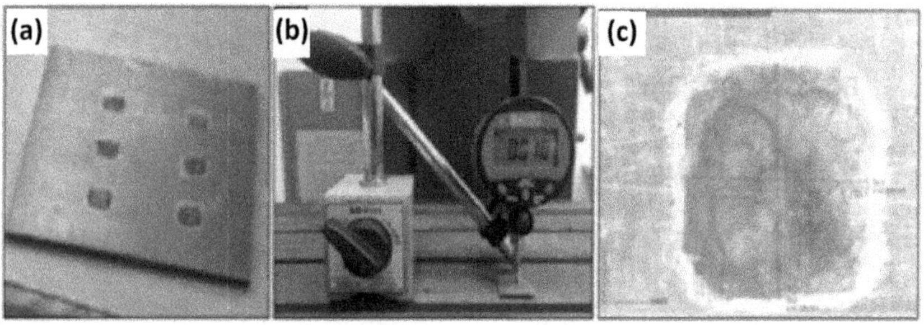

Figure 7.6 (a) Nickel deposition on copper (b) 10μm height of Ni was deposited on Cu (c) Closer view and Dimension of Nickel deposition on copper.

Masked ECAM experiments of Nickel deposition

Figure 7.6 illustrates the successful micro-deposition of nickel on a copper substrate, achieving a height of 10μm. This precise deposition was measured using a Mitutoyo Dial Indicator, a reliable instrument for such microscopic measurements. The uniformity and precision of the deposition underscore the potential of this method for various applications in material engineering and surface modification techniques.

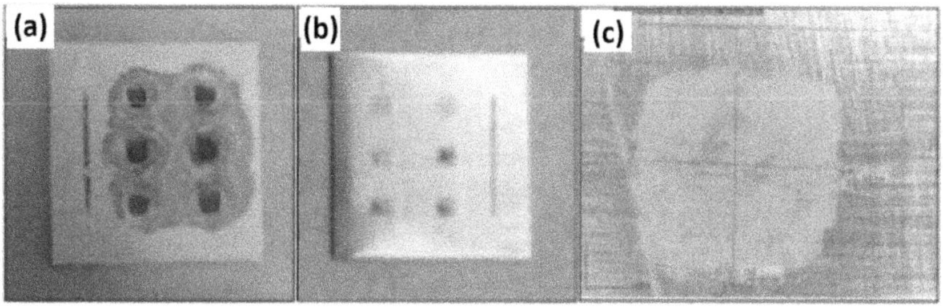

Figure 7.7 (a) Nickel deposition on brass (b) nickel deposition on stainless steel (c) Closer view nickel deposition on stainless steel.

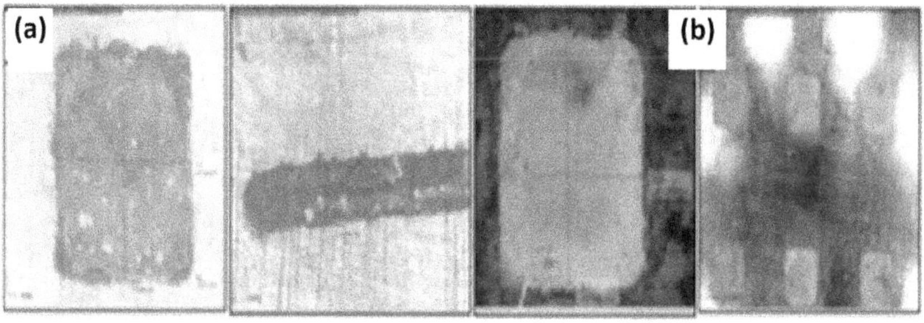

Figure 7.8 Copper deposition on brass (a) 0.1 A or above (b) 0.02 A – 0.05 A.

Nickel deposition on Brass and Stainless Steel

The images depict the results of nickel micro-deposition on brass Figure 7.7(a) and stainless-steel Figure 7.7(b) and (c) at a current above 0.1 A.

Masked ECAM experiments of copper deposition

Electroforming of copper:

When applying copper onto brass, it is noticed that because of the limited surface area, a substantial electric current is necessary to deposit the metal using the ECAM mask as shown in Figure 7.8. Hence, in the event that the electric current surpasses 0.1A, there will be no deposition and instead, a copper compound will be formed. On the other hand, if the current is less than 0.05 amperes, we can get an acceptable deposition.

Micro-Patterning using Masked ECAM

Intricate micro line and zig zag designs were created of copper on brass, with the goal of attaining the greatest possible elevation. The present electrical

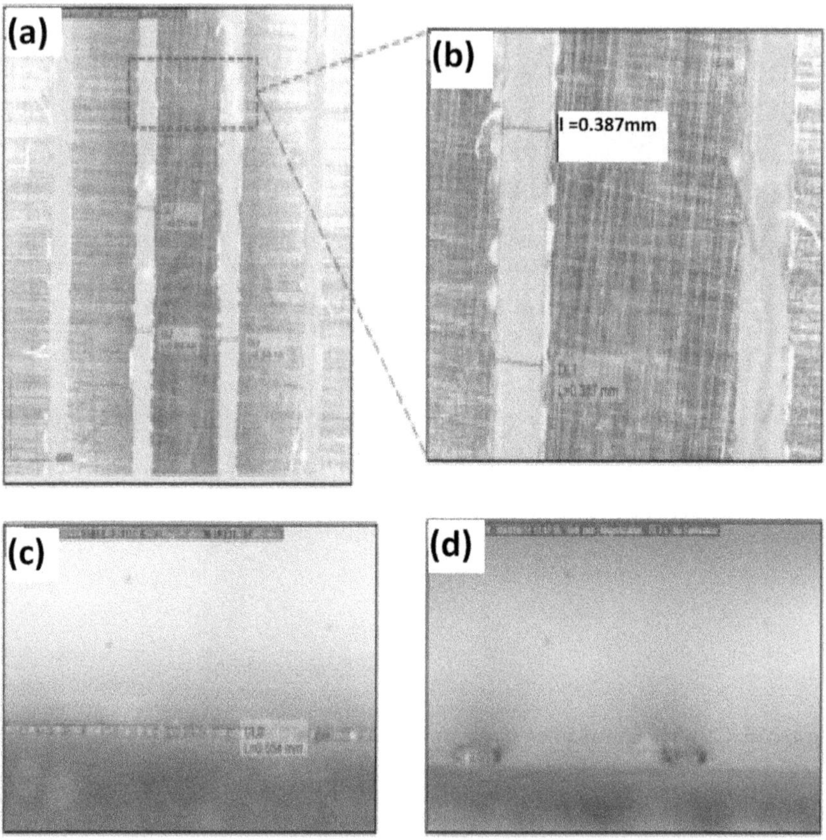

Figure 7.9 (a) and (b) Line deposition of copper on brass (min width achieved – 0.387 mm) (c) side cross section of lines deposited (d) front cross section of lines deposited.

current utilized was 0.02 A, leading to a maximum vertical distance of 54 μm and a minimum width of 387 μm for the line as shown in Figure 7.9 & 7.10.

7.3.1.1 Through-mask electroplating

Through-mask electroplating, also known as through-mask electrodeposition, is a specialized process that fabricates micro-scale solid geometries by electrodepositing metal materials into pre-patterned photoresist molds, referred to as through-masks. This process allows for the replication of intricate patterns with high precision, as the deposited metal inversely duplicates the shape of the through-mask.

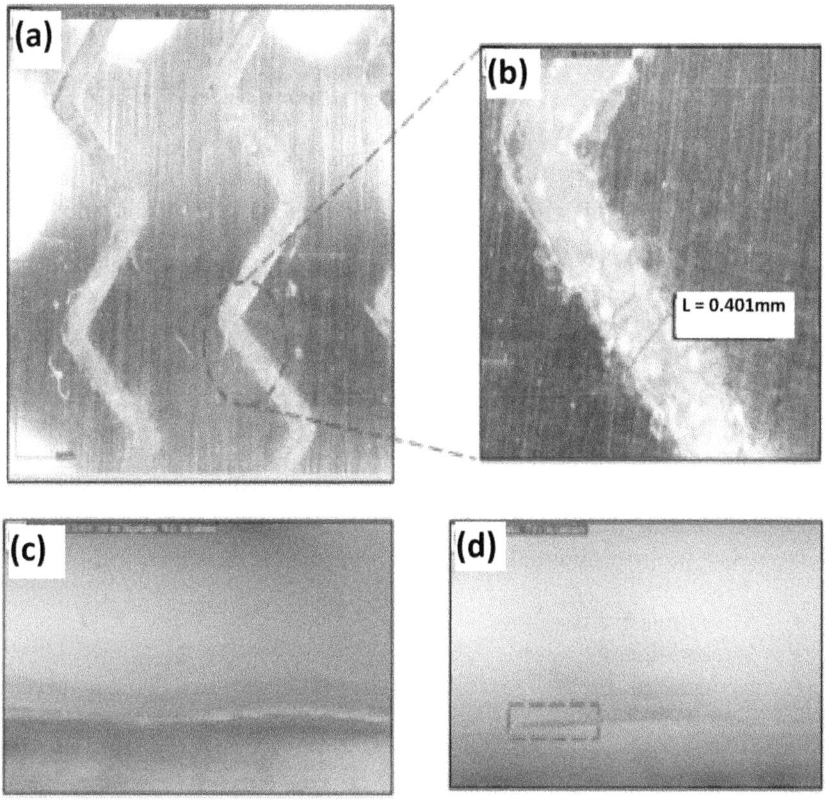

Figure 7.10 (a) and (b) Zig-zag pattern deposition of copper on brass (min width achieved – 0.401 mm) (c) side cross section of workpiece (d) front view of zig zag lines.

The quality of the resulting microstructures, including their geometric accuracy and dimensional stability, is highly dependent on the design and quality of the through-mask. Key applications of this technique include the manufacturing of high-precision components used in microelectronics, sensors, and micro-mechanical systems. By tailoring the properties of the electroplating bath and operating parameters, through-mask electroplating can achieve exceptional control over the deposited material's morphology and characteristics.

Electroplating of nickel on copper:
For the acquisition of fundamental knowledge, a series of straightforward experiments were conducted on nickel plating. These experiments provided valuable insights into the process and outcomes of nickel plating,

contributing to the foundational understanding of this technique. The results from these experiments is utilized to further explore and optimize the process of nickel plating in future studies.

7.3.1.2 Electrochemical fabrication (EFAB)

The **Electrochemical Fabrication** (**EFAB**) process was pioneered at the University of Southern California in 1996 and represents a significant advancement in microfabrication techniques. EFAB is a hybrid process that integrates additive and subtractive manufacturing principles to produce complex, high-precision metal devices.

The EFAB process enables the cost-effective and highly repeatable production of intricate structures ranging from millimeters to centimeters in overall size, with feature resolutions down to microns or tens of microns. Originally developed for electronics and defense applications, EFAB has expanded its utility into other fields, with some of the most promising advancements seen in medical applications.

In the **medical domain**, EFAB is employed to manufacture tools and devices that support **minimally invasive procedures**. Examples include:

- Microinvasive therapies.
- Microtissue debriders.
- Articulated biopsy forceps fabricated monolithically for precise operation.

EFAB's ability to create fully dense metal components with excellent mechanical properties and proven biocompatibility makes it particularly valuable in healthcare and biomedical engineering. Its precision and scalability continue to drive innovations in applications that require miniaturization and geometric complexity

7.3.2 Through mask-less additive manufacturing

Through mask-less additive manufacturing different technology used including, Localized electrochemical deposition used of fine anode or ultrafine anode and cathode growth guided by the anode. An ultra-high aspect ratio (AR up to 200) nickel micro-column was successfully fabricated, achieving a height of 600 μm and a diameter of 3 μm. Additionally, a complex 3D polypyrrole microstructure was produced using Localized Electrochemical Deposition (LECD). Unlike LECD, Jet Electrochemical Deposition (Jet ECD) employs an impinging electrolyte jet as the anode tool, instead of a solid ultrafine anode, to enable selective metal deposition at the cathode. Jet ECD achieves a significantly higher deposition rate, reaching up to 1 mm/

h, due to the application of extremely high current density (several hundred A/dm^2) facilitated by a high-speed electrolyte jet ejected from a nozzle connected to the positive terminal of the power supply and in Meniscus-confined electroplating use of nano-sized hollow anode, extremely small inter electrode gap. The schematic diagram of mask-less ECAM as shown in Figure 7.11.

Mask-less additive manufacturing eliminates the need for predefined masks or molds, allowing for greater flexibility and adaptability in the fabrication process. This approach enables the direct formation of microstructures by depositing materials in a highly localized manner. Mask-less methods are especially advantageous in applications requiring custom designs, rapid prototyping, or structures with intricate geometries. The working principle of mask-less ECAM as shown in Figure 7.12.

One prominent example of mask-less additive manufacturing is Localized Electrodeposition (LED), which has emerged as a reliable technique for producing high-resolution microstructures with excellent control over geometry and material composition.

7.3.2.1 Localized electrodeposition (LED)

Introduction and Process Principle

Localized Electrochemical Deposition (LECD), a typical mask-less micro-ECAM technique, was first reported by Madden and Hunter in 1995. The process operates on principles similar to electroplating but achieves a much higher degree of precision and control.

In LED, metallic ions move under the influence of an applied electric field, overcoming forces such as the negatively directed double-layer force (if present). The ions are then reduced to metal atoms at the cathode and deposited in a highly confined and controlled manner. The deposition is localized, occurring only where the anode makes contact with the cathode (either temporary or permanent).

Process Mechanism

- As the anode moves across the surface of the cathode, the metallic ions in the electrolyte receive electrons upon contact, transforming into metal atoms.
- These atoms deposit exclusively in the area around the anode-cathode contact point, allowing for precise control over the deposition process.
- This guided and localized mechanism enables the creation of intricate structures without the need for extensive post-processing or masking techniques.

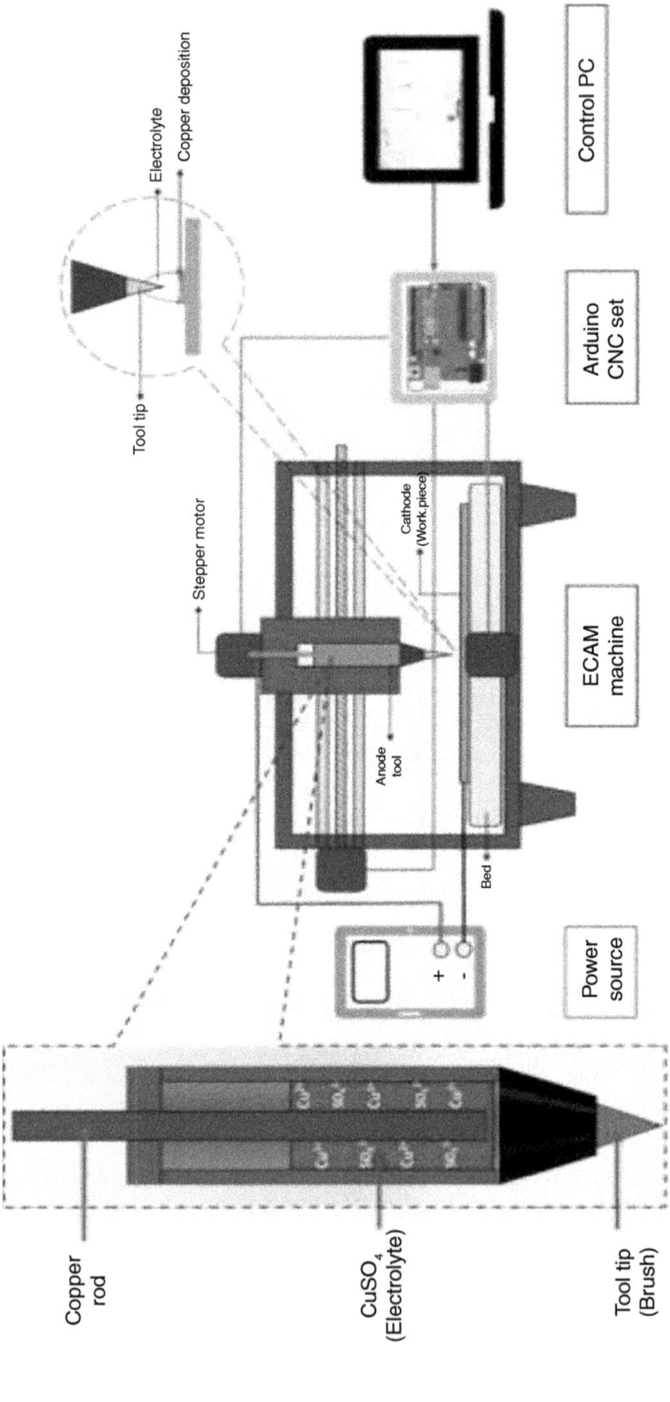

Figure 7.11 Schematic diagram of mask-less ECAM.

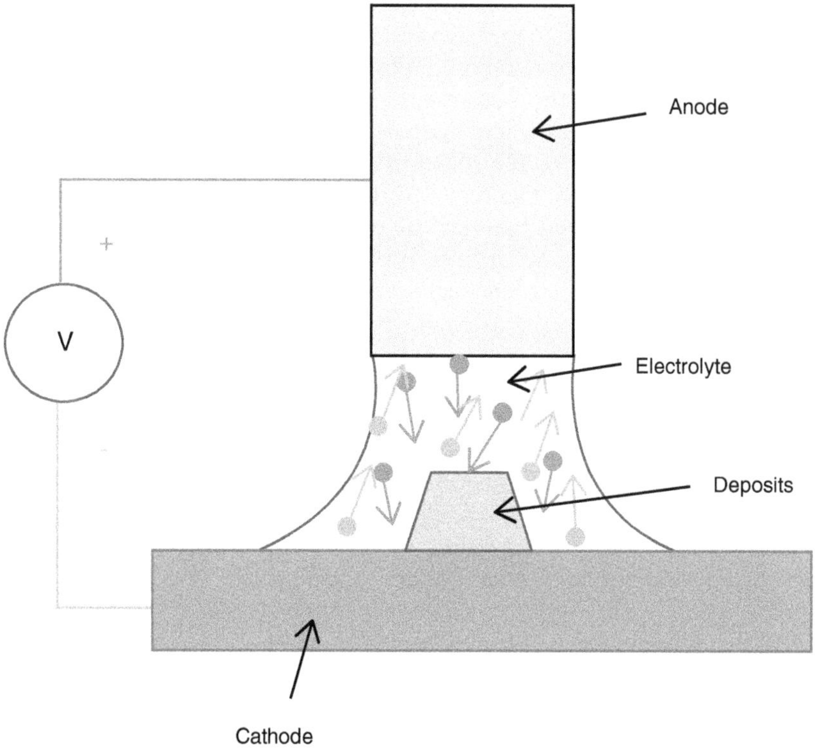

Figure 7.12 Mask-less ECAM principle.

Advantages

Localized Electrodeposition offers several benefits:

1. **Enhanced Microstructure Aspect Ratios:** The process can produce structures with high aspect ratios, suitable for complex geometries.
2. **Material Versatility:** It is capable of depositing multiple metals and is compatible with a variety of substrates.
3. **Defect-Free Fabrication:** Unlike heat-based additive manufacturing methods, LED avoids defects such as warping, residual stress, or material degradation caused by thermal effects, as heat is not involved.
4. **Precision and Control:** The ability to control deposition parameters ensures high accuracy and consistency in the final product.

Localized Electrodeposition is increasingly being recognized as a viable mask-less micro-ECAM technique for applications demanding precision, flexibility, and material diversity (Singh et al., 2023).

7.3.2.2 Numerical modelling and simulation

Numerical modelling of copper deposition on brass on 3D profile

An electrolyte solution, containing ions of the material intended for deposition, is applied over the substrate. The mask, already present on the cathode, defines the areas where material deposition is intended. An electric potential is applied across the substrate. The simulation model for copper deposition as shown in Figure 7.13. The mask prevents direct contact between the cathode and the electrolyte in covered areas, allowing electrochemical reactions to occur only in the exposed regions. In the exposed areas of the cathode, electrochemical reactions take place. Metal ions from the electrolyte are reduced, leading to the selective deposition of the desired material onto the cathode surface. Material deposition occurs exclusively in the regions exposed by the mask. The deposited material adheres to the cathode surface, conforming to the pattern or design defined by the mask. The key to the mechanism lies in the controlled exposure of specific areas on the cathode through the mask, allowing electrochemical reactions and material deposition only in the designated regions. This process is valuable for applications requiring precision, such as microfabrication, where intricate patterns or coatings are desired on a substrate.

Equations of importance of simulation

Electrodeposition

In the simulated process of electrodeposition, Faraday's Law of Electrolysis governs the overall deposition of material, dictating the quantity of substance deposited based on the amount of electric charge passed through the system. It using Laplace equation as the governing equation.

$$\nabla^2 .v = 0 \tag{1}$$

∇^2 is the Laplacian operator, which represents the divergence of the gradient of V and V is the electric potential. Furthermore, the physics of the electrodeposition process is intricately captured by the Butler-Volmer equation, which dictates the rate of charge transfer or local current density at the electrode-electrolyte interface. The cross-section of the work-piece as shown in Figure 7.14.

$$j = j0[\exp(\alpha \cdot F \cdot \eta / RT) - \exp(-(1-\alpha) \cdot F \cdot \eta)/RT] \tag{2}$$

j is the current density, j0 is the exchange current density, η is the overpotential, α is the charge transfer coefficient, F is the Faraday constant, R is the gas constant, T is the temperature. The 2D simulation domain is illustrated in Figure 7.15.

Cross section of work-piece and boundary conditions

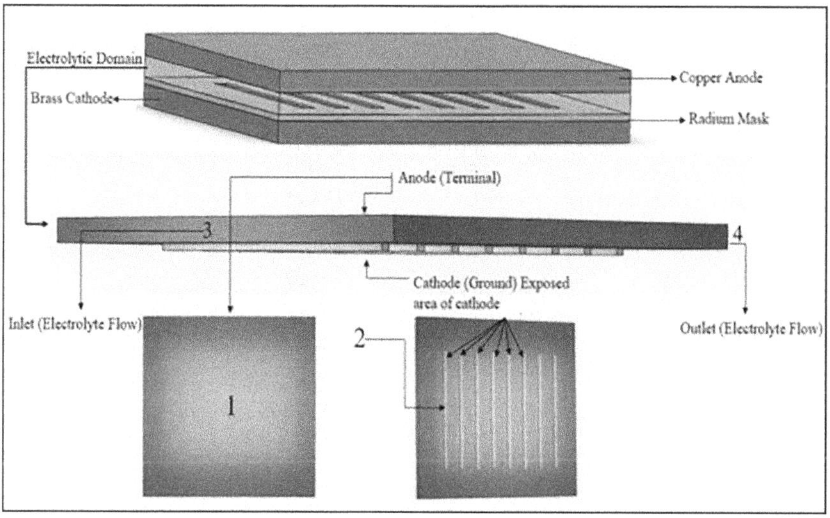

Figure 7.13 Model for copper deposition simulation.

Table 7.1 Boundary conditions

S.no.	*Boundary condition*	*Boundary*	*Equation*
For the charge conservation equation			
1.	Electric Potential	1	$I = A$
2.	Ground	2	$\varphi = 0$
3.	Insulation	Rest all boundaries	$\frac{d\varphi}{dn} = 0$
For deformation mesh			
1.	Prescribed mesh velocity	2	$v_y = -kjn$
2.	No deformation	Rest all boundaries	$v_x = 0$ $v_y = 0$

Results on numerical modelling of copper deposition on brass on 3D profile

Numerical simulation was performed on a 3D profile for copper deposition on brass using secondary current distribution for 1200s i.e. 20 mins same as experimental as shown in Figure 7.16. The image and graph presented provide a comprehensive view of the copper deposition process on brass over various time periods. The graph provides a quantitative representation of this process, plotting the height of the deposited material against the length of the cathode profile at different time intervals. It is observed that

Table 7.2 Parameters used for simulation

Parameter	*Symbol*	*Value*	*Units*
Electrolyte conductivity	A_l	24.6	S/m
Density	A_{Cu}	8960	kg/m^3
Molar mass	MCu	63.55	g/mol
Equilibrium potential	Eeq	0.34	V
Exchange current density	i_o	234.217	A/m^2
Anodic transfer coefficient	α_a	0.553	Dimensionless
Cathodic transfer coefficient	α_c	0.447	Dimensionless
Electrode thickness	s	2×10^{-7}	m
Electrical conductivity	A	3.8×10^{7}	S/m
Total current	Is, total	-34.6	A
Initial concentration	$C_{cu.0}$	250	mol/m^3
Diffusion coefficient	D_{cu}	6.404×10^{-10}	m^2/s
Density of electrolyte	A	1056.36	kg/m^3
Viscosity	μ	1.304×10^{-3}	Pa · s
Initial velocity	u_0	0.32	m/s

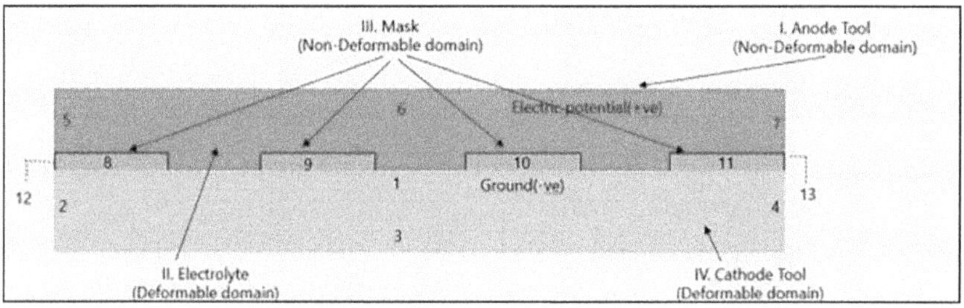

Figure 7.14 Cross-section of the workpiece.

as the time increases, there is a consistent rise in the height of the deposited material across all lengths of the cathode profile. This trend suggests a steady and uniform deposition process over time.

Numerical modelling of masked electrochemical additive manufacturing (Nickel)

The results obtained from the simulation, provide insightful observations about the deposition process at various time periods. One of the key observations made was the higher deposition rate at the edges of the mask compared to the center. This phenomenon can be attributed to the edge effect, a common occurrence in electrochemical processes. Figure 7.17 Height of deposition vs length of the exposed profile at cathode. The edge effect is caused by the uneven distribution of the electric field around the edges of the mask, leading to an increased deposition rate at these locations. The Figure 7.18 shows Nickel deposition on the exposed surface of the cathode. This

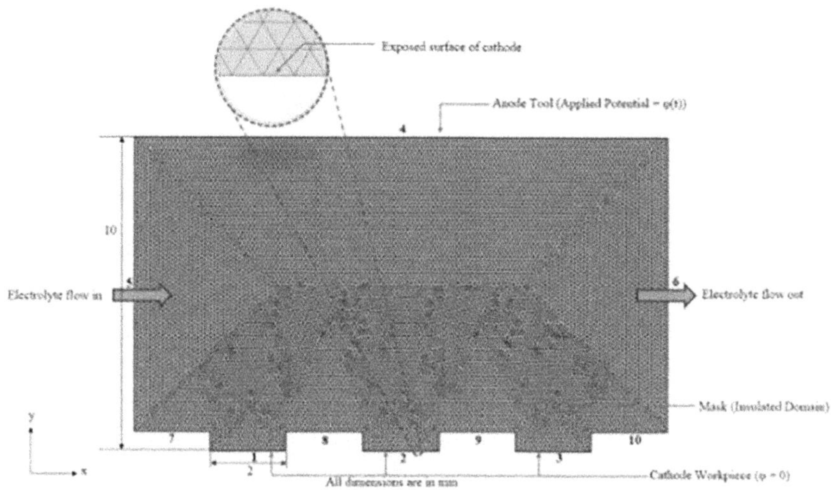

Figure 7.15 :Schematic diagram of the 2D simulation domain.

is further corroborated by the distribution of the electric field around the cathode, as shown in the simulation results. Furthermore, the concentration and distribution of ions near the cathode, as depicted in the simulation results, could also contribute to this observation. The Figure 7.19 (a) shows the potential distribution (b) concentration near cathode, and (c) electric field at various time periods. The flow of ions is influenced by the electric field, which is stronger at the edges of the mask. Consequently, a higher concentration of ions is observed at the edges, leading to an increased rate of deposition. The simulation results also indicate the effectiveness of the mask in creating the desired patterns on the workpiece. Despite the edge effect, the mask successfully restricts the deposition to the exposed areas, demonstrating the feasibility of the masked micro electrochemical additive manufacturing process for patterned deposition.

7.4 CONCLUSION

Over the past two decades, additive manufacturing (AM) technologies have undergone significant advancements, establishing themselves as a transformative force in the fabrication of high-quality 3D microcomponents for MEMS and microengineering applications. Among these, micro-additive electrochemical manufacturing (micro-AECM) stands out as a highly effective technology capable of producing complex, defect-free, and geometrically precise structures at the micro and nano scales.

This chapter reviewed the key micro-AM processes, emphasizing their evolution, principles, classifications, and practical applications. Micro-AM

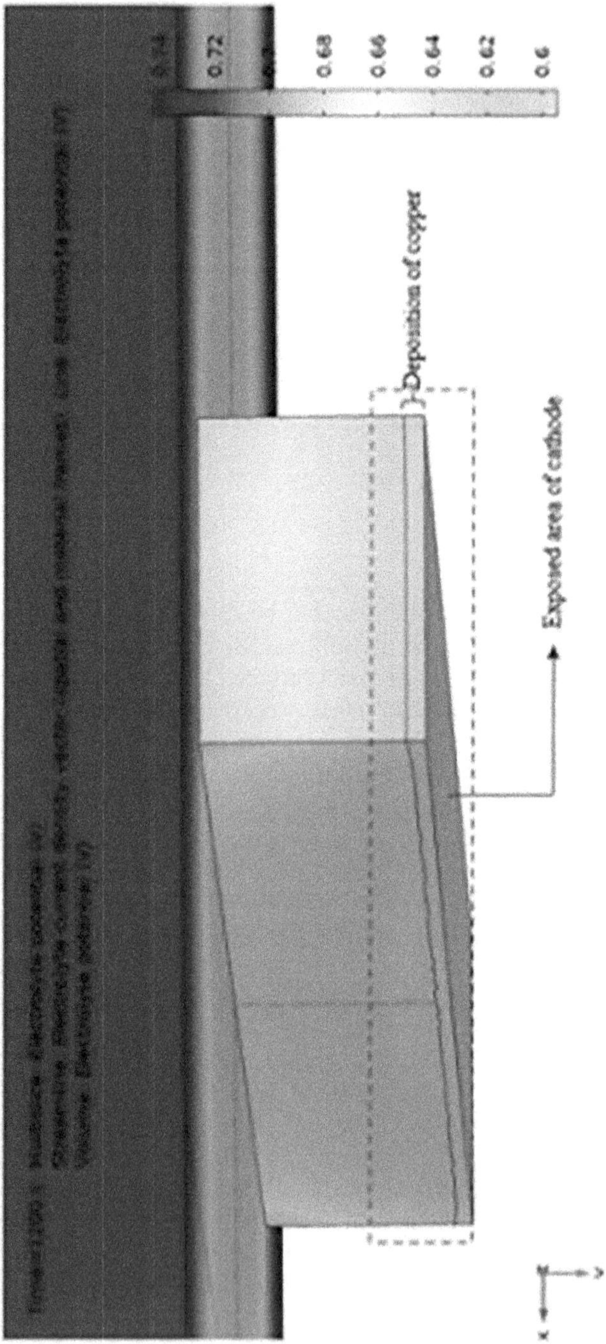

Figure 7.16 Potential distribution and deformation at cathode after 20 mins.

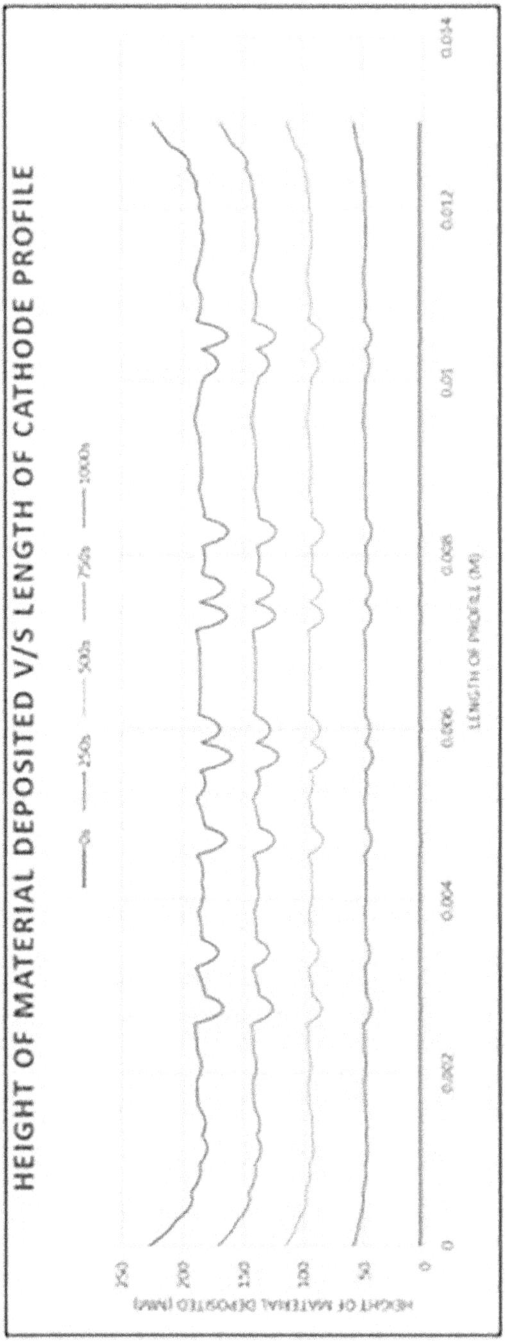

Figure 7.17 Height of deposition vs length of the exposed profile at cathode (13 mm).

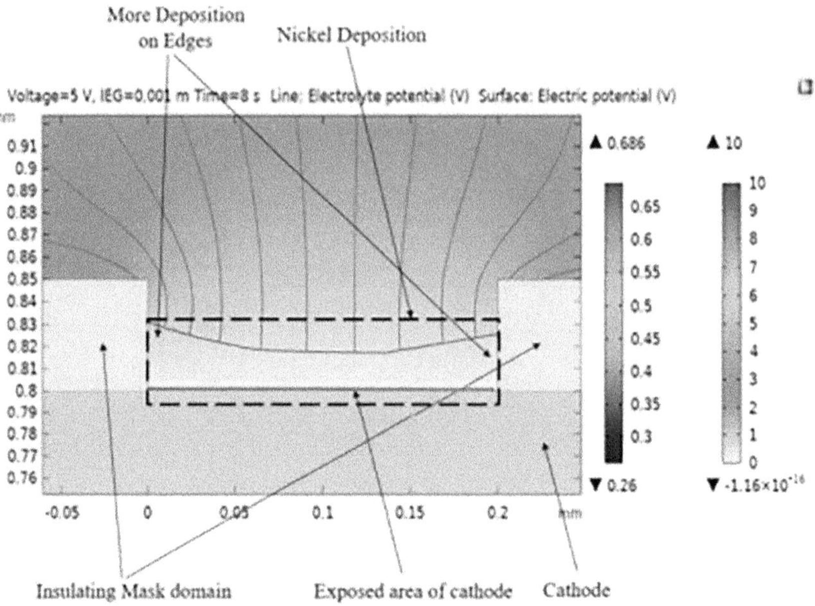

Figure 7.18 Nickel deposition on the exposed surface of the cathode.

systems have demonstrated immense potential for creating functional 3D microstructures, particularly in the biomedical and electronic domains, where high precision, material compatibility, and defect-free properties are critical. The flexibility of micro-A M, especially micro-A E C M, offers an unparalleled advantage in fabricating intricate geometries that are void-free, crack-free, and exhibit minimal internal stresses. Micro-AECM is categorized into mask-based and maskless techniques, both of which offer unique benefits and applications.

Despite the rapid progress in scalability, particularly in the development of biomedical and electronic microdevices, several challenges remain. These include achieving higher resolution, improving process efficiency, expanding material compatibility, and addressing the limitations of current fabrication methods in creating reproducible, high-quality microstructures. Additionally, the integration of advanced control systems and the development of environmentally friendly electrolytes for micro-AECM processes require further investigation to make the technology more sustainable and versatile.

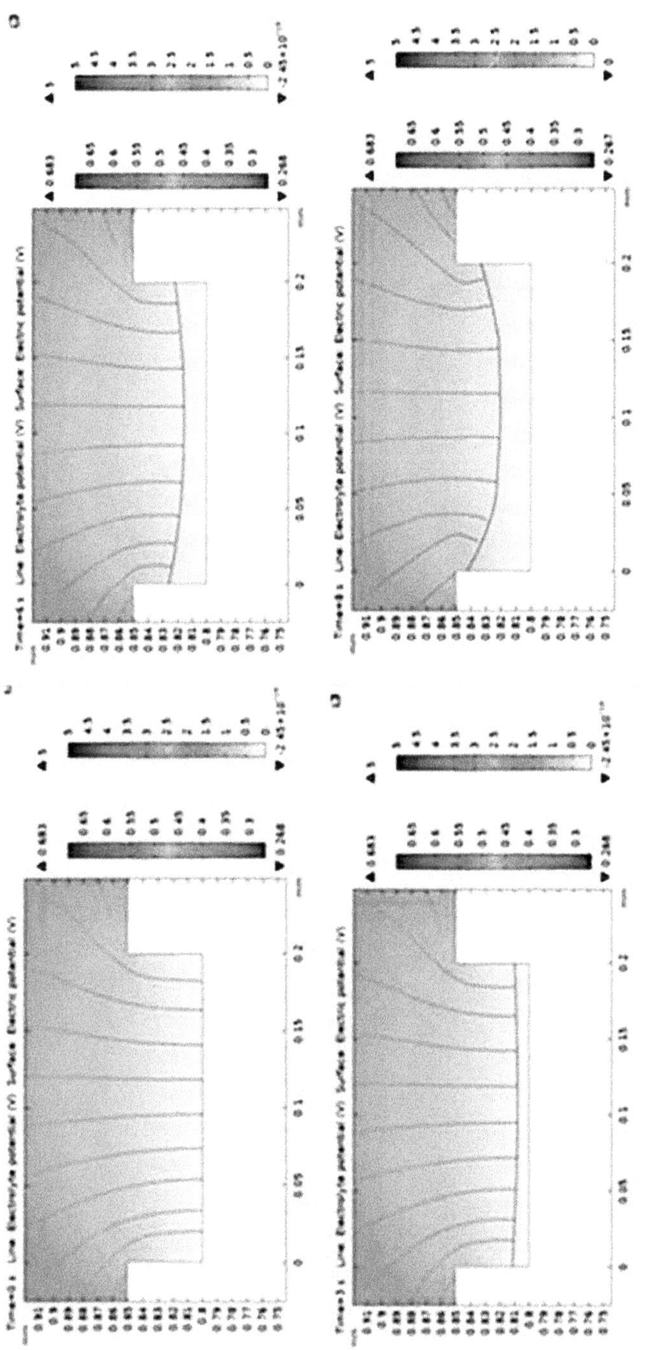

(a)

Figure 7.19 (a) Potential distribution and electrodeposition of nickel (c) Concentration and distribution of ions near the cathode (d) Distribution of electric field around the cathode, at various time periods at 0s, 3s, 6s, 8s.

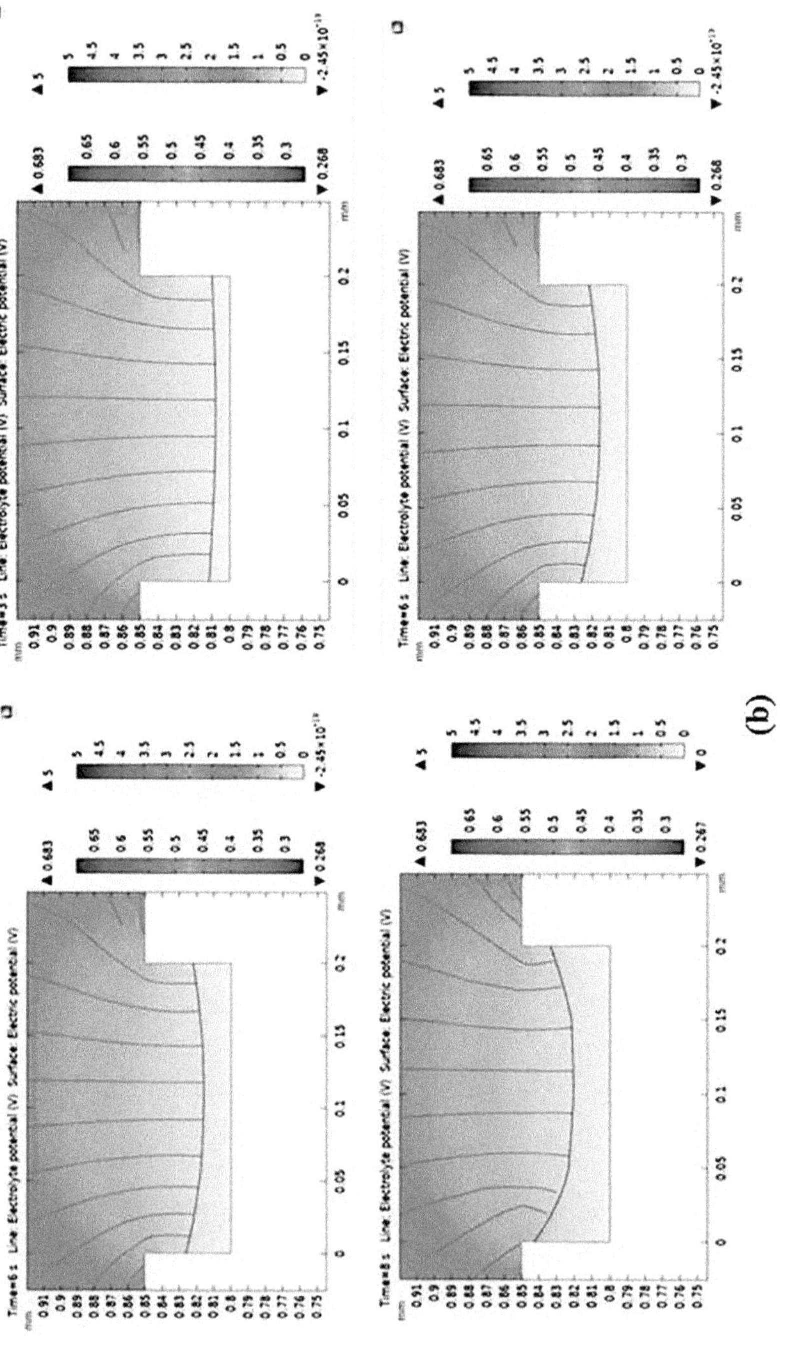

Figure 7.19 Continued

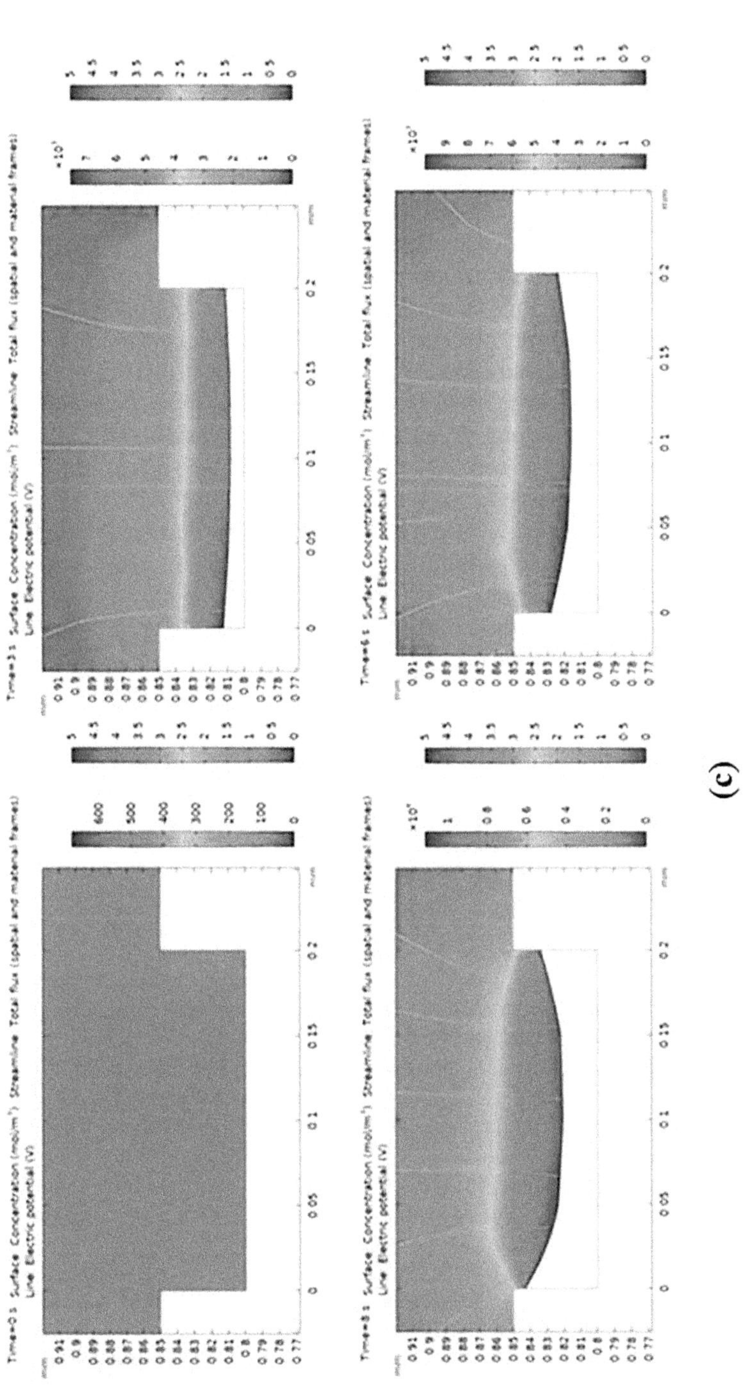

Figure 7.19 Continued

Research Opportunities

1. **Optimization and Automation:** Developing advanced automation systems to enhance precision, efficiency, and throughput while minimizing human intervention.
2. **Material Advancements:** Exploring novel alloys, composites, and functional materials to expand the range of applications and improve the performance of microdevices.
3. **Hybrid Technologies:** Integrating micro-AM with other advanced manufacturing methods, such as lithography or nanoprinting, to achieve multifunctional structures with tailored properties.
4. **Environmental Sustainability:** Designing greener electrolytes and reducing waste to make micro-AM technologies environmentally friendly.
5. **Biomedical Applications:** Enhancing biocompatibility and customization capabilities for personalized medical devices, such as implants and minimally invasive surgical tools.
6. **Quality Control and Metrology:** Developing non-destructive testing and in-situ monitoring techniques to ensure defect-free production at the micro and nano scales.
7. **Scalability to Nano-Fabrication:** Pushing the limits of AM technologies to enable true nanoscale fabrication, bridging the gap between micro and nanotechnology.

By addressing these research opportunities, micro-AM technologies, particularly micro-AECM, have the potential to revolutionize industries, including electronics, healthcare, and aerospace, while also inspiring future innovations in micro and nanofabrication.

REFERENCES

Afridi, A., Al Rashid, A., & Koç, M. (2024). Recent advances in the development of stereolithography-based additive manufacturing processes: A review of applications and challenges. *Bioprinting*, 36, e00360.

Aufa, A. N., Hassan, M. Z., Ismail, Z., Ramlie, F., Jamaludin, K. R., Daud, M. Y. M., & Ren, J. (2024). Current trends in additive manufacturing of selective laser melting for biomedical implant applications. *Journal of Materials Research and Technology*, 30

Ayalew, A. A., Han, X., & Sakairi, M. (2023). A critical review of additive material manufacturing through electrochemical deposition techniques. *Additive Manufacturing*, 71, 103796.

Balázs, B. Z., Geier, N., Takács, M., & Davim, J. P. (2021). A review on micro-milling: Recent advances and future trends. *The International Journal of Advanced Manufacturing Technology*, *112*, 655–684.

Cao, X., Maharjan, S., Ashfaq, R., Shin, J., & Zhang, Y. S. (2021). Bioprinting of small-diameter blood vessels. *Engineering*, 7(6), 832–844.

Cohen, A., Chen, R., Frodis, U., Wu, M. T., & Folk, C. (2010). Microscale metal additive manufacturing of multi-component medical devices. *Rapid Prototyping Journal*, *16*(3), 209–215.

Diba, M., Koons, G. L., Bedell, M. L., & Mikos, A. G. (2021). 3D printed colloidal biomaterials based on photo-reactive gelatin nanoparticles. *Biomaterials*, *274*, 120871.

Hasan, M., Zhao, J., & Jiang, Z. (2017). A review of modern advancements in micro drilling techniques. *Journal of Manufacturing Processes*, *29*, 343–375.

Hengsteler, J., Kanes, K. A., Khasanova, L., & Momotenko, D. (2023). Beginner's guide to micro-and nanoscale electrochemical additive manufacturing. *Annual Review of Analytical Chemistry*, *16*(1), 71–91.

Khalid, M. Y., Arif, Z. U., Tariq, A., Hossain, M., Khan, K. A., & Umer, R. (2024). 3D printing of magneto-active smart materials for advanced actuators and soft robotics applications. *European Polymer Journal*, *205*, 112718.

Li, X., Ming, P., Ao, S., & Wang, W. (2022). Review of additive electrochemical micro-manufacturing technology. *International Journal of Machine Tools and Manufacture*, *173*, 103848.

Mbugua, N. S., Kang, M., Zhang, Y., Ndiithi, N. J., V. Bertrand, G., & Yao, L. (2020). Electrochemical deposition of Ni, NiCo alloy and NiCo–ceramic composite coatings—A critical review. *Materials*, *13*(16), 3475.

Muldoon, K., Song, Y., Ahmad, Z., Chen, X., & Chang, M. W. (2022). High precision 3D printing for micro to nano scale biomedical and electronic devices. *Micromachines*, *13*(4), 642.

Qin, G., Han, L., Li, S., Niu, S., Liu, H., Zheng, X., & Ming, P. (2024). Enhancing microscale additive manufacturing: Electrolyte-column localized electrochemical deposition for microwire and microdevice substrate connection. *International Journal of Electrochemical Science*, 19, 100683.

Raj, D., Reddy, B. V. R., Maity, S. R., & Pandey, K. M. (2019). Laser beam micromachining of metals: A review. *Materials Today: Proceedings*, *18*, 98–103.

Saxena, K. K., Qian, J., & Reynaerts, D. (2018). A review on process capabilities of electrochemical micromachining and its hybrid variants. *International Journal of Machine Tools and Manufacture*, *127*, 28–56.

Singh, N., Siddiqui, H., Koyalada, B. S. R., Mandal, A., Chauhan, V., Natarajan, S., ... & Kumar, S. (2023). Recent advancements in additive manufacturing (AM) techniques: A forward-looking review. *Metals and Materials International*, *29*(8), 2119–2136.

Vaezi, M., Seitz, H., & Yang, S. (2013). A review on 3D micro-additive manufacturing technologies. *The International Journal of Advanced Manufacturing Technology*, *67*, 1721–1754.

Wang, M., Xu, J., Ren, W., & Yang, Z. (2024). Fabrication of microstructure arrays via localized electrochemical deposition. *Nanomanufacturing and Metrology*, *7*(1), 15.

Wang, P., Sin, W. J., Nai, M. L. S., & Wei, J. (2017). Effects of processing parameters on surface roughness of additive manufactured Ti-6Al-4V via electron beam melting. *Materials*, *10*(10), 1121.

Chapter 8

Novel bioimplant fabrication strategies

Advances in incremental sheet forming and additive manufacturing

Sharad Singh Thakur and Parnika Shrivastava

8.1 INTRODUCTION

Bioimplants, such as artificial joints, dental prostheses, and surgical instruments, are critical components in modern healthcare, playing a vital role in restoring function, improving quality of life, and enhancing patient outcomes. These medical devices require high strength, corrosion resistance, and biocompatibility, to ensure long-term functionality and safety within the human body [1], [2]. Traditionally, bioimplants have been manufactured using conventional techniques like casting, forging, and machining. However, these methods often result in significant material waste, high manufacturing costs, and limited design flexibility, hindering the ability to produce the intricate geometries and patient-tailored designs required for advanced medical devices.

The rapid progress in materials science and manufacturing technologies has led to the development of innovative techniques for bioimplant fabrication, revolutionizing the production of these critical medical devices. Two particularly promising approaches are incremental sheet forming and additive manufacturing, also known as 3D printing [3]. Incremental sheet forming, a flexible and cost-effective metal forming process, allows for the fabrication of custom-fit implants with complex geometries, reduced material usage, and improved mechanical properties [4]. Similarly, 3D printing has enabled the creation of personalized bioimplants with intricate internal structures, enhanced bio integration, and superior mechanical performance, overcoming the limitations of traditional manufacturing methods.

These advanced manufacturing techniques offer several advantages over conventional processes, including improved material efficiency, enhanced design flexibility, and the ability to create highly customized devices tailored to the unique needs and anatomical characteristics of individual patients. By leveraging the capabilities of incremental sheet forming and 3D printing, medical professionals can now deliver more effective and personalized solutions, ultimately leading to better patient outcomes and improved overall well-being.

 DOI: 10.1201/9781003581192-8

8.2 INCREMENTAL SHEET FORMING (ISF) IN BIOIMPLANTS MANUFACTURING

8.2.1 Process overview

Incremental Sheet Forming is an advanced forming process that allows for the creation of complex geometries from sheet metal with minimal tooling requirements. This process can be understood better with the help of the diagram displayed in Figure 8.1. In bioimplant applications, ISF has proven to be an effective method for shaping titanium and other biocompatible metals commonly used in implants. This flexibility and customization offered by ISF make it a valuable technique for manufacturing patient-specific bioimplants that can be tailored to the unique anatomical needs of each individual, leading to improved fit, functionality, and overall patient outcomes.

The key advantages of using incremental sheet forming for bioimplant manufacturing include:

- Improved material utilization and reduced waste compared to traditional subtractive manufacturing techniques like machining [5].
- Ability to produce complex and intricate geometries that are difficult or impossible to achieve with conventional forming methods [4].
- Reduced tooling requirements, resulting in lower production costs and easier automation.
- Enhanced design flexibility, allowing for the creation of customized, patient-specific implants that better integrate with the patient's anatomy.

Several studies have investigated the application of incremental sheet forming to the production of various bioimplants, including orthopedic devices, dental prosthetics, and cardiovascular stents [1], [2]. One study focused on the use of ISF for the fabrication of titanium-based cranial implants, highlighting the process's ability to create complex, asymmetric shapes while maintaining the material's biocompatibility and mechanical properties [1]. Another study explored the use of ISF to manufacture patient-specific hip implants, demonstrating the potential for this technique to improve the fit and function of orthopedic devices.

While incremental sheet forming has shown promise in the bioimplant manufacturing field, there are still some challenges that need to be addressed, such as improving surface finish, enhancing mechanical properties, and ensuring consistent product quality. Ongoing research and development in these areas will be crucial to further advancing the capabilities of ISF and expanding its applications in the healthcare industry.

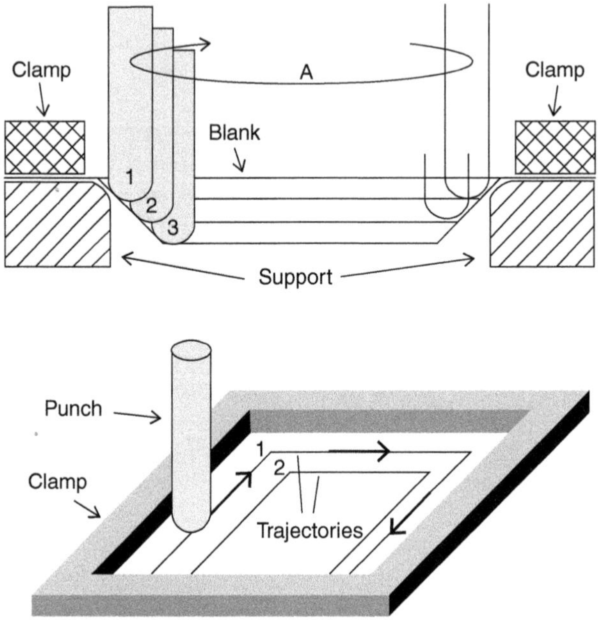

Figure 8.1 Principle of incremental step forming [6].

8.2.2 Advancements in ISF

Recent advancements in ISF for bioimplants include:

8.2.2.1 Automation and robotics

The use of automated and robotic systems in incremental sheet forming has significantly enhanced the precision of the manufacturing process. This increased accuracy has enabled the fabrication of bioimplants with more intricate geometries and complex designs, allowing for the creation of customized medical devices that better match the unique anatomical requirements of individual patients. Robotic ISF systems, for instance, can precisely control the forming tool movements and apply localized forces, enabling the production of patient-specific implants with intricate features and contours that closely mimic the patient's anatomy. This advancement in ISF technology has been crucial for improving the fit, integration, and overall functionality of bioimplants, leading to enhanced patient outcomes and quality of life [1].

8.2.2.2 Hybrid ISF

Researchers have explored the use of hybrid ISF techniques that combine incremental forming with other manufacturing processes to further enhance the capabilities of bioimplant production. The integration of ISF with other advanced manufacturing techniques, such as laser forming and friction stir processing, has significantly improved the material properties of bioimplants, including enhanced fatigue strength and corrosion resistance. These hybrid ISF approaches have been extensively explored to further enhance the mechanical and surface characteristics of bioimplants, effectively addressing common challenges related to long-term implant performance and durability. By combining ISF with complementary processes, researchers have been able to develop bioimplants with superior mechanical integrity, improved surface finishes, and increased resistance to wear and degradation, ultimately contributing to better long-term outcomes for patients. One of the primary motivations for developing hybrid ISF processes is to enhance the mechanical properties of bioimplants, particularly fatigue strength and corrosion resistance, which are crucial for long-term implant success [4].

8.2.2.3 Laser forming

Integrating ISF with laser forming offers a unique advantage by introducing controlled heat input during the forming process. This localized heating can refine the microstructure of the material, leading to increased strength and ductility. Studies have demonstrated that laser-assisted ISF can significantly enhance the fatigue life of titanium implants, making them more resistant to cyclic loading conditions experienced within the body [7–10].

8.2.2.4 Friction stir processing

Friction stir processing is a solid-state joining technique that can also be employed to modify the microstructure and properties of materials. When integrated with ISF, FSP can refine the grain structure and introduce beneficial compressive residual stresses in the implant, enhancing both fatigue strength and corrosion resistance [11].

8.2.2.5 Ultrasonic vibration-assisted ISF

Introducing ultrasonic vibrations during ISF can reduce forming forces and improve surface finish. The vibrations help to distribute the material more evenly, leading to more uniform wall thickness and reduced risk of defects. This process has shown promise for the fabrication of thin-walled bioimplants with complex geometries, as the ultrasonic vibrations can facilitate the local deformation of the material, enabling the creation of intricate features and contours [12].

8.2.3 Tailoring surface characteristics for improved biocompatibility

Beyond mechanical properties, surface characteristics play a critical role in bioimplant performance, influencing protein adsorption, cell adhesion, and ultimately, the integration of the implant with the surrounding tissue. Hybrid ISF processes offer promising avenues for tailoring surface properties to enhance biocompatibility.

8.2.3.1 Laser surface modification

Laser-based techniques can be employed to create micro- and nano-scale surface textures on ISF-formed implants. These textures can mimic the topography of natural tissues, promoting cell adhesion and guiding tissue growth. Studies have shown that laser-treated titanium surfaces exhibit enhanced osteoblast (bone-forming cell) adhesion and proliferation, indicating improved osseointegration potential [13–19].

8.2.3.2 Friction stir processing for surface modification

FSP can be utilized to modify the surface composition and properties of bioimplants. By incorporating bioactive particles into the surface layer during FSP, researchers have demonstrated enhanced bioactivity and bone-forming potential in titanium implants. The integration of ISF with advanced surface modification techniques, such as laser processing and friction stir processing, has enabled the development of bioimplants with enhanced mechanical properties, improved corrosion resistance, and tailored surface characteristics for improved bio compatibility [11].

8.2.3.3 Material research

Research into biocompatible materials, such as titanium and nickel-titanium (NiTi) alloys, has enhanced the applicability of ISF in bioimplants. These materials exhibit desirable properties like high strength-to-weight ratio, corrosion resistance, and biocompatibility, making them well-suited for use in medical implants. Ongoing material research aims to further improve the mechanical, physical, and biological properties of ISF-formed bioimplants, enabling them to better mimic the natural tissues they are designed to replace or support. Titanium and its Alloys: Optimizing for ISF. Titanium and its alloys remain the preferred choice for bioimplants due to their biocompatibility, corrosion resistance, and favorable mechanical properties. However, their inherent properties require careful consideration when applied to ISF. While titanium exhibits good ductility, its high strength can pose challenges for ISF, potentially leading to sheet tearing or springback during forming. Research is exploring modified ISF parameters, such as optimized toolpaths and localized heating, to improve the formability of titanium sheets [20], [21].

8.2.4 Nickel-titanium alloys: Leveraging unique properties in ISF

The unique properties of nickel-titanium alloys, specifically their shape memory effect and superelasticity, open up exciting possibilities for bioimplants manufactured using incremental sheet forming techniques. The shape memory effect of NiTi alloys allows for the creation of complex structures that can be formed in their martensitic state using ISF. These structures can then be implanted and, upon exposure to body heat, utilize the shape memory effect to return to their pre-determined form. This self-expanding capability could revolutionize medical procedures by eliminating the need for invasive surgical expansion techniques, leading to more minimally invasive approaches. Furthermore, the superelasticity of NiTi alloys makes them highly suitable for ISF-fabricated implants that require flexibility and adaptability to conform to complex anatomical contours. This characteristic is particularly beneficial for applications such as cranial plates or spinal cages, where the ability to closely match the implant to the patient's unique anatomy is crucial for successful implantation and long-term stability within the body. The use of NiTi alloys in ISF-fabricated bioimplants offers additional advantages beyond their shape memory and superelastic properties. These alloys exhibit excellent biocompatibility, making them well-suited for direct contact with living tissues without adverse biological reactions. Furthermore, NiTi alloys demonstrate superior corrosion resistance, which is critical for long-term implant performance and safety within the human body. Ongoing research is focused on optimizing the composition, processing, and surface treatments of NiTi alloys to further enhance their compatibility and performance in incremental sheet forming of bioimplants [20–22].

8.3 3D PRINTING IN BIOIMPLANT MANUFACTURING

3D printing, also known as additive manufacturing, has revolutionized the bioimplant sector. By enabling the creation of highly customized and complex designs previously unattainable with traditional methods, 3D printing is driving innovation and improving patient outcomes [23], [24].

8.3.1 Process overview

Unlike subtractive manufacturing that removes material from a larger block, 3D printing constructs bioimplants layer by layer from a digital model. This additive approach offers unparalleled customization and the ability to produce intricate geometries with high precision. Various 3D printing technologies are employed, depending on the material and desired outcome, which are displayed in Figure 8.2.

8.3.1.1 Selective laser sintering

In the selective laser sintering process, a high-powered laser is utilized to selectively fuse powdered materials, such as polymers or metals, layer by layer. This additive manufacturing technique enables the fabrication of intricate geometries and highly customized designs that can be tailored to the unique requirements and anatomical features of individual patients. By building the bioimplant in a layer-by-layer fashion, SLS allows for the creation of complex structures and shapes that would be difficult or impossible to achieve through traditional subtractive manufacturing methods. This flexibility and customization offered by SLS are particularly beneficial for the development of patient-specific bioimplants, ensuring a precise fit and optimal integration with the surrounding tissues [25].

8.3.1.2 Fused deposition modeling

In the fused deposition modeling process, a thermoplastic filament is heated and extruded through a nozzle. As the molten filament is deposited, it solidifies layer by layer, building up the desired object. This additive manufacturing technique allows for the creation of complex geometric shapes and customized designs. FDM is commonly used for the fabrication of bioimplants due to its ability to produce patient-specific structures that closely match the patient's unique anatomy. The versatility of FDM enables the printing of a wide range of biocompatible thermoplastic materials, including polymers such as polylactic acid, polyetheretherketone, and polycaprolactone. These materials can be tailored to exhibit the necessary mechanical properties, degradation rates, and biological compatibility required for successful implantation. The layer-by-layer approach of FDM also allows for the incorporation of additional features, such as internal porosity or surface textures, which can enhance bone ingrowth and integration of the implant with the surrounding tissues. The customization and versatility of FDM make it a valuable tool in the field of bioimplant manufacturing, enabling the production of patient-specific devices that optimize fit, function, and long-term performance [26–34].

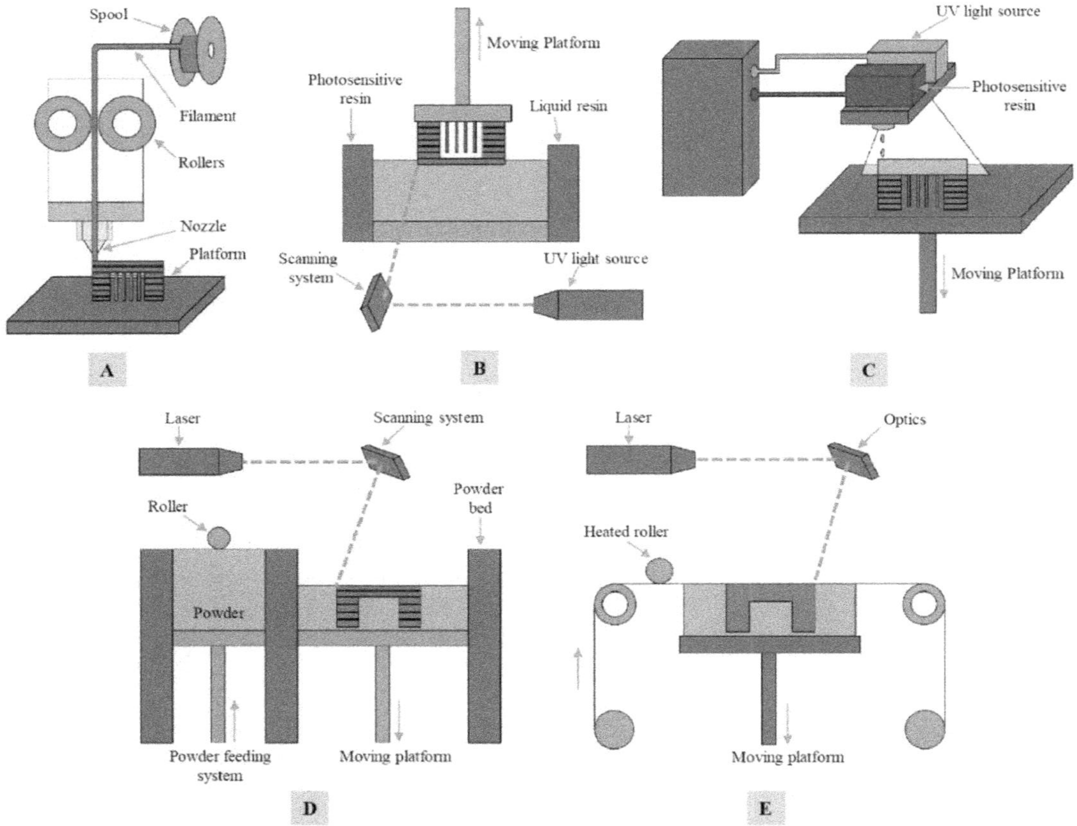

Figure 8.2 Schematic diagram of popular additive manufacturing processes: (A) fused deposition modeling (FDM); (B) stereolithography (SLA); (C) PolyJet printing; (D) selective laser sintering (SLS); (E) laminated object manufacturing (LOM) [35].

8.3.1.3 Direct metal laser sintering

Similar to SLS, but specifically designed for metal powders, DMLS uses a laser to melt and fuse the metal particles, creating highly dense and complex metal implants [25].

8.3.2 Advancements in 3D printing for bioimplants

The field of 3D printing for bioimplants is rapidly evolving, with ongoing advancements pushing the boundaries of what's possible:

8.3.2.1 Bioprinting

This cutting-edge technology enables the printing of living cells and biomaterials, paving the way for the creation of functional tissues and organs. Bioprinting holds immense potential for regenerative medicine, offering the possibility of replacing damaged tissues with lab-grown counterparts [36–38].

8.3.2.2 Multi-material printing

Advanced 3D printers can now combine multiple materials within a single printing process. This capability allows for the fabrication of functionally graded implants, where different regions of the implant possess distinct properties tailored to their specific function. For instance, an orthopedic implant could combine a strong, load-bearing metal core with a porous, biocompatible coating to encourage bone ingrowth [39–42].

8.3.2.3 Surface modification

3D printing processes can be carefully optimized to engineer specific surface characteristics on bioimplants, which is crucial for their successful integration and long-term performance within the human body. For instance, by precisely controlling the surface roughness of 3D-printed implants, researchers can enhance the process of osseointegration—the seamless fusion of the implant with the surrounding bone tissue. This improved integration leads to enhanced implant stability and longevity, ultimately benefiting the patient's overall health and quality of life. Advanced 3D printing techniques allow for the tailoring of surface topography, porosity, and other parameters to create an optimal interface between the implant and the host tissue, minimizing the risk of complications and maximizing the implant's functional lifespan [43].

8.3.3 Applications

The applications of 3D printing in bioimplant manufacturing are vast and continue to expand:

8.3.3.1 Orthopedic implants

Custom-designed hip, knee, and spinal implants can be created using 3D printing, ensuring an optimal fit for each patient's unique anatomy. This personalized approach leads to improved implant stability, reduced recovery times, and better long-term outcomes [43–45].

8.3.3.2 Dental prosthetics

3D printing has revolutionized the production of dental implants, crowns, and bridges. The technology allows for the creation of highly accurate and aesthetically pleasing dental restorations that seamlessly integrate with the patient's existing teeth. This personalized approach enables the fabrication of customized prosthetics that closely match the individual's unique dental anatomy, resulting in a natural-looking and comfortable fit. Furthermore, 3D printing facilitates the rapid and efficient production of these dental restorations, reducing the overall treatment time and improving the patient's overall experience [46–50].

8.3.3.3 Cranial and maxillofacial implants

3D printing has revolutionized the manufacturing of patient-specific cranial plates and facial reconstruction implants. This advanced technology enables the creation of highly customized implants that are tailored to precisely match the unique anatomy of each individual patient. By leveraging 3D scanning and computer-aided design, these implants can be designed to seamlessly integrate with the patient's natural bone structure, restoring both the form and functional integrity of the affected areas. This personalized approach is particularly beneficial for complex craniofacial deformities or injuries, where the ability to accurately replicate the patient's unique anatomical features is crucial for achieving optimal surgical outcomes and improving the patient's quality of life. The customization afforded by 3D printing in this field has revolutionized the way cranial and maxillofacial reconstructions are performed, leading to enhanced implant stability, improved aesthetic results, and faster recovery times for patients [51–55].

The ability to tailor-make implants based on patient-specific data obtained from CT or MRI scans is a key advantage of 3D printing in bioimplant manufacturing. This personalized approach ensures an optimal fit, leading to improved clinical outcomes, faster recovery times, and a reduced risk of complications. As 3D printing technologies continue to advance, we can expect even more innovative applications and breakthroughs in the field of bioimplants, ultimately improving the lives of patients worldwide.

8.4 4D PRINTING IN BIOIMPLANT MANUFACTURING

8.4.1 Process overview

4D printing, an emerging field that builds upon the remarkable capabilities of 3D printing, holds immense promise for the future of biomedical implants. This revolutionary technology incorporates the fourth dimension of time, enabling printed objects to dynamically change their shape or functionality in response to external stimuli such as temperature, moisture, or light. In the realm of biomedicine, 4D printing primarily utilizes innovative smart materials, such as shape memory polymers and hydrogels, that exhibit programmable transformations after the printing process is complete [56]. The advancements of 4D printing over 3D printing can be clearly understood via diagrammatic presentation of 3D and 4D printing, shape memory materials for 4D printing—displayed in Figure 8.3.

The potential applications of 4D printing in biomedical implants are truly remarkable and hold immense promise for transforming personalized medicine. Imagine a bioresorbable stent that can autonomously expand upon deployment within a blocked artery, gradually opening up the passageway and promoting natural healing. This dynamic capability could significantly

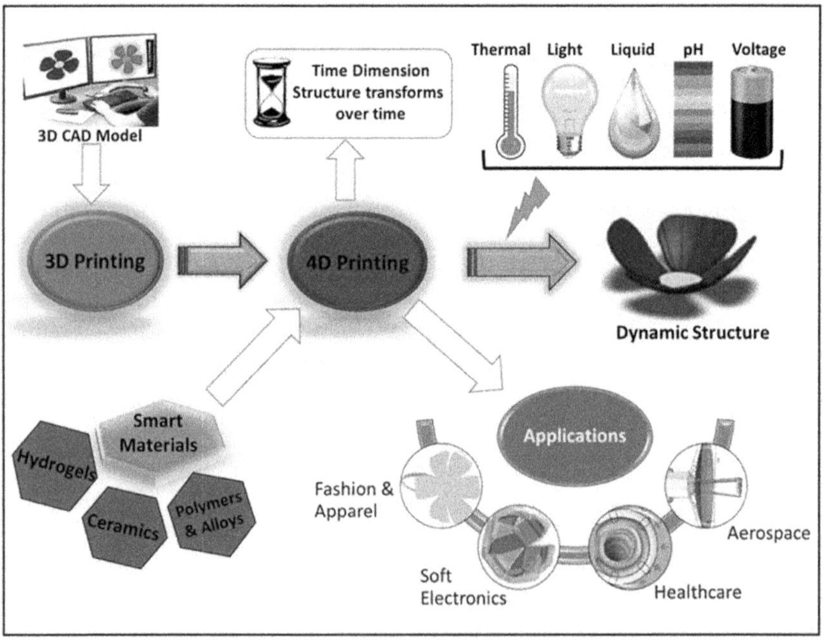

Figure 8.3 Diagrammatic presentation of 3D and 4D printing, shape-memory materials for 4D printing [57].

improve patient outcomes by facilitating the restoration of blood flow without the need for invasive procedures. Similarly, a customized bone scaffold fabricated using 4D printing could gradually adapt its shape to match the unique contours of a healing fracture, providing optimal structural support and seamlessly guiding the natural bone regeneration process. These are just a few captivating examples of how 4D printing can create dynamic, responsive implants that can adapt to the complex and ever-changing environment of the human body, ultimately revolutionizing the way we approach personalized medical treatments and enhance patient care [56], [58], [59].

While 4D printing is still in its early stages, the technology is attracting significant research interest from the scientific community. As it continues to evolve and mature, the translation of 4D printing into clinical applications holds the promise to revolutionize personalized medicine, enabling the development of highly customized and adaptive implants that can dramatically improve patient care and outcomes.

While ISF, 3D, and 4D printing hold immense promise for revolutionizing bioimplant fabrication, several challenges need to be addressed to unlock their full potential and facilitate widespread clinical adoption.

8.5 CHALLENGES

8.5.1 Material development

A key challenge lies in developing biocompatible and mechanically robust materials suitable for long-term implantation. While significant progress has been made, there's a constant need for new materials that can mimic the complex mechanical properties and biological functions of native tissues. This is particularly crucial for 4D printing, which relies heavily on smart materials with predictable and reliable shape-changing behaviors.

8.5.2 Scalability and cost

Scaling up production to meet clinical demands while maintaining cost-effectiveness remains a significant hurdle. Current ISF, 3D, and 4D printing processes can be time-consuming and resource-intensive—limiting their widespread accessibility.

8.5.3 Process control and reproducibility

Ensuring consistent process control and reproducibility is essential for producing reliable and high-quality implants. Variations in material properties, process parameters, and equipment can all impact the final product—necessitating stringent quality control measures.

8.5.4 Regulatory approval

Navigating the regulatory landscape for new manufacturing technologies and materials in the medical device sector can be complex and time-consuming. Meeting stringent safety and efficacy standards is crucial for clinical translation.

8.6 FUTURE SCOPE

8.6.1 Advanced bioprinting

The future of bioprinting lies in developing more sophisticated bioinks that can incorporate multiple cell types and growth factors to create complex, functional tissues. Integrating bioprinting with ISF, 3D, and 4D printing techniques could lead to the fabrication of personalized implants with enhanced bioactivity and regenerative capabilities.

8.6.2 Artificial intelligence and machine learning

AI and ML algorithms can be leveraged to optimize process parameters, predict material behavior, and personalize implant designs based on patient-specific data. This data-driven approach can significantly improve implant performance and reduce development time.

8.6.3 In-situ printing and biofabrication

Research into in-situ printing aims to develop technologies that can directly print or biofabricate implants within the body, minimizing invasiveness and reducing the need for complex surgical procedures.

8.6.4 Hybrid manufacturing

Combining the strengths of ISF, 3D, and 4D printing with other manufacturing techniques, such as biomimetic surface modifications or microfluidic integration, can lead to the development of next-generation implants with enhanced functionality and performance.

Addressing these challenges and pursuing these future directions will pave the way for ISF, 3D, and 4D printing to revolutionize the field of bioimplant manufacturing, leading to more personalized, effective, and accessible treatments for patients worldwide.

8.7 CONCLUSION

The advancements in incremental sheet forming, 3D printing, and 4D printing have opened up unprecedented possibilities for the development of personalized and adaptive biomedical implants. These transformative technologies offer unparalleled capabilities in creating highly customized, intricate, and responsive implants that hold immense potential to improve patient care and outcomes. The ability to tailor implants to the unique anatomical requirements of individual patients, combined with the potential to incorporate smart materials that can dynamically adapt to the body's environment, promises a future where medical interventions are more effective and less invasive. However, realizing the full potential of these technologies requires overcoming significant challenges. Developing novel biocompatible materials with enhanced properties, ensuring scalable and cost-effective production processes, maintaining stringent quality control, and navigating the complex regulatory landscape are all critical hurdles that must be addressed. Despite these challenges, the future of bioimplant fabrication is promising. Ongoing research in advanced bioprinting, the incorporation of artificial intelligence and machine learning for optimized design and fabrication, and the exploration of in-situ printing and hybrid manufacturing techniques, all point towards a future where personalized implants can seamlessly integrate with the human body—promoting healing, restoring function, and ultimately enhancing the quality of life for patients worldwide. As these technologies continue to evolve and mature, a future where the boundaries between biology and engineering become increasingly blurred, leading to truly revolutionary advancements in healthcare, can be anticipated.

REFERENCES

[1] Cheng, Z., Li, Y., Xu, C., Liu, Y., Ghafoor, S., & Li, F. (2020). Incremental sheet forming towards biomedical implants: A review. *Journal of Materials Research and Technology*, 9(5), 11571–11584. https://doi.org/10.1016/j.jmrt.2020.04.096.

[2] C. W. Kang and F. Z. Fang, "State of the art of bioimplants manufacturing: Part I," *Adv Manuf*, vol. 6, no. 1, pp. 20–40, Mar. 2018, doi: 10.1007/s40436-017-0207-4.

[3] H. N. Chia and B. M. Wu, "Recent advances in 3D printing of biomaterials," *J Biol Eng*, vol. 9, no. 1, Mar. 2015, doi: 10.1186/s13036-015-0001-4.

[4] R. Araújo, P. Teixeira, M. B. Silva, A. Reis, and P. A. F. Martins, "Single point incremental forming of a medical implant," in *Key Engineering Materials*, Trans Tech Publications Ltd, 2013, pp. 1388–1393. doi: 10.4028/www.scientific.net/KEM.554-557.1388.

[5] B. Lu *et al.* Yang, Y., Ma, Z., Chen, L., & Wang, J. (2014). *Mechanism investigation of friction-related effects in single point incremental forming using a developed oblique roller-ball tool.* International Journal of Machine Tools and Manufacture, 85, 14–29. https://doi.org/10.1016/j.ijmachtools.2014.04.007

[6] Emmens, W. C., Sebastiani, G., & van den Boogaard, A. H. (2010). The technology of incremental sheet forming—A brief review of the history. *Journal of Materials Processing Technology*, 210(8), 981–997. https://doi.org/10.1016/j.jmatprotec.2010.02.014

[7] P. J. McGrath and C. J. Hughes, "Experimental fatigue performance of laser-formed components," *Opt Lasers Eng*, vol. 45, no. 3, pp. 423–430, Mar. 2007, doi: 10.1016/j.optlaseng.2006.09.004.
[8] Araghi, B. T., et al. (2011). Review on the development of a hybrid incremental sheet forming system for small batch sizes and individualized production. *Production Engineering*, 5(3), 353–362. https://doi.org/10.1007/s11740-011-0325-y
[9] A. Göttmann *et al.*, "Laser-assisted asymmetric incremental sheet forming of titanium sheet metal parts," *J. Prod. Eng*, vol. 5, no. 3, pp. 263–271, Jun. 2011, doi: 10.1007/s11740-011-0299-9.
[10] G. Dearden and S. P. Edwardson, "Some recent developments in two-and three-dimensional laser forming for 'macro' and 'micro' applications," 2003. [Online]. Available: http://iopscience.iop.org/1464-4258/5/4/352
[11] C. Zhu *et al.*, "Microstructures, mechanical, and biological properties of a novel Ti-6V-4V/zinc surface nanocomposite prepared by friction stir processing," *Int J Nanomedicine*, vol. 13, pp. 1881–1898, Mar. 2018, doi: 10.2147/IJN.S154260.
[12] V. Satpute, D. Huo, J. Hedley, and M. Elgendy, "Design of a novel 2D ultrasonic transducer for 2D high-frequency vibration–assisted micromachining," *Int J Adv Manuf Tech*, vol. 126, no. 3–4, pp. 1035–1053, May 2023, doi: 10.1007/s00170-023-11154-1.
[13] R. Olsson, J. Powell, A. Palmquist, R. Brånemark, J. Frostevarg, and A. F. H. Kaplan, "Formation of osseointegrating (bone integrating) surfaces on titanium by laser irradiation," *J Laser Appl*, vol. 31, no. 2, May 2019, doi: 10.2351/1.5096075.
[14] J. I. Rosales-Leal *et al.*, "Effect of roughness, wettability and morphology of engineered titanium surfaces on osteoblast-like cell adhesion," *Colloids Surf A Physicochem Eng Asp*, vol. 365, no. 1–3, pp. 222–229, 2010, doi: 10.1016/j.colsurfa.2009.12.017.
[15] R. Motzfeld, C. Covarrubias, L. Gómez, F. Bastias, and M. Maureira, "A comparative study on the microstructural and antibacterial properties of Laser – textured and SLA dental implants," *Int J Interdiscip Dent*, vol. 14, no. 3, pp. 222–225, Dec. 2021, doi: 10.4067/s2452-55882021000300222.
[16] M. Marticorena, G. Corti, D. Olmedo, M. B. Guglielmotti, and S. Duhalde, "Laser surface modification of Ti implants to improve osseointegration," *J Phys Conf Ser*, vol. 59, no. 1, pp. 662–665, Apr. 2007, doi: 10.1088/1742-6596/59/1/139.
[17] F. A. Shah, M. L. Johansson, O. Omar, H. Simonsson, A. Palmquist, and P. Thomsen, "Laser-modified surface enhances osseointegration and biomechanical anchorage of commercially pure titanium implants for bone-anchored hearing systems," *PLoS One*, vol. 11, no. 6, pp. 1–24, Jun. 2016, doi: 10.1371/journal.pone.0157504.
[18] Souza, J. C. M., et al. (2019). Nano-scale modification of titanium implant surfaces to enhance osseointegration. *Acta Materialia Inc Biomaterialia*, 94, 112–131. https://doi.org/10.1016/j.actbio.2019.05
[19] S. Allegrini Jr, M. Yoshimoto, M. Barbosa Salles, and A. H. de Almeida Bressiani, "Biologic response to titanium implants with laser-treated

surfaces," *Int J Oral Maxillofac Implants*, vol. 29, no. 1, pp. 63–70, 2014, doi: 10.11607/jomi.3213.
[20] Elahinia, M. H., Hashemi, M., Tabesh, M., & Bhaduri, S. B. (2012). Manufacturing and processing of NiTi implants: A review. *Progress in Materials Science*, 57(5), 911–946. 2012, Elsevier Ltd. doi: 10.1016/j.pmatsci.2011.11.001.
[21] Mantripragada, V. P., Lecka-Czernik, B., Ebraheim, N. A., & Jayasuriya, A. C. (2013). An overview of recent advances in designing orthopedic and craniofacial implants. *Journal of Biomedical Materials Research Part A*, 101(11), 3349–3364. https://doi.org/10.1002/jbm.a.34605.
[22] K. V. Sergienko *et al.*, "Investigation of static properties of medical alloys Ti-(20-30)Nb-(10-13)Ta-5Zr," in *IOP Conference Series: Materials Science and Engineering*, Institute of Physics Publishing, Apr. 2018. doi: 10.1088/1757-899X/347/1/012049.
[23] Sanicola, H. W., et al. (2020). Guidelines for establishing a 3-D printing bio fabrication laboratory. *Biotechnology Advances*, 46, 107652. doi: 10.1016/j.biotechadv.2020.107652.
[24] Ghofa, A. A., & Önöral, Ö. (2023). An assessment of the passivity of the fit of multiunit screw-retained implant frameworks manufactured by using additive and subtractive technologies. *The Journal of Prosthetic Dentistry*, 129(3), 440–446. https://doi.org/10.1016/j.prosdent.2021.06.022
[25] Duan, B., & Wang, M. (2011). Selective laser sintering and its application in biomedical engineering. *MRS Bulletin*, 36(12), 998–1005. https://doi.org/10.1557/mrs.2011.270
[26] Winarso, R., Anggoro, P. W., Ismail, R., Jamari, J., & Bayuseno, A. P. (2022). Application of fused deposition modeling (FDM) on bone scaffold manufacturing process: A review. *Heliyon*, 8(11), e11701. https://doi.org/10.1016/j.heliyon.2022.e11701.
[27] Sathies, T., Senthil, P., & Anoop, M. S. (2020). A review on advancements in applications of fused deposition modelling process. *Rapid Prototyping Journal*, 26(4), 669–687. https://doi.org/10.1108/RPJ-08-2018-0199.
[28] V. Dhinakaran, K. P. M. Kumar, P. M. B. Ram, M. Ravichandran, and M. Vinayagamoorthy, "A review on recent advancements in fused deposition modeling," in *Materials Today: Proceedings*, Elsevier Ltd, Jan. 2020, pp. 752–756. doi: 10.1016/j.matpr.2019.12.036.
[29] M. Cicciù *et al.*, "Prosthetic and mechanical parameters of the facial bone under the load of different dental implant shapes: A parametric study," *Prosthesis*, vol. 1, no. 1, pp. 41–53, Dec. 2019, doi: 10.3390/prosthesis1010006.
[30] P. Szarlej *et al.*, "Composite polyurethane-polylactide (Pur/pla) flexible filaments for 3d fused filament fabrication (fff) of antibacterial wound dressings for skin regeneration," *Materials*, vol. 14, no. 20, Oct. 2021, doi: 10.3390/ma14206054.
[31] D. Bourell *et al.*, "Fused deposition modeling of patient'specific polymethylmethacrylate implants," *Rapid Prototyp J*, vol. 16, no. 3, pp. 164–173, Apr. 2010, doi: 10.1108/13552541011034825.
[32] A. Alafaghani, A. Qattawi, B. Alrawi, and A. Guzman, "Experimental optimization of fused deposition modelling processing parameters: A

design-for-manufacturing approach," in *Procedia Manufacturing*, Elsevier B.V., 2017, pp. 791–803. doi: 10.1016/j.promfg.2017.07.079.

[33] E. Ceretti, P. Ginestra, P. I. Neto, A. Fiorentino, and J. V. L. Da Silva, "Multi-layered scaffolds production via fused deposition modeling (FDM) Using an open source 3D printer: Process parameters optimization for dimensional accuracy and design reproducibility," in *Procedia CIRP*, Elsevier B.V., 2017, pp. 13–18. doi: 10.1016/j.procir.2017.04.042.

[34] W. Z. Wu, P. Geng, J. Zhao, Y. Zhang, D. W. Rosen, and H. B. Zhang, "Manufacture and thermal deformation analysis of semicrystalline polymer polyether ether ketone by 3D printing," *Materials Research Innovations*, vol. 18, pp. S5–12–S5-16, Aug. 2014, doi: 10.1179/1432891714Z.000000000898.

[35] Mobarak, M. H., et al. (2023). Recent advances of additive manufacturing in implant fabrication – A review. *Additive Manufacturing Letters*, 7, 100462. https://doi.org/10.1016/j.apsadv.2023.100462

[36] A. Skardal, "Bioprinting essentials of cell and protein viability," in *Essentials of 3D Biofabrication and Translation*, Elsevier Inc., 2015, pp. 1–17. doi: 10.1016/B978-0-12-800972-7.00001-3.

[37] S. Banudevi, "Current perspectives on printing technology for biomedical applications," *Biochemistry & Physiology: Open Access*, vol. 05, no. 03, 2016, doi: 10.4172/2168-9652.1000e154.

[38] B. Shokoohian, B. Negahdari, and M. Vosough, "Bio-printing damaged tissues: A novel approach in regenerative medicine," *Modern Medical Laboratory Journal*, vol. 2, no. 2, pp. 113–117, Jun. 2019, doi: 10.30699/mmlj17.2.1.1.

[39] S. Arabnejad Khanoki and D. Pasini, "The fatigue design of a bone preserving hip implant with functionally graded cellular material," 2013. [Online]. Available: www.asme.org/about-asme/terms-of-use.

[40] Van Hengel, I. A. J., et al. (2020). Functionality-packed additively manufactured porous titanium implants. *Materials Today Bio*, 7, 100060. https://doi.org/10.1016/j.mtbio.2020.100060

[41] Putra, N. E., Mirzaali, M. J., Apachitei, I., Zhou, J., & Zadpoor, A. A. (2020). Multi-material additive manufacturing technologies for Ti-, Mg-, and Fe-based biomaterials for bone substitution. *Acta Biomaterialia*, 108, 3–22. https://doi.org/10.1016/j.actbio.2020.03.037

[42] Parthasarathy, J. C. M., Starly, B., & Raman, S. (2011). A design for the additive manufacture of functionally graded porous structures with tailored mechanical properties for biomedical applications. *Journal of Manufacturing Processes*, 13(2), 160–170. https://doi.org/10.1016/j.jmapro.2011.01.004

[43] N. Nagarajan, A. Dupret-Bories, E. Karabulut, P. Zorlutuna, and N. E. Vrana, "Enabling personalized implant and controllable development through 3D printing. *Biotechnology Advances*, 36(5), 1121–1130. doi: 10.1016/j.biotechadv.2018.02.004.

[44] S. H. Woo, M. J. Sung, K. S. Park, and T. R. Yoon, "Three-dimensional-printing technology in hip and pelvic surgery: Current landscape. *Hip &*

Pelvis, 32(1), 1–7," Mar. 01, 2020, *The Korean Hip Society*. doi: 10.5371/hp.2020.32.1.1.

[45] O. Okolie, I. Stachurek, B. Kandasubramanian, and J. Njuguna, "3d printing for hip implant applications: A review. *Polymers*, 12(11), 2682," Nov. 02, 2020, MDPI AG. doi: 10.3390/polym12112682.

[46] T. Graf, K. J. Erdelt, J. F. Güth, D. Edelhoff, O. Schubert, and J. Schweiger, "Influence of pre-treatment and artificial aging on the retention of 3D-printed permanent composite crowns," *Biomedicines*, vol. 10, no. 9, Sep. 2022, doi: 10.3390/biomedicines10092186.

[47] Javaid, M., & Haleem, A. (2019). Current status and applications of additive manufacturing in dentistry: A literature-based review. *Journal of Oral Biology and Craniofacial Research*, 9(3), 179–185. https://doi.org/10.1016/j.jobcr.2019.04.004

[48] Oberoi, G., Nitsch, S., Edelmayer, M., Janjic, K., Müller, A. S., & Agis, H. (2018). 3D printing—encompassing the facets of dentistry. *Frontiers in Bioengineering and Biotechnology*, 6, 172. https://doi.org/10.3389/fbioe.2018.00172

[49] A. Kessler, R. Hickel, and M. Reymus, "3D printing in dentistry-state of the art," *Oper Dent*, vol. 45, no. 1, pp. 30–40, Jan. 2020, doi: 10.2341/18-229-L.

[50] Schweiger, J., Edelhoff, D., & Güth, J. F. (2021). 3D printing in digital prosthetic dentistry: An overview of recent developments in additive manufacturing. *Journal of Clinical Medicine*, 10(9), 2010. https://doi.org/10.3390/jcm10092010.

[51] M. Matias, H. Zenha, and H. Costa, "Three-dimensional printing: Custom-made implants for craniomaxillofacial reconstructive surgery," *Craniomaxillofac Trauma Reconstr*, vol. 10, no. 2, pp. 089–098, Jun. 2017, doi: 10.1055/s-0036-1594277.

[52] A. De La Peña, J. De La Peña-Brambila, J. Pérez-De La Torre, M. Ochoa, and G. J. Gallardo, "Low-cost customized cranioplasty using a 3D digital printing model: A case report," *3D Print Med*, vol. 4, no. 1, Dec. 2018, doi: 10.1186/s41205-018-0026-7.

[53] E. K. Park *et al.*, "Cranioplasty enhanced by three-dimensional printing: Custom-made three-dimensional-printed titanium implants for skull defects," *J. Craniofacial Surg*, vol. 27, no. 4, pp. 943–949, 2016, doi: 10.1097/SCS.0000000000002656.

[54] Jindal, S., Manzoor, F., Haslam, N., & Mancuso, E. (2020). 3D printed composite materials for craniofacial implants: Current concepts challenges and future directions. *The International Journal of Advanced Manufacturing Technology*, 108, 2373–2392. https://doi.org/10.1007/s00170-020-06397-1

[55] F. Ebel *et al.*, "Clinical and patient-reported outcome after patient-specific 3D printer-assisted cranioplasty," *Neurosurg Rev*, vol. 46, no. 1, Dec. 2023, doi: 10.1007/s10143-023-02000-9.

[56] Piedade, A. P. (2019). 4D printing: The shape-morphing in additive manufacturing. *Journal of Functional Biomaterials*, 10(1), 9. https://doi.org/10.3390/jfb10010009,"

[57] Mahmood, A., Akram, T., Shenggui, C., & Chen, H. (2023). Revolutionizing manufacturing: A review of 4D printing materials, stimuli, and cutting-edge applications. *Composites Part B: Engineering*, 266, 110952. https://doi.org/10.1016/j.compositesb.2023.110952
[58] Bajpai, A., Baigent, A., Raghav, S., Ó Brádaigh, C., Koutsos, V., & Radacsi, N. (2020). 4D printing: Materials, technologies, and future applications in the biomedical field. *Sustainability*, 12(24), 10628. https://doi.org/10.3390/su122410628
[59] V. Serpooshan, J. B. Hu, O. Chirikian, D. A. Hu, M. Mahmoudi, and S. M. Wu, "4D printing of actuating cardiac tissue," in *3D Printing Applications in Cardiovascular Medicine*, Elsevier, 2018, pp. 153–162. doi: 10.1016/B978-0-12-803917-5.00008-0.

Chapter 9

Revolutionizing breast cancer treatment with 2.45 GHz microwave hyperthermia and phased array technology

Ajay Kumar, Nitesh Kashyap, Ashish Raman, and Swapnil Shrivastava

9.1 INTRODUCTION

Hyperthermia has emerged as a revolutionary modality in breast cancer treatment, leveraging precise thermal energy to enhance the effectiveness of traditional therapies such as chemotherapy and radiotherapy. Among the various technologies available, microwave hyperthermia using phased array systems operating at 2.45 GHz has gained prominence due to its ability to deliver targeted and controlled heating to malignant tissues. This frequency strikes an optimal balance between tissue penetration and selective energy deposition, making it highly effective for deep-seated tumor treatment. Phased array antenna systems allow dynamic beamforming through amplitude and phase adjustments of individual antenna elements. This enables the precise focusing of microwave energy on tumor sites while minimizing damage to surrounding healthy tissues. Coupled with advanced thermal monitoring and feedback mechanisms, these systems ensure consistent maintenance of therapeutic temperatures (42–45°C) for effective treatment with minimal side effects. Recent advancements in phased array configurations have significantly improved specific absorption rate (SAR) localization, uniform energy distribution, and patient safety. Integrating real-time feedback systems further enhances treatment precision, paving the way for broader clinical adoption. This study explores the potential of a 2.45 GHz phased array system for microwave hyperthermia, emphasizing its precision, adaptability, and safety in breast cancer therapy.

9.2 ADVANCEMENTS IN CANCER THERAPY USING MICROWAVE HYPERTHERMIA

In recent years, microwave hyperthermia has emerged as a transformative approach in cancer treatment, leveraging the unique ability of electromagnetic waves to heat cancerous tissues selectively. Unlike conventional methods, hyperthermia enhances the therapeutic outcomes of radiotherapy and chemotherapy by increasing tumor oxygenation, improving drug

DOI: 10.1201/9781003581192-9

delivery, and stimulating anti-tumor immune responses. Among the microwave frequencies, 2.45 GHz has proven to be highly effective, offering a balance between penetration depth and energy absorption. By utilizing phased array systems, microwave hyperthermia achieves precise energy targeting, enabling focused heating of tumor sites while sparing surrounding healthy tissues. This innovation marks a significant step forward in non-invasive cancer treatment, offering a safer and more adaptable alternative to traditional invasive therapies.

Hyperthermia has emerged as a groundbreaking adjunct to conventional cancer therapies, leveraging localized heating to target malignant tissues while preserving healthy cells. By raising the temperature of tumor regions to 42–45°C, this approach disrupts cancer cell growth, enhances drug efficacy, and improves radiotherapy outcomes by increasing tumor oxygenation and promoting cellular sensitivity. In this context, microwave hyperthermia, particularly at the 2.45 GHz frequency, has garnered attention due to its ability to penetrate deeper tissues effectively while providing precise energy control. Integrating phased array antenna systems into hyperthermia treatments marks a pivotal advancement in this field. These systems utilize dynamic beamforming capabilities, enabling the fine-tuning of energy delivery to specific tumor sites. By adjusting the phase and amplitude of each antenna element, they achieve focused heating patterns that align with the tumor's geometry and anatomical location. This precision reduces the risk of overheating adjacent healthy tissues, ensuring safer and more effective treatments.

Moreover, recent innovations in real-time feedback and thermal monitoring technologies have significantly enhanced treatment safety and efficiency. These advancements enable continuous adjustments to energy delivery, ensuring that therapeutic temperatures are maintained throughout the procedure. With patient-specific treatment planning, such as adaptive phased array configurations and SAR optimization, microwave hyperthermia represents a paradigm shift in non-invasive cancer therapy. Its adaptability to diverse tumor sizes, locations, and minimal side effects positions it as a cornerstone in modern oncological care.

The phased array antenna system operates at a frequency of 2.45 GHz, chosen for its optimal penetration depth and heating efficacy in biological tissues. Each antenna element is designed using advanced simulation tools like CST Microwave Studio and HFSS, ensuring accurate modeling of electromagnetic behavior. The phased array system employs dynamic beamforming by adjusting the phase and amplitude of each antenna element. This approach allows precise targeting of the tumor site, ensuring focused energy delivery. Thermal feedback mechanisms monitor temperature distributions in real-time, adjusting parameters to maintain therapeutic temperatures. The phased array antenna system operating at 2.45 GHz is a state-of-the-art technology designed to revolutionize medical therapeutics, particularly hyperthermia treatments for cancer. This frequency, widely recognized for its optimal penetration and heating characteristics in biological tissues, ensures precise energy delivery to targeted regions while minimizing harm to surrounding healthy tissues. Each antenna element is meticulously designed using advanced electromagnetic simulation tools such as CST Microwave Studio and HFSS, ensuring accurate modeling and optimization of key parameters like gain, radiation patterns, and Specific Absorption Rate (SAR). A cornerstone of this system is its dynamic beamforming capability, which allows the electromagnetic beam to be steered and focused with exceptional precision, by controlling the phase and amplitude of individual elements. This adaptability is crucial for addressing patient-specific anatomical variations and ensuring effective tumor targeting. Complementing this is an integrated thermal feedback mechanism that monitors real-time temperature distributions, dynamically adjusting power levels to maintain therapeutic temperatures and prevent overheating. Moreover, the phased array system is often integrated with imaging technologies like MRI or ultrasound, providing detailed anatomical data and enabling real-time treatment visualization. This multimodal approach enhances precision, safety, and efficacy, making the phased array system a powerful tool for modern medical interventions. As research progresses, these systems are expected to play an even greater role in personalized medicine, offering solutions for targeted drug delivery, non-invasive surgery, and beyond.

9.3 LITERATURE REVIEW

This chapter reviews the ongoing development of these systems, emphasizing the critical parameters that influence the effectiveness of 2.4 GHz microwave-based hyperthermia treatment. Topics such as the optimization of phased array configurations, the role of frequency selection, and the integration of real-time temperature feedback for treatment adjustments are discussed.

Table 9.1 summarizes diverse research on antenna technology, showcasing significant variations in design and application. Antenna dimensions range from compact designs such as 11×16.7 mm to larger setups like 170×250 mm. These variations align with their intended purposes, with smaller antennas often suited for space-constrained medical applications, while larger designs address broader coverage or higher power requirements.

Performance metrics such as S_{11}, SAR, and gain reflect the antennas' efficiency and application-specific optimizations. For instance, low S_{11} values, commonly below -10 dB, indicate strong impedance matching and minimal signal loss, with some designs achieving impressive figures like <-30 dB. The SAR values differ markedly, with minimal levels around 0.3 W/kg for safety-critical applications and higher values, like 230.75 W/kg, for concentrated energy delivery in therapeutic contexts. Gain also varies significantly;

Table 9.1 Comparative analysis of antenna designs

Ref.	*Dim.(mm)*	*S11*	*SAR(W/kg)*	*Gain*	*Attributes*
[1]	30×40	<-50dB	0.8	NA	Microwave hyperthermia using 2.45 GHz phased array antennas offers precision, adaptability, and safety, revolutionizing breast cancer treatment and paving the way for improved outcomes and broader clinical adoption.
[2]	32 ×32× 3.27	<-25	18.90	NA	The spiral FSS lens applicator improves power deposition and electric field distribution for cancer treatment. It increases PD to 38 mm and EFS to 40×40 mm^2, with minimal heating of healthy tissue. Integrated with a water bolus, it targets deep tumors and provides uniform temperature distribution, resonating at 2.45 GHz.
[3]	1.6×240×150	<-30dB	0.3	NA	The research highlights a significant advancement in antenna technology for medical applications, particularly cancer treatment, by focusing on flexibility, efficiency, and thermal management. The innovative design and thorough simulations underscore this technology's potential impact in improving patient therapeutic outcomes.
[4]	38.393×29.1	<-16dB	NA	NA	This paper provides valuable insights into a microstrip antenna array's design and practical implementation, emphasizing educational applications and cost-effective manufacturing.
[5]	75.85× 57.23×1.6	-38.86	NA	3.121 dBi	The 2.4 GHz Microstrip Patch Antenna is a well-designed component for wireless communication, characterized by its low return loss, excellent VSWR, adequate bandwidth, compact size, and reliable material choice, making it suitable for various applications in modern communication systems.

Table 9.1 (*Cont.*)

Ref.	*Dim.(mm)*	*S11*	*SAR(W/kg)*	*Gain*	*Attributes*
[6]	54 × 54	NA	Na	21.4dBi	The near-field focused folded transmit array antenna is a promising advancement in medical technology, combining a compact design with effective power-focusing capabilities. Its innovative features and validated performance make it a suitable candidate for various therapeutic applications, particularly in targeted heating treatments.
[7]	11×16.7	<-15dB	95.3	NA	The paper highlights the MR-compatible antenna's innovative design and potential applications in enhancing cancer treatment methodologies through hyperthermia.
[8]	37.6×29.15	<-18dB	2.873	NA	This paper highlights the innovative approach to designing and applying the microstrip patch antenna (MSA) for breast cancer treatment, focusing on efficiency, precision, and safety.
[9]	170×250	<-14dB	2.97	NA	These attributes collectively enhance the system's capability to deliver effective hyperthermia treatment for breast cancer, ensuring that the tumor is heated to therapeutic levels while protecting healthy tissues.
[10]	26×26×1.6	-17.46 dB	230.75	-5.1dBi	This work highlights the T-slot antenna's potential in medical applications, particularly for hyperthermia therapy, while ensuring safety and effectiveness in treatment delivery.
[11]	25.04×3.95	<-10 dB	1.68	8dBi	These attributes collectively enhance the multi-resonance applicator (MRA) effectiveness as a treatment tool, making it a promising option for improving outcomes in microwave hyperthermia therapy.
[12]	50×2	NA	1.86	NA	The approach collectively enhances the understanding of how electromagnetic hyperthermia can be effectively applied in breast cancer treatment, particularly through optimized dipole antenna arrays.

(*continued*)

Table 9.1 (Cont.)

Ref.	*Dim.(mm)*	*S11*	*SAR(W/kg)*	*Gain*	*Attributes*
[13]	65.6×3.6	<-14dB	2.96	NA	The hyperthermia treatment method using a grid array antenna for breast cancer is compact, wideband, and easy to deploy. It delivers high power density to the tumor with minimal impact on healthy tissue, ensuring selective energy absorption within safe SAR limits.
[14]	65×65×1.6	<-10dB	NA	4.70dB	The study designs compact, cost-effective microstrip antennas for 2.4 GHz using a copper-coated FR-4 substrate and a 50-ohm microstrip feed. A three-slot patch antenna was optimized via CST Microwave Studio for high gain and efficiency.

some antennas exhibit negative values (e.g., -5.1 dBi), while others achieve substantial positive gains, such as 21.4 dBi, catering to applications that demand directional power focus. Many antennas emphasize medical applications, particularly in hyperthermia treatments for cancer. These designs prioritize precision, safety, and efficiency, leveraging compact geometries and advanced materials. Examples include antennas optimized for MR compatibility or those designed for selective energy delivery to tumors, thereby protecting healthy tissues. Communication antennas, in contrast, focus on features like low return loss and bandwidth adequacy, ensuring reliable performance in wireless systems. Additionally, some designs highlight cost-effectiveness and ease of manufacturing, making them suitable for educational or mass-market deployment. Across the studies, a clear trend toward innovation and miniaturization emerges, with efforts to optimize materials, such as FR-4 substrates, and employ advanced simulation tools like CST Microwave Studio. These advancements align with the dual goals of enhancing performance and ensuring practical applicability across varied technological domains. This diversity in design underscores the versatility of antenna technology and its capacity to meet specific demands in medical and communication fields.

Figure 9.1(a) represents an 8-element monopole antenna array with a numerical breast phantom to optimize energy distribution for hyperthermia treatment. The S-parameter graph (S_{11}) (Figure 9.1(b)) evaluates the antenna's reflection coefficient to determine radiation efficiency and

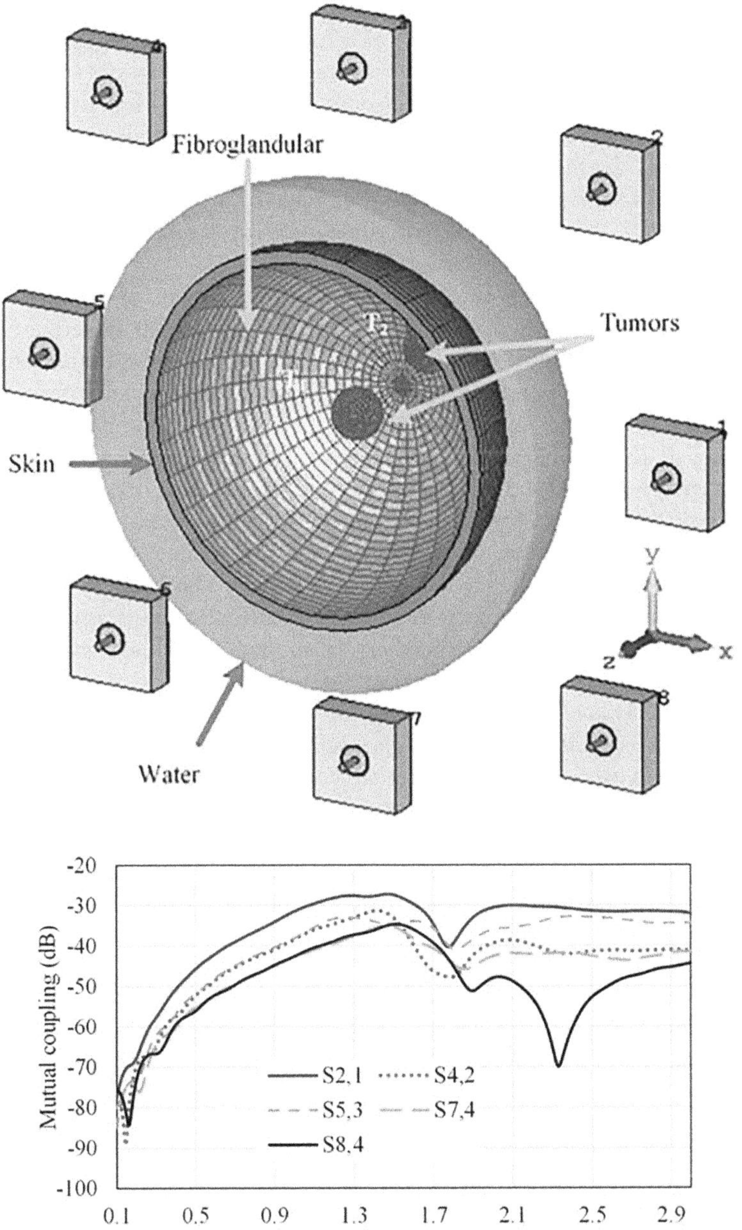

Figure 9.1 (a) Numerical breast phantom surrounded by monopole antennas, (b) The mutual coupling between the adjacent elements in the 8-elements antenna array [1].

impedance matching. Low S_{11} values (below -10 dB) across frequencies (e.g., 0.5–2.4 GHz) confirm effective energy transmission into the medium with minimal reflection. The graph also highlights how changes in medium properties, like saline content, impact antenna performance. Overall, the results demonstrate excellent efficiency and suitability for hyperthermia applications. This study [1] introduces an advanced system for microwave hyperthermia treatment of breast tumors, aiming to achieve precise heating of cancerous tissues while minimizing damage to healthy tissues. The work involves the design of a novel experimental setup supported by numerical modeling and practical experimentation.

A significant aspect of this study is the development of a foam-based, water-immersed monopole antenna designed to radiate effectively in a water-coupling medium. The choice of this medium facilitates efficient energy transfer and patient safety during treatment. The antenna's design prioritizes flexibility, lightweight construction, and compatibility with human soft tissues, particularly the breast. To achieve optimal operation, the antenna was modeled and analyzed for its resonating capabilities across a range of frequencies, focusing on 2.4 GHz. The antenna demonstrated a well-matched S-parameter (S_{11}) response at this frequency, indicating minimal signal reflection and efficient energy radiation. The S_{11} value at 2.4 GHz showed significant energy coupling to the surrounding medium, validating the antenna's suitability for hyperthermia applications. The system's design includes a numerical breast phantom developed using CST Microwave Studio Suite. This phantom replicates the multi-layered structure of human breast tissue, including skin, fibro glandular tissue, and tumors. The dielectric properties of each layer were set to match realistic frequency-dependent values. Tumors were embedded in the phantom strategically, allowing the study to evaluate SAR (specific absorption rate) distribution and energy localization. Using a phased array tool implemented in MATLAB enabled energy delivery optimization. By calculating precise phase shifts, the system achieved constructive interference at tumor sites while reducing unintended energy absorption in healthy tissues. Experimental validation was conducted in a controlled laboratory setup. A saline-filled tank simulated the tissue medium, with the water-immersed antenna operating at multiple frequencies, including 2.4 GHz. The S-parameter analysis confirmed that the antenna maintained efficient energy transfer under these conditions, with S_{11} results indicating strong resonance and minimal energy loss. Temperature rise measurements showed a controlled increase, with the medium's temperature elevating by approximately 6°C over ten minutes. This result highlighted the antenna's effectiveness in focusing energy on the target area. The phased array configuration demonstrated enhanced energy localization. When operating at 2.4 GHz, the SAR distribution maps revealed well-focused energy deposition at tumor locations, preventing overheating in adjacent healthy tissues. This was further supported by simulation results showing optimized E-field patterns and SAR values at this frequency.

In conclusion, the study successfully demonstrates the feasibility of the proposed hyperthermia system for breast tumor treatment. The well-designed monopole antenna and phased array system achieved efficient energy coupling and precise thermal effects. Future work will focus on refining the setup with realistic physical phantoms, incorporating multi-channel operations, and integrating non-invasive imaging systems for improved accuracy and clinical applicability.

The spiral antenna (Figure 9.2(a)), designed on an FR4 substrate, provides aperture coupling for improved bandwidth and efficient energy radiation. The S-parameter graph (Figure 2(b)) shows the applicator's reflection coefficient (S_{11}), demonstrating effective impedance matching at the target frequency of 2.4 GHz. This study [2] presents the design and performance evaluation of a metasurface-based hyperthermia lens applicator optimized

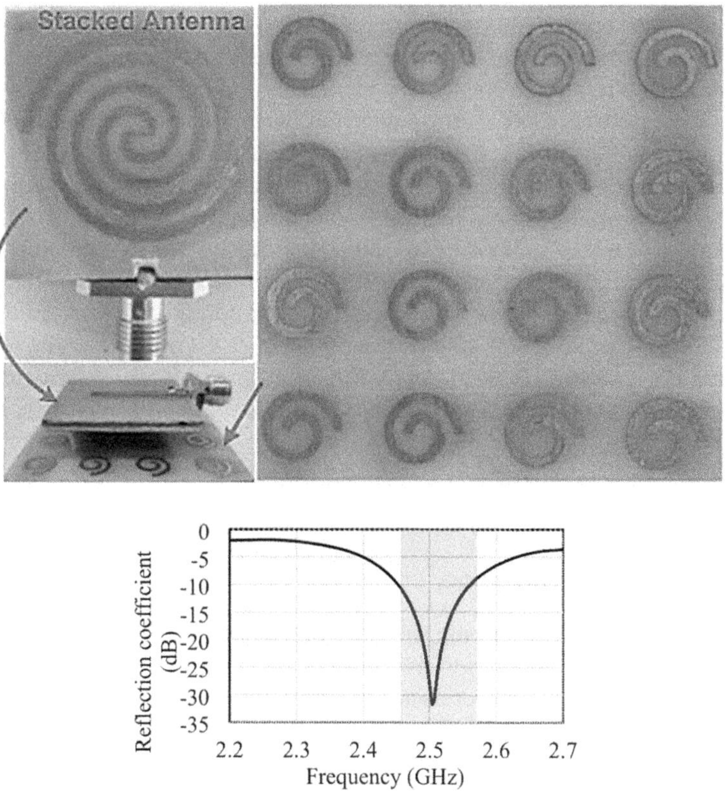

Figure 9.2 (a) Fabricated prototype of the proposed applicator, (b) S-parameter result [2].

for cancer treatment at a frequency of 2.4 GHz. The primary objective is to provide precise and uniform heating of cancerous tissues while minimizing the effect on surrounding healthy tissues. The novel approach combines a spiral antenna with a frequency-selective surface (FSS) metasurface for enhanced performance.

The design features a compact double-spiral antenna constructed on an FR-4 substrate with a dielectric constant 4.4. The antenna's structure ensures aperture coupling, which improves bandwidth and simplifies impedance matching. The spiral antenna is coupled with an FSS metasurface optimized for 2.4 GHz to focus energy and enhance penetration depth. The FSS structure consists of compact spiral unit cells that enhance the directionality of the radiated field and increase the effective field size. The metasurface and antenna are separated by an optimized distance to achieve maximum energy coupling. The system's performance was evaluated in various configurations using simulated and experimental setups. The S-parameter analysis demonstrated effective impedance matching for the simulated heterogeneous phantom (skin, fat, and muscle layers), with the resonance frequency observed at approximately 2.4 GHz. The experimental validation corroborated these findings, showing close agreement between the measured and simulated reflection coefficients (S_{11}). Thermal analysis revealed that the applicator achieves a penetration depth of 38 mm and a specific absorption rate (SAR) sufficient for hyperthermia applications. When operated with an input power of 1.9 W, the applicator raised the tumor's temperature to 44.7°C while maintaining healthy tissue temperatures within safe limits. Integrating a water bolus further improved the system by preventing skin overheating and enhancing energy transfer to deeper tissues. This paper uses the metasurface-based hyperthermia lens applicator to offer an innovative solution for targeted cancer treatment at 2.4 GHz. Its compact size, focused energy delivery, and efficient heating make it suitable for clinical applications, providing an effective alternative for non-invasive hyperthermia treatments.

9.4 CONCLUSION

9.4.1 Simulation results

The microwave hyperthermia system simulation results highlight significant advancements in energy distribution, SAR localization, and temperature control within the target tissues. Numerical modeling demonstrated the capability of the system to deliver precise energy to specific tumor sites while minimizing absorption in surrounding healthy tissues. The simulations showed uniform energy deposition with maximum SAR values concentrated within malignant tissues, ensuring effective heating without overheating adjacent areas. E-field analysis confirmed that beamforming at 2.45 GHz achieved deep penetration into the modeled breast tissue, with field distribution enhancing treatment precision through constructive interference at the target sites. Simulated temperature profiles demonstrated the system's ability to maintain therapeutic heating (42–45°C) within tumor regions over a sustained period while keeping the surrounding healthy tissue below critical thresholds. The system effectively minimized hotspots in non-target areas, improving the overall safety and efficacy of the treatment.

9.4.2 Experimental results

Laboratory experiments validated the simulation findings, confirming the system's efficacy in energy transmission, SAR distribution, and temperature control. The S-parameter analysis demonstrated excellent impedance matching, with S_{11} values consistently below -10 dB across tested frequencies (0.5, 0.9, 1.8, and 2.45 GHz), indicating minimal signal reflection and optimal energy coupling. The antennas used in the experiments maintained stable performance in saline-based mediums, ensuring efficient energy delivery. Real-time temperature monitoring recorded a controlled rise in the medium's temperature over 10 minutes. The experiments also confirmed that energy delivery was focused on the target regions, preventing excessive heating in non-target areas. Experimental SAR measurements closely aligned with the simulation results, further validating the system's ability to deliver focused energy effectively while adhering to safety limits.

9.4.3 System performance

The combined simulation and experimental results illustrate the robust performance of the proposed microwave hyperthermia system. The system achieved precise energy delivery and effective SAR localization, enhancing energy absorption in tumor regions while protecting healthy tissues. Thermal feedback mechanisms ensured consistent therapeutic temperatures without compromising surrounding areas. The modular and adaptable design of the system allows for potential future enhancements, such as multi-channel operations and integration with advanced imaging techniques. Overall, the findings validate the feasibility and effectiveness of the 2.45 GHz microwave hyperthermia system for breast cancer treatment, demonstrating its potential as a safe and precise therapeutic solution.

9.4.4 Clinical implications

Microwave hyperthermia offers a transformative, non-invasive solution for breast cancer treatment, enhancing precision and safety while complementing existing therapies. The 2.45 GHz phased array system enables focused energy delivery to tumors, minimizing damage to healthy tissues and allowing personalized treatment plans, based on tumor size and location. Its integration with real-time temperature monitoring ensures consistent therapeutic effects, reducing complications. Hyperthermia's interaction with radiotherapy and chemotherapy enhances tumor oxygenation and drug sensitivity, potentially improving outcomes while lowering required doses. Beyond breast cancer, this adaptable technology shows promise for treating other malignancies like head and neck cancers, or deep-seated tumors. With further advancements in system design, clinical trials, and standardized protocols, microwave hyperthermia is poised to become a cornerstone of modern oncology, offering safer, more effective, and patient-friendly cancer care. Microwave hyperthermia, driven by advancements in phased array technology, represents a significant leap forward in the non-invasive breast cancer treatment. Operating at 2.45 GHz, this technique provides precise and controlled energy delivery, ensuring targeted heating of malignant tissues while safeguarding healthy surrounding structures. Through dynamic beamforming and SAR localization, it achieves uniform energy distribution and effective temperature control—key factors in enhancing therapeutic outcomes. Integrating microwave hyperthermia with traditional therapies like radiotherapy and chemotherapy offers synergistic benefits, including improved tumor oxygenation, enhanced drug delivery, and sensitization of cancer cells. These capabilities position hyperthermia as a powerful adjunctive therapy that can reduce the required doses of conventional treatments, minimizing the side effects and improving the patient's quality of life. Beyond its application in breast cancer, microwave hyperthermia demonstrates versatility in treating a range of malignancies, including head and neck cancers, cervical tumors, and deep-seated lesions. Its adaptability to diverse anatomical and clinical contexts, and its modular and scalable design, highlight its potential as a universal tool in oncological care. Future advancements, such as integrating multi-channel operations, real-time imaging, and machine learning for energy optimization, will further elevate the precision and efficacy of this technology.

In conclusion, microwave hyperthermia exemplifies the next generation of cancer therapies, bridging the gap between innovation and clinical application. Combining precision, safety, and adaptability can redefine the standard of care in oncology, offering hope for improved patient outcomes and a better quality of life. As research continues to evolve, microwave hyperthermia is poised to become integral to personalized and effective cancer treatment strategies.

REFERENCES

[1] Nizam-Uddin, Abdulkawi, W. M., Elshafiey, I., & Sheta, A.-F. A. (2022). Towards an efficient system for hyperthermia treatment of breast tumors. *Biomedical Signal Processing and Control, 71*, 103084. https://doi.org/10.1016/j.bspc.2021.103084

[2] Sharma, Nitika, et al. "Development of metasurface based hyperthermia lens applicator for heating of cancerous tissues." *Biomedical Engineering Letters 14*.1 (2024): 1–12.

[3] Hossain, S., Alam, T., Rawshan, F., Nahid, M. R., Alam, S., & Rana, M. S. (2024). *Design and analysis of microstrip patch* antenna *for breast tumor detection*. In 2024 International Conference on Advances in Computing, Communication, Electrical, and Smart Systems (iCACCESS), pp. 1–4.

[4] Rojas, Jeanette Mejia, Mario Reyes-Ayala, Edgar Alejandro Andrade-Gonzalez, Sandra Chavez-Sanchez, Hilario Terres-Peña, and Rene Rodriguez-Rivera. "2 x 1 rectangular-patch antenna array at 2.4 GHz." *WSEAS Transactions on Communications 22 (*2023*)*: 49–57. 10.37394/23204.2023.22.5.

[5] Abdulhussein, A. M., Khidhir, A. H., & Naser, A. A. (2021). *2.4 GHz microstrip patch antenna for S-band wireless* communications. Journal of Physics: Conference Series, 2114(1), 012029 (pp. 1–7). IOP Publishing. https://doi.org/10.1088/1742-6596/2114/1/012029

[6] Zainud-Deen, Saber H., Walaa M. Hassan, and Hend A. Malhat. "Near-field focused folded transmitarray antenna for medical applications." *The Applied Computational Electromagnetics Society Journal (ACES*) (2016): 31(3), 315–320.

[7] Raaijmakers, Elles AL, et al. "An MR-compatible antenna and application in a murine superficial hyperthermia applicator." *International Journal of Hyperthermia 34*.6 (2018): 697–703.

[8] Shehata, Rana M., Mohamed I. Badawi, and Nour Eldin Ismail. "Hyperthermia for breast cancer treatment using a slotted microstrip patch antenna array." *Journal of Al-Azhar University Engineering Sector 16*.61 (2021): 1135–1155.

[9] Suseela, Sreekala, and Parveen Wahid. "Breast cancer hyperthermia using a grid array applicator." *2020 SoutheastCon*. pp. 310–313. IEEE., 2020.

[10] Khan, Azharuddin, Satya Kesh Dubey, and Amit Kumar Singh. "Corner T-slot antenna at 2.45 GHz for hyperthermia application." *Journal of Electromagnetic Waves and Applications 38*.4 (2024): 508–521.

[11] Mahmoud, Korany R., and Ahmed M. Montaser. "Design of multiresonance flexible antenna array applicator for breast cancer hyperthermia treatment." *IEEE Access 10* (2022): 93338–93352.

[12] Gas, Piotr, Arkadiusz Miaskowski, and Mahendran Subramanian. "In silico study on tumor-size-dependent thermal profiles inside an anthropomorphic female breast phantom subjected to multi-dipole antenna array." *International Journal of Molecular Sciences 21*.22 (2020): 8597.

[13] Suseela, Sreekala. "Investigations on the use of hyperthermia for breast cancer treatment." (2020).

Sahu, A. K., Misra, N. K., Mounika, K., & Sharma, P. (2022). *Design and performance analysis of MIMO patch antenna using CST* microwave *Studio*. In Smart Systems: Innovations in Computing (Smart Innovation, Systems and Technologies), Springer, pp. 431–441. https://doi.org/10.1007/978-981-16-2877-1_39.

Chapter 10

IoT-based smart health monitoring system with sensor and electronics integration

Navneet Singh, Neha Kumari, and Nikhil Tiwari

INTRODUCTION

Often when someone gets sick, a doctor in the hospital orders to do a number of tests. Being ill makes it challenging for the patient to travel to several locations to undergo the testing. These issues must be eliminated, for which some devices have also been invented.

Nowadays, the health care system is developing to give people better facilities, and technology has played a significant role in this marathon of progress. Technology often makes life simpler for people when applied intelligently. In the Technological integration with patient health monitoring, the technology involved to make this project are:

The technological integration of patient health monitoring systems involves the use of various sensing and communication technologies to enable real-time and efficient monitoring of patients' health conditions. The technologies incorporated in this project include temperature sensors, heart rate sensors, oximeter sensors, ECG sensors, and blood pressure sensors for measuring vital health parameters. In addition, IoT-based communication modules are employed to facilitate the transmission and monitoring of health data. The integration of these technologies enables continuous health monitoring, improves accessibility to patient information, and facilitates effective collaboration between patients and healthcare professionals.

In our research, a system of five different health indices, including body temperature, Blood Pressure, heart rate, pulse oximeter, and ECG can now be measured by a single medical device. IoT based patient health monitoring systems were created so that the condition of the patient may be accurately tracked in real-time and Health care providers are able to do the necessary thing for the good health of the patient.

IoT gives us access to a variety of technologies and modules to focus on or enhance the healthcare system [2], introducing the technology to keep patients safe and healthy, and giving supervisors opportunity to continuously monitor it.

Though, these modules' uses are widespread and have the potential to go even further in the future. In order to effectively monitor health care,

DOI: 10.1201/9781003581192-10

it is also true that many other technical developments may take place in tandem with IoT but not at minimal cost [1]. As a result, since the patient is constantly being monitored by the system, this work can be employed in hospitals as well as for patients who can be continuously monitored while moving from one location to another.

LITERATURE REVIEW

Various reviews about Health Care or monitoring systems have been given. In the past, sensors techniques have also been used in research papers and technical reports about IoT-based health monitoring systems.

Piogea: Effective healthcare promotion can be achieved with the help of IOT technologies. Interaction with doctors in an emergency regarding health-related information is possible, even while working with doctors who are in an emergency, or when there is no doctor available for the patient [3]. The human users may receive alerts based on their health, fitness, and previous medical or genetic history —Brian Blake had said.

Bazzani et al.: has provided details on the Internet of Things (IoT) technology, which he uses to autonomously and continually monitor the patient's activity from a distance [7]. Additionally, a patient can be managed utilizing an IoT paradigm when they activate from home. The IoT idea in this context is tied to the middleware-based architecture layer. Virtus was an event-driven middleware that discussed e-health IoT principles.

Page et al.: has said that there is no accurate way to forecast chronic heart failure; for this reason, a panoramic monitoring system is needed, which is necessary for efficient clinical diagnosis. Additionally, this system will enable ongoing patient monitoring, providing feedback via an automatic alarm for a status report on the patient[5]. A revolutionary virtualization method in this system also enables the doctor to monitor several patients in real-time. This system is highly beneficial for patients with low risk of mortality, including those who are receiving ECG monitoring [9]. As a result, it is necessary to implement transmitting the data to an appropriate database that is well-managed and has an automatic update from the actual data itself.

Harshavardhan B. Patil: The article "Wireless Biomedical Parameter Monitoring System" was published in April 2015 in the International Journal of Engineering Research (IJERT) and Applications. This review paper discusses a ZigBee-based wireless system for monitoring biological parameters. The system can be used to track physiological values for a human subject, including temperature, pulse rate, and blood pressure (whether systolic or diastolic)[6]. The person is electronically monitored in his own home or elsewhere using a variety of sensors to measure various vital signs. To detect falls, impact sensors have been employed. The device transmits an alarm to a receiver unit that is connected to a computer if a person is in medical crisis. This caused an alarm, enabling assistance to be given to the user. For outdoor use, a battery-powered gadget is required. Wireless sensors and communication modules are used in the wireless biological parameter monitoring systems [8].

IoT is used in a variety of ways by both the public and private sectors:
Apple: Applications and gadgets were introduced to help us take care of our health while still at work, such as the Apple Watch, which displays the accelerometer and heart rate of the person. Health apps can provide data on the body's performance.

Sunshine: User data is gathered through smartphone usage and crowdsourcing. Sunshine enables individuals to make the best life decisions in comparison to the rest of the world.

We reviewed some research work on health monitoring systems and looked at previous work on the issue, which used Zigbee technology, Web-services, and other technologies. The keywords for our suggested system are pulse rate sensor, temperature sensing device, blood pressure monitoring unit, and an adaptive part that we will utilize is ESP 32, because it has an inbuilt Wi-Fi module that enables connecting to the internet easier. Additionally, we employed SIM GSM to track patients in real-time. Health parameters without electronic sensors can also be tracked by measurement with conventional tools and observation—only through this system, which benefits patients and those providing healthcare.

SCOPE OF THE PROJECT

In this project, we are connecting the patient to IoT (Internet of Things) and one step ahead, in this present era of internet. In recent days, the population of India has crossed 1.4 Billion and the total number of hospitals are around 8 lakh, and this number is very low when compared to the population. In this situation, the availability of a free bed in the hospital is surplus. If a patient has a normal Blood Pressure problem or Heartbeat problem, then he or she needs 24*7 diagnosis, then the doctor has to admit him/her to the hospital for a few days or a week, and it will occupy a bed. But using this project, the doctor can keep his/her eyes on the patient 24*7—anytime, anywhere; using the internet, the data will upload on thingspeak website using ESP32 as ESP 32, which consist of an inbuilt Wi-Fi module. It has alarm system which will alert, and it will notify the doctor, as well as the family member or loved ones during an emergency: only when Blood Pressure, temperature, and heartbeat will go high. Otherwise, in normal conditions, it has SIM GSM module, which sends a message directly to the family as well as the doctor, that will help them to keep patience for the recovery of the patient in the absence of Internet.

Table 10.1 Literature review of various studies related to patient health monitoring system

Author's name	*Title*	*Year of Publishing*	*Proposed Work*
Emilio Zhuma, Byron Oviedo, and Jorge J. Gómez.	Patient Monitoring System Based on Internet of Things	2016	In order to assist patients with chronic conditions, this study describes a substitute called Internet of Things-based patient monitoring.
J. Jansi Rani, B. Vidhya, and H. Aritha are C. Senthamilarasi.	A Smart Patient Health Monitoring System.	2018	The paper describes a patient monitoring system that uses an Arduino Uno to track several patient health indicators. The Arduino Uno is connected to a cloud database system, which serves as a server, after being connected to the internet.
Shivam Gupta, Shivam Kashaundhan, Prakhar Pratap Singh Gaur, and Divesh Chandra Pandey.	IoT Based Patient Health Monitoring System.	2017	This study demonstrates how to calculate results relating to health conditions in less than one minute. Due to the integration of several medical devices on a single chip, size is also reduced in comparison to the conventional system.
Shola Usha Rani, Bala Vishnu V J, Bhava Vyasa Hari, and Antony Ignatous.	IoT Patient Monitoring System	2017	This study demonstrates how sensor readings are utilized to keep track of any state changes, and when a change occurs, the new state is relayed to AWS IOT through MQTT. It has a simple, incredibly straightforward, and light design.
Md. Kawrshik Shikder, Yousuf, and Rifat Rahman Akash.	IoT Based Real-time Health Monitoring System	2020	In order to run the medical tests digitally and present the results on an OLED display and on their mobile phone app, the device requires five inputs from the patient. By delivering quick results, this technology will cut patient waiting times.
G. Jogar Rao, J. Durg Prasad, P. Karthik, G. Sai Sameer Kumar K, N. Ajay, and K. Anil Kumar.	Health Monitoring System of Patient Using IoT	2020	This study demonstrates that the sensors employed here are essentially accurate and suitable for analytical purposes. As a result, we are using the Thingspeak cloud and the Thingview android app.
Prof. Mini Sreejeth, Richa, Anwesha Das, and Ajeet Kumar Kushwaha.	An IoT based Health Monitoring System using Arduino Uno	2021	Since they may be tracked daily, noted, and saved as a database, the suggested patient health monitoring system can be used extensively in an emergency situation. Based on the Arduino Uno Board, this system.

(continued)

Table 10.1 (*Cont.*)

Author's name	*Title*	*Year of Publishing*	*Proposed Work*
Vikrant Halikar, Pranav Jadhav, Sanket More, S.D.Patil .	Patient Health Monitoring System Using IoT Devices	2022	In this study, a mobile physiological monitoring system that can continually track a patient's heart rate, blood pressure, and other vital signs inside a hospital is described.
Ms. Prachi Patil, Mr. Swapnil Patil, Mr. Gaurav Parab, Ms. Mugdha Salvi	IoT Based Patient Health Monitoring System.	2020	The suggested solution has been put into place, and the Thingspeak cloud channel is now receiving real-time patient information. When the patient's body is fitted with contemporary sensors. A doctor can view the patient's status. The database contains the patient's prior information, which aids the doctor in providing the right care.
Mohit Yadav, Aditya Vardhan, Amarjeet Singh Chauhan, Sanjay Saini	Iot Based Health Monitoring System.	2022	Using Raspberry Pi, a health monitoring system for the Internet of Things was created. Using sensors, the system kept track of body temperature, pulse rate, and the temperature and humidity of the environment. This data is also shown on an IoT dashboard. IoT platform, so the doctor may determine the patient's health and diagnose the patient's ailment using the information received.
Tanmay Patil, Tanish Meshram, Ankit Rai, Manav Dadwal, Prof. N. Narkhede.	Remote Health Monitoring System	2022	The system used sensors to monitor the environment's temperature and humidity as well as the user's body temperature and heart rate. An IoT dashboard also displays this data. IoT platform, allowing the doctor to use the data obtained to assess the patient's health and identify their illness.
E. R. GANESH	Health Monitoring System using Raspberry Pi and IoT	2019	In this paper, a system using a Raspberry Pi and a Pi camera is described. If the threshold value is achieved that instructs patients to consult a doctor, an emergency alert email is sent to the patients.

PROPOSED WORK

Our system will overcome some drawbacks. An ESP 32, a Wi-Fi module, will be used by the suggested system for real-time communication between the patient and the doctor, which is a novel way to employ ESP 32 instead of any Arduino, which does not have an in-built internet system past the current system. The systems already discussed include a health monitoring system that makes use of a raspberry pi, Zigbee, etc. The suggested system will address the shortcomings of the prior system, which prevented real-time communication between patients and doctors. The proposed approach will be beneficial and helpful for patients in the village who do not receive timely care or an appropriate prescription. Although the doctors in villages are likely aware of the prescription, they nevertheless refer patients to specialists, just because of lack of technology or machine for measuring the necessary rates, like pulse rate, ECG, etc., so, at that time, this system will be very helpful.

Even while it aids in providing a patient's family and doctor with instantaneous knowledge of their health status, it also alerts and notifies them.

The major objective of making this device is to monitor the patients and inform the doctors and loved ones. Therefore, we are putting out a creative proposal that makes use of a Patient Health Monitoring system to prevent sudden death rates; that's why we will use sensor & the internet to notify or alert the doctors and patients as well. To track a patient's health, this system uses a temperature sensor, a heart rate sensor, an oxygen sensor, an ECG sensor, and a blood pressure sensor. The sensors are linked with ESP-32 (Wi-Fi-module). To track the patient's health ESP 32 leads to send the data on Thingspeak and to transmit the data, it is connected to an OLED display and a wireless network. Whenever, there will be a greater value than the threshold of any sensor, then in that situation, a patient-related warning via IoT is sent. Then, the doctor or any nurse who is connected with this system, seeing the patient's health, will come soon and treat or take care of the patient as soon as possible. As a result, the patient health monitoring system based on the Internet of Things uses the internet to efficiently monitor patient health.

It also assists users in keeping an eye on the patients and their loved ones, which ultimately saves lives.

Advantages:

- Increases & improves virtual access to care and treatment: Patients are able to reach the facilitation they require nearly anywhere; they will be able to see the temperature, blood pressure, heartbeat rate, pulse at any place, and won't need to stay in the hospital for check-ups.

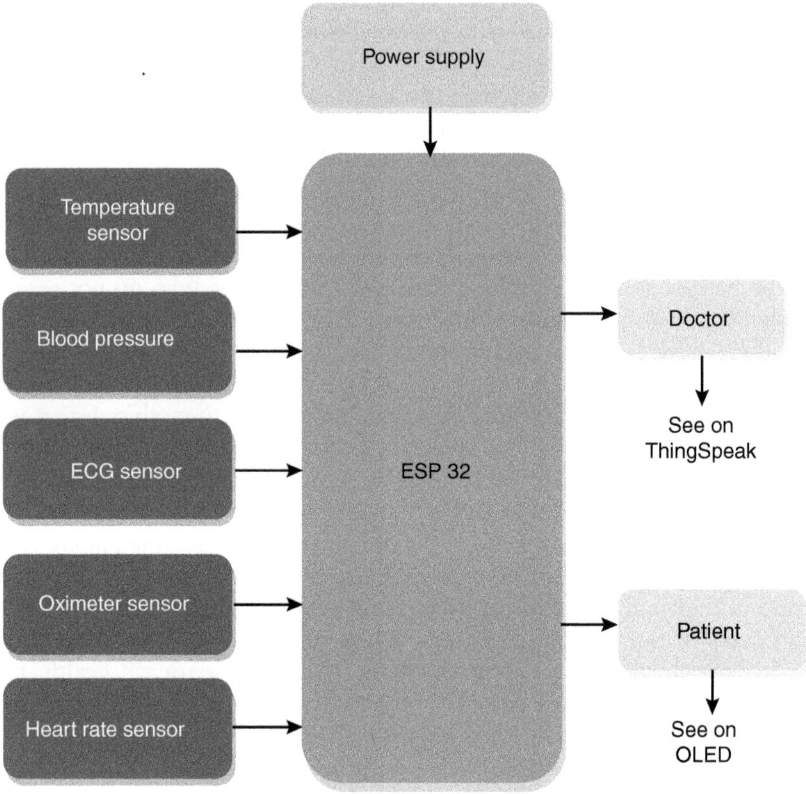

Figure 10.1 Block diagram of patient health monitor system.

- Minimize the costs for both parties: Because this system supports virtual care, it reduces the need for in-person doctor and hospital visits.
- Strengthens patient engagement & experience: Streamlining a system, i.e., easier and more convenient to access—overall, it improves the customer satisfaction. Patients can feel more at ease monitoring their health in the comfort of their homes.

METHODOLOGY

Illustrated diagram of our proposed system is given in Figure 10.1.

Major Components:

Several components will be needed to create a patient health monitoring system; their descriptions are provided below:

ESP 32

The term "**Internet of Things**" refers to the global network made up of billions of physically connected internet-connected gadgets that are all gathering, processing, and sharing data. Now that IoT-based technology has advanced, everything can be transformed into an IoT-enabled application. Despite the market's abundance of IoT-enabled hardware, the ESP32 Module is one of the models that experts and amateurs most frequently employ.

With ESP32, you may use Wi-Fi in station and access point modes.

The benefits of using ESP32 is that it also has high price-performance ratio, compact volume, simple integration with other goods, powerful functionality with lwip protocol support, freertos supporting three modes: Ap, sta, and ap+sta supporting program, simply developable.

Temperature sensor

Temperature is one of the most widely used metrics in a wide range of sectors, including the food, pharmaceutical, medical and life science, machinery and equipment, and almost every other industry.

Patient information is analyzed using a variety of sensors. The carer can offer suitable advice on medical matters.

A temperature sensor is used to gauge how cold or hot an object is and notifies management if there is a temperature disparity. The voltage applied across the diode determines how it functions. The resistance of the diode is exactly proportional to the temperature change. It converts the resistance across the diode into readable units, such as degrees Celsius, Fahrenheit, and centigrade. It is simple to measure once it has been converted to readable units.

ECG sensor

To determine the electrical activity of the human heart, a commercial board called the ECG sensor is employed. An analogue readout can be obtained from this action by creating a chart similar to an electrocardiogram. Electrocardiograms can be highly loud, so the AD8232 chip can be used to cut down on the noise. The ECG sensor functions similarly to an operational amplifier, to assist in receiving a clear signal from the intervals quickly.

Oximeter Sensor

A pulse oximeter sensor is a sensor that measures changes in skin-blood volume and the oxygen saturation of a patient's blood indirectly rather than directly through a blood sample. This results in a photoplethysmogram, which can then be processed to produce further readings.

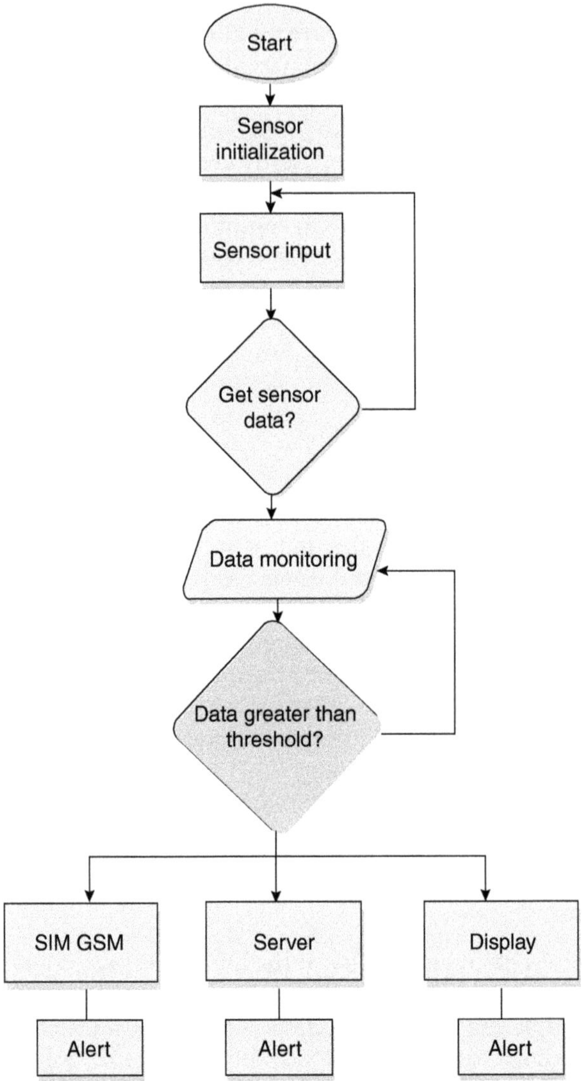

Figure 10.2 Flow chart of the patient health monitoring system.

An electronic processor and two tiny light-emitting diodes (LEDs) facing a photodiode through a translucent area of the patient's body—typically a fingertip or earlobe—make up a conventional pulse oximeter. The wavelength of one LED is red, while the wavelength of the other LED is infrared.

Heart rate sensor

Heart rate sensors monitor the activity of the heart rate.

Your heart's rate is the number of times it beats each minute.

Data about heart rate will be extracted using this sensor.

The electrocardiography method is used by the heart rate sensor:

Electrical (electrocardiography): With each beat, your heart produces a tiny electrical current. Electrically capable heart rate monitors can find and measure that current.

OLED

This OLED is used to see all the details which have been measured by all the sensors added with the patient health monitoring system.

An OLED is a solid-state device that emits light when electricity is applied via nearby electrodes. It is made of a thin, carbon-based semiconductor layer. One of the electrodes must be transparent in order for light to exit the gadget. The electrodes' application of electric current regulates how much light is produced, and the emissive material's choice affects the hue of the light. The majority of devices use a combination of red, green, and blue emitters that can be configured in a variety of ways to produce white light.

FLOW CHART

Any electronic device needs the power supply to start the function. So, in this project, ESP32 will be connected to the power supply, and all sensors, such as those for blood pressure, heart rate, temperature, ECG sensor, and oximeter sensor, will take input from the body in different forms and convert it into electric form, which will be as output to ESP32, and then it will evaluate and send the data to the server displayed on OLED to the user's side. If the value of data (output of all sensors) is more than the threshold, then it sends an alert message to SIM GSM module, and also on the server of the hospital on thingspeak or another website which is made for seeing the data.

CONCLUSION

IoT (Internet of Things) based patient health monitoring system has the ability to measure many health indices by oneself. It would make life easier for all patients, doctors, and family members—thanks to patient health monitoring systems. Both patients and doctors will be able to view the device's outcomes without actually visiting the hospital. The device's goal is to reduce the risk of health problems arising from travel in addition to saving money and time.

To execute the medical tests digitally, the device requires five inputs from the patient using sensor technology. The results are displayed on an OLED display and on Thingspeak. By providing instant results, this device also cuts down on patients' waiting times. With this, the device produces quick results and is inexpensive, so it is affordable to everyone.

The system is also user-friendly and appropriate for the entire human body.

REFERENCES

1. M. Marathi and D. Preethi, "IoT Based Patient Health Monitoring System," *International Journal of Engineering Research & Technology*, Vol. 7,1–5 2019.
2. S. Gupta, S. Keshaun, and D. C. Pandey, "IoT Based Patient Health Monitoring System," *International Research Journal of Engineering and Technology*, Vol. 4, pp. 2016–2019, March 2017.
3. Mariya Chithra Mary, A., Veerakumar, S., & Babu, R. (2018). Health Monitoring *Systems Using IoT*. International Journal of Engineering Research & Technology (IJERT), Volume 6, Issue 7 (ICONNECT – 2018).
4. R. Jegadeesan, G. Vennila, and M. P. Ramya, "Health Monitoring System Using Internet of Things," *International Journal of Engineering Research and Advanced Technology (IJERAT)*, E-ISSN: 2454-6135, Vol. 4, Issue 3, 21–26, March 2018.
5. P. Kumar, S. V. Prasad, and A. Patak, "Design and Implementation of an M-Health System Using Cloud Computing," *International Journal of Innovative Research in Science, Engineering and Technology*, Vol. 5, pp. 2319–8753, 2016.
6. Prasad, N. R., Rokale, V. M., & Prasad, R. J. (2011). A Cooperative Internet of Things (IoT) for Rural Healthcare Monitoring and Control. In Proceedings of the 2nd International Conference on Wireless Communication, Vehicular Technology, Information Theory and Aerospace & Electronic Systems Technology (Wireless VITAE), pp. 1–6. River Publishers.
7. M. Viswas, "A Raspberry Pi-based System for Wireless Sensor Nodes-Based Patient Monitoring. 1693–1696," *International Research Journal of Engineering and Technology (IRJET)*,3(4), 1693–1696. April 2016.
8. S. N. Malodkar and S. D. Mali, "Patient Monitoring System Based on Internet of Things Using Raspberry Pi: Key Features," *Application, and Open Issues, Computer Communication,* Vol. *54,* 2016.
9. J. Gomez, "Patient Monitoring System Based on Internet of Things: A Survey in Computer Networks," Vol. *54*, 2787–2805.
10. B. Giovanni, "Design of IOT Based Smart Health Monitoring and Alert System," *Center for TeleIn Frastuktr*, Aalborg University, Denmark. 2787–2805. Volume 54 (2016)

Chapter 11

Tailoring bioimplants for regenerative medicine

Focus on bone tissue engineering

Amey Dukle and M. Ravi Sankar

11.1 INTRODUCTION

Bone is a vital organ responsible for critical functions such as maintaining shape and posture, protecting vital organs, supporting movements, and acting as a reservoir for essential minerals [1]. Bones are also important for red blood cell production and maintaining the balance of electrolytes in the body [2]. However, despite its strength, it is highly susceptible to damage due to various factors such as trauma, disease, ageing, and congenital defects [3]. Fractures and bone loss can occur when the bone's structural integrity is compromised [4]. Conditions like osteoporosis weaken bone by reducing bone density, making it more prone to fractures [5]. Bacterial infections such as osteomyelitis and bone tumours can also lead to substantial bone loss, leading to severely impaired bone health and function [6]. In the case of healthy individuals, bone tissues are capable of regenerating on their own through the internal mechanism [7], [8]. However, in a case of the defect being larger than the critical defect size (the size of the defect is 2-2.5 times the diameter of the affected bone) or an individual suffering from diseases, external surgical intervention in the form of bone grafts is needed [9].

Bone grafts are bone tissues that are inserted at the defect site to fill the lost bone mass. These grafts provide a conducive environment for triggering the bone regeneration process that typically occurs in three overlapping stages (i.e., inflammation, repair, and remodelling) and also provide mechanical support at the defect site [10], [11]. Typically, three types of bone grafts have been studied for bone regeneration applications, i.e., autografts, allografts, and xenografts [12]. Autografts are bone tissues harvested from one site in the patient's body and transplanted to the damaged site. Autografts are considered the gold standard for bone repair due to their osteogenic, osteoconductive, and osteoinductive properties. However, the need for a secondary surgical site increases the risk of complications such as infection, donor site morbidity, and chronic pain. The amount of bone that can be harvested is also limited, making it unsuitable for the repair of larger bone defects [13]. To address the issue, allografts and xenografts have been

DOI: 10.1201/9781003581192-11

explored. Allografts are the bone grafts obtained from other human donors. These grafts are typically available in wide quantities. However, they lack osteoinductive properties and also carry the risk of immune rejection and disease transmission [14]. Xenografts are bone tissues extracted from an animal species. Although xenografts are more readily available, there is an even higher risk of immune rejection and disease transmission. The limitations of these grafting techniques, along with the increasing demand for bone scaffolds, led researchers to explore synthetic alternatives in the form of scaffolds [15], [16].

Various synthetic materials such as metals, ceramics, polymers, and composites have been explored for the fabrication of artificial bone scaffolds [17]. Traditionally, metal alloys were the most widely used due to the availability of machining techniques. However, due to the elastic modulus mismatch, the stress shielding effect (reduction in bone density due to the removal of typical stress from the bone by an implant) was observed, leading to the weakening of the surrounding bones [18]. Since metal implants are non-biodegradable, there was no space available for bone regrowth, leading to a need for revision surgery for the removal of implants [18]. These limitations led to the exploration of various other materials. Implants fabricated using wide range of e-polymers and ceramics have also been explored for bone scaffold applications. However, these implants displayed poor fatigue strength, making them unsuitable for long-term applications. [19]. Despite these advancements, autografts remain the gold standard in bone regeneration due to their inherent biological properties. Being a cell-laden tissue, autograft promotes the proliferation and adhesion of the stem cells, leading to the regeneration of the bone tissue [20]. Due to these reasons, it was hypothesized that due to the unique microarchitecture of the human bone, the bone scaffolds that closely match the biological, chemical, and physical properties of the human bone will show better treatment outcomes [21], [22]. There are various approaches that have been adopted to ensure better implant integration with the human body. We can broadly classify these interventions into material, fabrication, and surface-level. These interventions aim to promote bone regeneration by promoting interactions between the scaffold and the cells (Figure 11.1).

Material-level interventions involve the use of bioactive materials for the fabrication of the implants [23]. These bioactive materials provide the necessary biological signals that promote cell proliferation, leading to faster bone regeneration [24]. Fabrication-level interventions involve the fabrication of scaffolds with optimal pore size, porosity, and architecture that mimic the natural bone structure to ensure lower chances of immune rejection and allow higher surface area for cell adhesion and proliferation [25], [26]. Surface-level interventions involve modifications like plasma treatment, chemical etching, and bioactive coatings to improve the scaffold's bioactivity by enhancing cell adhesion, proliferation, and osteogenic

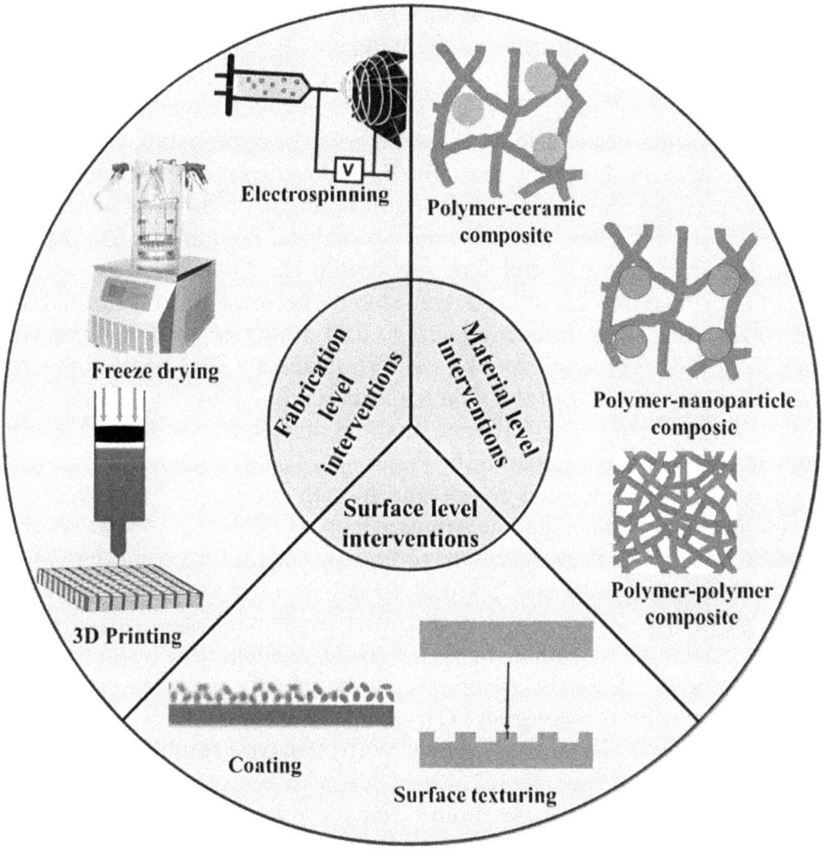

Figure 11.1 Schematic representation of the different interventions adopted to enhance the bioactivity of bioimplants.

differentiation [27], [28]. The following sections discuss in detail the three levels of interventions that have been used in the development of regenerative bone implants.

11.2 MATERIAL INTERVENTIONS IN REGENERATIVE BONE IMPLANTS

Traditionally, bone implant materials were fabricated using metals such as titanium, stainless steel (SS316L), etc. [29]. These materials were bioinert in nature and did not take an active part in the bone regeneration process. A fibrous tissue would be formed around the implant, isolating it from the other tissues, leading to a need for revision surgery for their removal [30].

This led to the development of bioactive biomaterials for tissue regeneration applications. These materials chemically and biologically interact with the surrounding tissues and promote the bone regeneration process [31], [32]. However, a single material cannot effectively achieve the mechanical and biological functions required from a bone scaffold; composite materials – combining properties of two or more materials have been explored [33].

Composite scaffolds combining different bioactive materials have shown promise in enhancing the mechanical and biological properties of scaffolds [34]. Such combinations aim to mimic the natural bone matrix, thus facilitating better integration and function within the biological environment [35], [36]. Bioactive glasses are considered the most promising material due to their excellent osteoconductivity and ability to form a bond with bone [37], [38]. The work by Fu et al. fabricated a 13-93 borate bioactive glass foam as a bone scaffold. The scaffold exhibited mechanical strengths comparable to human cortical bone, making them suitable for load-bearing applications in bone regeneration. Figure 11.2 shows the surface morphology of the bioactive glass foams and human trabecular bone. It can be found that after immersion in simulated body fluids, the bioactive glass foams acquires morphology similar to human bone. [39]. In another study, gelatin and sodium alginate-based hydrogels were incorporated with bioactive glass. The hydrogels demonstrated improved osteogenic differentiation of stem cells leading to faster tissue regeneration [40]. Bioactive glasses can also release therapeutic ions that enhance osteogenesis, thereby promoting new bone formation [41].

The functionalization of scaffolds with bioactive molecules, such as growth factors and therapeutic agents, has also been explored [42], [43]. Quinlan et al., in their study, found that the incorporation of bone morphogenetic proteins (BMPs) into scaffolds significantly enhances osteogenic differentiation and promotes bone healing [44]. The integration of bioactive materials in bone regeneration scaffolds represents a dynamic area of research with substantial implications for clinical practice [45]. As advancements continue in material science and engineering technologies, the potential for developing highly effective scaffolds that not only support bone repair but also enhance biological activity will likely lead to improved outcomes in the treatment of bone defects and injuries [46].

11.3 FABRICATION INTERVENTIONS OF REGENERATIVE BONE IMPLANTS

Bioactive bone scaffolds for regeneration applications are designed to mimic the structure of ECM of bone to promote cell attachment, growth, and differentiation. Various methods, such as additive manufacturing, electrospinning, and freeze-drying, have been used for the fabrication of bone scaffolds.

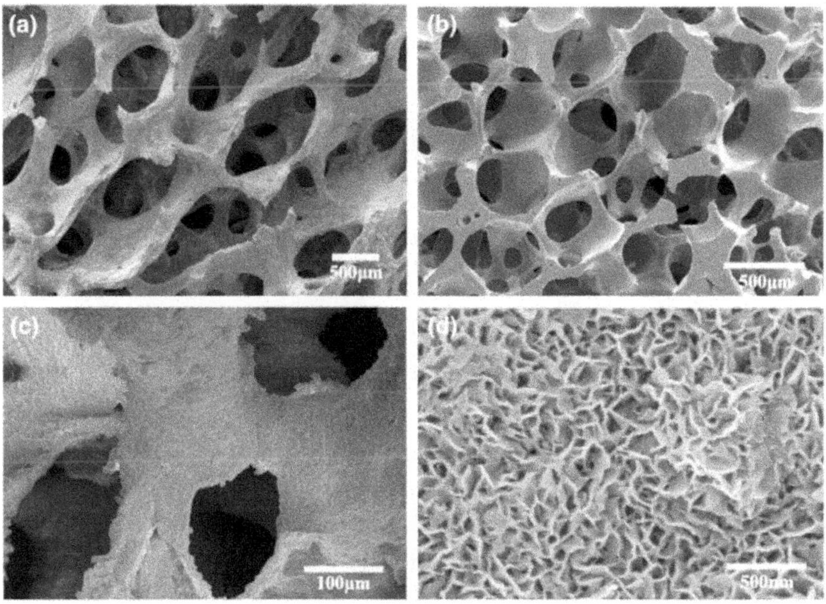

Figure 11.2 Surface morphology of (a) trabecular bone, (b) 13-93 borate bioactive glass scaffold (c),(d) bioactive glass foam after immersion of potassium phos[phate scaffold in 7 days. (Reproduced with permission from [39].)

11.3.1 Additive manufacturing

Additive manufacturing allows for precise control over scaffold architecture, porosity, and mechanical properties. The use of 3D printing has enabled the fabrication of intricate scaffold designs that can be tailored to specific anatomical requirements [47]. Additive manufacturing is capable of fabricating scaffolds with the microarchitecture that closely replicates the bone. Various lattice structures that were impossible to fabricate using traditional manufacturing techniques are now being fabricated using additive manufacturing techniques [48]. Figure 11.3 shows various Triply periodic minimum surfaces-based lattice structures that can be fabricated using additive manufacturing for bone tissue engineering applications.

Additive manufacturing has also evolved into 3D bioprinting for fabrication of tissues. 3D bioprinting allows for the fabrication of cell-laden scaffolds [49]. These scaffolds are characteristically similar to autografts as they contain cells that proliferate inside the human body and lead to new bone formation [50]. Although the development of the right material combination to be used for 3D Bioprinting remains a challenge, the technology holds potential to completely replace autografts in future [51].

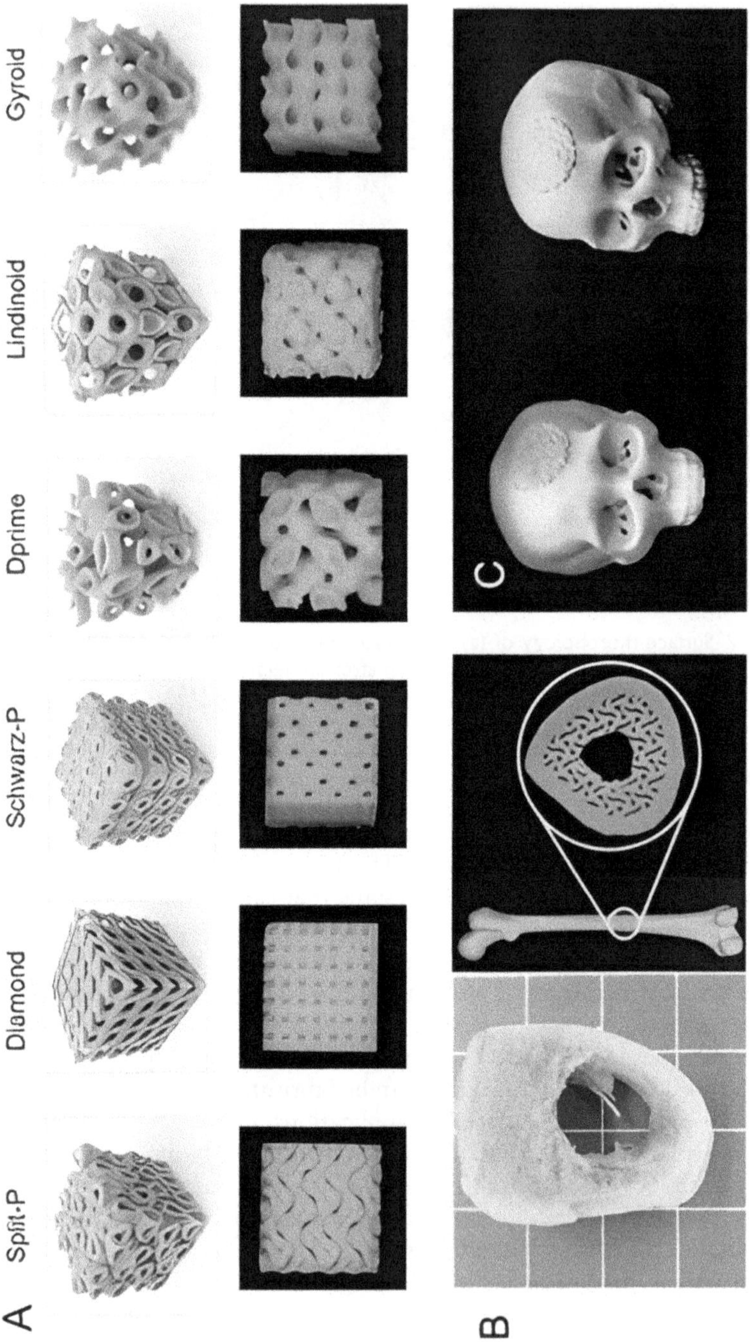

Figure 11.3 (A) 3D-printed HAp scaffolds with different types of TPMS lattice structures. (B, C) Application of TPMS lattics structures in bone scaffolding applications. (Reproduced with permission for [48].)

11.3.2 Electrospinning

Electrospinning is a widely used technique for fabricating nanofibrous scaffolds that replicate the extracellular matrix (ECM) of bones [52], [53]. This method produces fibres with diameters in the nanometer range that provide higher surface area to enhance cell attachment and proliferation [54]. Electrospun scaffolds often incorporate biocompatible polymers such as PLGA or PCL with bioactive materials like HA or bioactive glasses [55], [56]. The incorporation of these materials can enhance the mechanical properties and bioactivity of the scaffolds, promoting osteogenesis.

Studies have demonstrated that electrospun scaffolds support enhanced osteogenic differentiation of stem cells, facilitating effective bone healing and regeneration [56]. The tunable properties of electrospun fibres allow for the optimization of scaffold architecture, which is critical for successful integration into bone tissue [55]. Lima et al. [57] in their study developed an electrospun Polycaprolactone/HA composite Scaffold for bone tissue engineering applications. The composite scaffolds were found to promote new bone formation on rat models, compared to pure PCl scaffolds used as control (Figure 11.4) .

11.3.3 Freeze-drying

The fundamental principle behind freeze-drying involves freezing a material and then reducing the surrounding pressure to allow the frozen water to sublimate directly from solid to gas. This process results in the formation of high porosity and interconnected pore structures, which are crucial for nutrient and cell migration in bone tissue engineering. The high porosity enhances the scaffold's ability to support osteoconductive and osteoinductive properties, thereby facilitating bone healing and remodelling.

Recent studies have explored various composite materials, including chitosan, gelatin, and polycaprolactone, combined with bioactive ceramics like tricalcium phosphate and nano-hydroxyapatite. Kazimierczak et al., in their study, developed freeze-dried chitosan-agarose and hydroxyapatite composite scaffolds with a hydroxyapatite loading of 70 wt.%. It was found that the scaffolds promoted cell adhesion and proliferation of various osteoblast cell lines making them suitable in bone regeneration applications [58]. Figure 11.5 shows the surface norphology and cellular activity of the freeze-dried scaffolds.

11.4 SURFACE-LEVEL INTERVENTIONS OF REGENERATIVE BONE IMPLANTS

Surface interventions typically focus on facilitating surface-level cell scaffold interactions to promote bone regrowth. Two main strategies that have

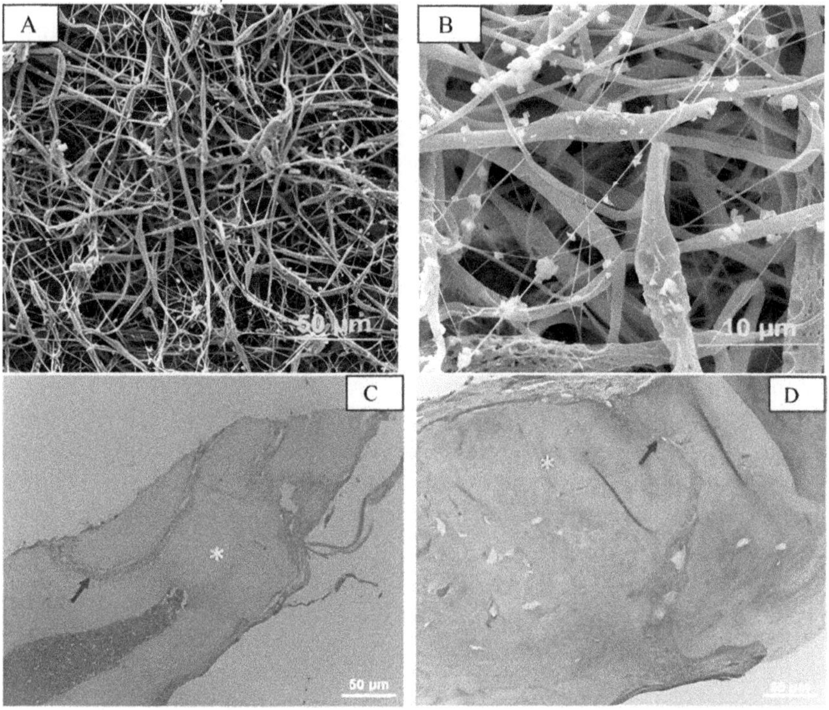

Figure 11.4 (A,B) Surface morphology of electrospun polycaprolactone/HA composite Scaffolds. Histopathological cross section analysis of the rat model implanted with the composite scaffold for 30 days. (C) confirmation of osteoid presence (asterisk) and fibrous cord (arrow). (D) confirms mature bone tissue (asterisk). (Reproduced with permission from [57] under CC-BY-4.0.)

been used to enhance surface-level interactions are surface topography modifications and bioactive coatings. These interventions aim to optimize the biocompatibility, bioactivity, and functionality of the implant.

11.4.1 Surface topography modification

Cells are highly sensitive to their surrounding area in range of 100µm to 10nm. The surface topography plays an important role in cellular responses such as adhesion, orientation, motility, antigen activity, and activation of signaling cascades [59], [60]. By controlling the micro- and nanoscale features of an implant surface, it is possible to mimic the natural extracellular matrix (ECM) leading to higher cellular activity [61], [62]. Surface topographies such as channels, pillars, ridges, and pits are commonly achieved using techniques such as machining, etching, laser texturing, and

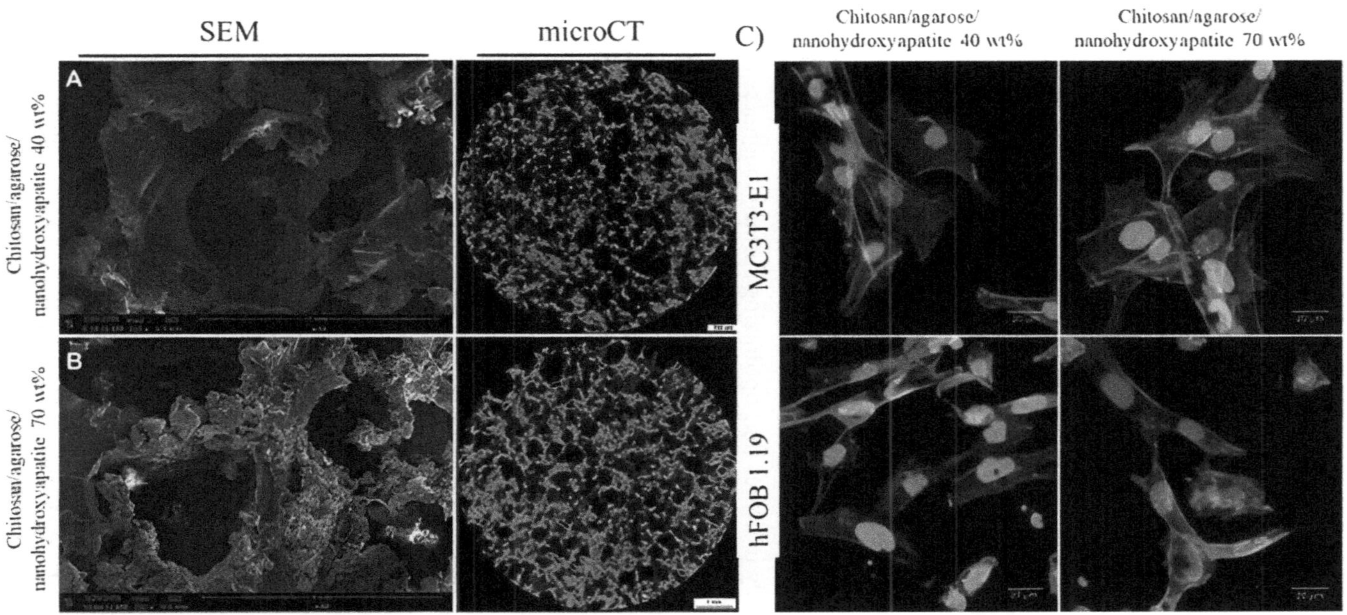

Figure 11.5 Surface horphology of the freeze dried dried scaffolds evaluated through scanning electron micrography and micro-computed tomography for scaffolds with (A) 40 wt.% hydroxyapatite loading and (B) 70 wt.% hydroxyapatite loading. (C) cellular activity of the composite freeze-dried scaffolds against preosteoblast (MC3T3-E1) and human fetal osteoblastic (hFOB 1;19) cell lines. (Reproduced from [58] under CC-BY.)

3D printing [63]. It has been observed that increasing the surface roughness using patterning techniques increases the ECM secretion, compared to the relatively smooth surface.

Various techniques, such as laser surface texturing, sandblasting, and chemical etching, are employed to achieve desired surface characteristics. Each method produces unique micro- and nanoscale topographies that can significantly impact bone cell behaviour. Tiainen et al. [64] found that laser-textured surfaces exhibited enhanced wettability which is critical for protein adsorption and cellular attachment. The study found that micropatterns improve the primary stability of implants, thereby facilitating better integration with bone. Villapún et al. [65], in their study, evaluated the influence of different nano- and micro-level surface textures on 3D printed Ti-6Al-4V titanium implants. It found that the micro-level surface patterns were more effective compared to nanoscale textures (Figure 11.6).

Surface roughness also enhances cell-material interactions by stimulating collagen secretion [66]. Zhang et al. [67] investigated the effects of surface roughness on osteoclastogenesis and found that varying roughness levels significantly influenced the morphology and differentiation of osteoclasts, thereby affecting the balance between bone resorption and formation. The study indicates that optimizing surface roughness can enhance osseointegration by regulating cellular behaviors that are critical for bone remodelling. Liu et al. [68] demonstrated that different surface treatments, such as sandblasting and femtosecond laser treatment, resulted in varying wettability and biomineralization activity — directly impacting cellular responses. Their findings suggest that surface properties not only promote osteoblast proliferation but also modulate macrophage polarization, which is crucial for reducing inflammation and promoting tissue integration.

11.4.2 Surface coatings

Surface coatings can modify the physicochemical properties of scaffolds, such as hydrophilicity, surface roughness, and chemical functionality [27]. Such modifications can enhance cellular responses, which are crucial for tissue regeneration. Various materials have been explored for coating applications.[69] These range from natural and synthetic polymers, bioceramics, antibiotics, nanofilms, etc. Polydopamine is the most widely used polymer for coating applications [70], [71]. In a study by Sun et al., [72] polydopamine (PDA) coatings on 3D-printed β-tricalcium phosphate (β-TCP) scaffolds have been shown to increase surface roughness (Figure 11.7), which in turn promotes the adhesion and osteogenic differentiation of bone marrow mesenchymal stem cells (BMSCs). This study indicates that the enhanced surface characteristics facilitate better cellular interactions, leading to improved osteogenesis via multiple signalling pathways such as TGF-beta.

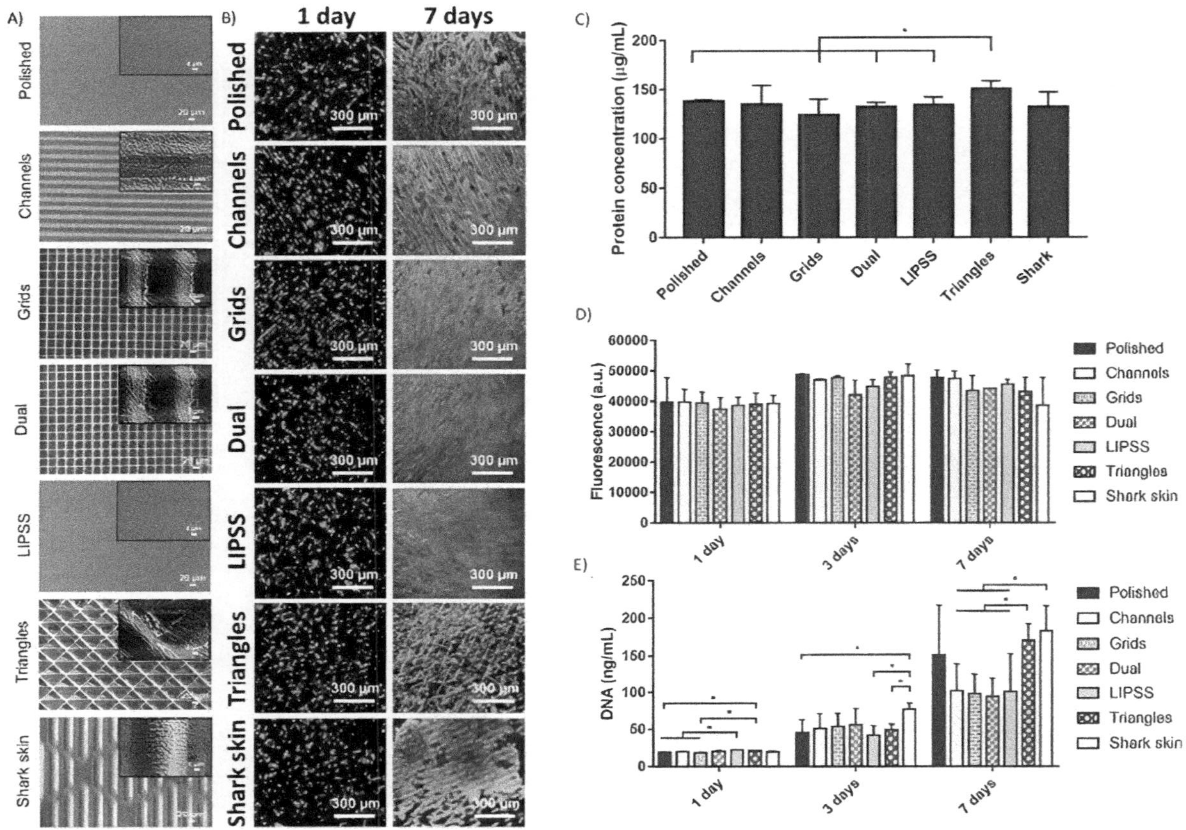

Figure 11.6 (A) Surface morphology of different laser textured surface of 3D-printed titanium implants, Results of (B) cellular proliferation, (C) protein adsorption, (D) cell viability, and (E) DNA quantification studies conducted on laser textured implants. (Reproduced from [65] under CC-By-4.0.)

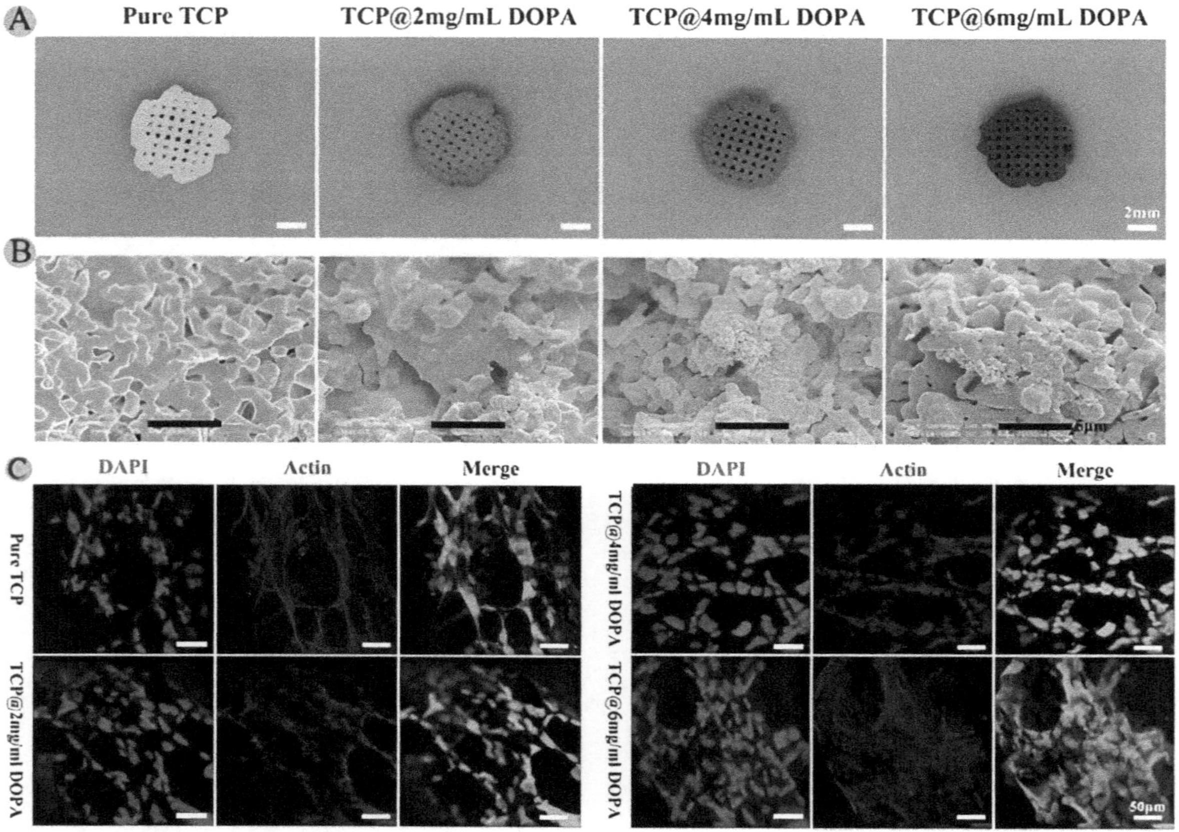

Figure 11.7 (A) Optical micrographs and (B) surface morphology of PDA coated β-TCP scaffolds. (C) Cellular activity of BMSCs on the coated scaffolds. (Reproduced with permission from [72].)

The above studies provide some insights into various approaches that can be adopted for enhancing the bioactivity of bone implants. As can be observed from the above studies, a single strategy may not be sufficient in efficiently enhancing the bioactivity of the implant. One may need to develop a highly bioactive material with desirable mechanical properties to ensure that the implant provides sufficient mechanical support to the patient. Using an efficient fabrication process the implant microarchitecture could be tailored to enhance the strength-to-weight ratio and provide higher surface area for cell adhesion and proliferation. The surface cellular activity can be enhanced by using surface level interventions eventually leading to better regenerative capabilities.

11.5 CONCLUSION AND FUTURE OUTLOOK

The field of regenerative medicine has witnessed significant progress in developing bone implants tailored for tissue regeneration. This progress is driven by the need to address limitations associated with traditional bone treatments [73]. Bone implants tailored for regenerative medicine aim to overcome these challenges by providing biocompatible and biodegradable scaffolds that promote bone regrowth [74]. However, several challenges still exist in translating these technologies into clinically effective solutions.

The selection of appropriate biomaterials for bone implants remains a significant challenge . While various materials, including metals, ceramics, polymers, and composites, are currently employed, there is no consensus on a universal material that can effectively meet all requirements for bone regeneration [74]. The ideal biomaterial should exhibit biocompatibility, biodegradability, mechanical strength, and osteoconductivity to facilitate bone ingrowth and integration [75]. Scaffold architecture also plays a crucial role in bone regeneration by providing structural support and facilitating cell proliferation and vascularization [76]. The scaffold's pore size and interconnectedness must be optimized to allow for nutrient diffusion, waste removal, and cell migration, while maintaining mechanical integrity [76]. Achieving the optimal balance between mechanical properties and porous architecture is a critical challenge. The interaction between cells and the scaffold material is also crucial for successful bone regeneration [77]. The ideal scaffold should promote cell adhesion, proliferation, and differentiation into osteoblasts: the cells responsible for bone formation [77], [78]. However, achieving controlled cell behaviour and directing cell differentiation towards specific lineages within the scaffold remains a significant challenge [79].

The translation of bone implant technologies from laboratory research to clinical applications is often slow and challenging [80]. This is mainly attributed to the complex regulatory processes. The regulatory landscape for novel bone implants can be complex and requires careful consideration of ethical and safety concerns [46], [77]. The development of bone implants tailored for regenerative medicine is a rapidly evolving field with significant potential to improve the treatment of bone defects and enhance the quality of life for patients. While significant progress has been made, several challenges remain, including material selection, scaffold design, cellular interactions, hypoxia, drug delivery, and clinical translation. The future of bone implants holds exciting possibilities with the emergence of advanced materials, innovative manufacturing techniques, stem cell therapies, and personalized medicine approaches [74], [81]. Continued research and collaboration among scientists, engineers, clinicians, and industry professionals are essential to overcome these challenges and achieve the full potential of bone implants in regenerative medicine.

REFERENCES

[1] M. Dermience, G. Lognay, F. Mathieu, and P. Goyens, "Effects of thirty elements on bone metabolism," *J Trace Elem Med Biol*, vol. 32, pp. 86–106, Oct. 2015, doi: 10.1016/j.jtemb.2015.06.005.

[2] Y.-H. Chen *et al.*, "In anemia zinc is recruited from bone and plasma to produce new red blood cells," *J Inorg Biochem*, vol. 210, p. 111172, Sep. 2020, doi: 10.1016/j.jinorgbio.2020.111172.

[3] Z. Seref-Ferlengez, O. D. Kennedy, and M. B. Schaffler, "Bone microdamage, remodeling and bone fragility: How much damage is too much damage?," *Bonekey Rep*, vol. 4, p. 644, 2015, doi: 10.1038/bonekey.2015.11.

[4] N. L. Fazzalari, "Bone fracture and bone fracture repair," *Osteoporosis International*, vol. 22, no. 6, pp. 2003–2006, Jun. 2011, doi: 10.1007/s00198-011-1611-4.

[5] T. Sözen, L. Özışık, and N. Ç. Başaran, "An overview and management of osteoporosis," *Eur J Rheumatol*, vol. 4, no. 1, pp. 46–56, Mar. 2017, doi: 10.5152/eurjrheum.2016.048.

[6] I. Brook, "Microbiology and management of joint and bone infections due to anaerobic bacteria," *J Orthop Sci*, vol. 13, no. 2, pp. 160–169, Mar. 2008, doi: 10.1007/s00776-007-1207-1.

[7] R. Dimitriou, E. Jones, D. McGonagle, and P. V Giannoudis, "Bone regeneration: Current concepts and future directions," *BMC Med*, vol. 9, no. 1, p. 66, Dec. 2011, doi: 10.1186/1741-7015-9-66.

[8] K. Arvidson , Abdallah, B. M., Applegate, L. A., Baldini, N., Cenni, E., Gomez-Barrena, E., Granchi, D., Kassem, M., Konttinen, Y. T., Mustafa, K., Pioletti, D. P., Sillat, T., & Finne-Wistrand, A. (2011). Bone regeneration and stem cells. *Journal of Cellular and Molecular Medicine*, 15(4), 718–746. https://doi.org/10.1111/j.1582-4934.2010.01224.x

[9] E. H. Schemitsch, "Size matters: Defining critical in bone defect size!," *J Orthop Trauma*, vol. 31, no. 5, pp. S20–S22, Oct. 2017, doi: 10.1097/BOT.0000000000000978.

[10] E. Gibon, L. Y. Lu, K. Nathan, and S. B. Goodman, "Inflammation, ageing, and bone regeneration," *J Orthop Translat*, vol. 10, pp. 28–35, Jul. 2017, doi: 10.1016/j.jot.2017.04.002.

[11] F. Loi, L. A. Córdova, J. Pajarinen, T. Lin, Z. Yao, and S. B. Goodman, "Inflammation, fracture and bone repair," *Bone*, vol. 86, pp. 119–130, May 2016, doi: 10.1016/j.bone.2016.02.020.

[12] J. W. Alexander, "Bone grafting," *Vet Clin North Am Small Anim Pract*, vol. 17, no. 4, pp. 811–819, Jul. 1987, doi: 10.1016/S0195-5616(87)50078-X.

[13] P. Baldwin, D. J. Li, D. A. Auston, H. S. Mir, R. S. Yoon, and K. J. Koval, "Autograft, allograft, and bone graft substitutes: Clinical evidence and indications for use in the setting of orthopaedic trauma surgery," *J Orthop Trauma*, vol. 33, no. 4, pp. 203–213, Apr. 2019, doi: 10.1097/BOT.0000000000001420.

[14] C. Laurencin, Y. Khan, and S. F. El-Amin, "Bone graft substitutes," *Expert Rev Med Devices*, vol. 3, no. 1, pp. 49–57, Jan. 2006, doi: 10.1586/17434440.3.1.49.

[15] S. T. Kao and D. D. Scott, "A review of bone substitutes," *Oral Maxillofac Surg Clin North Am*, vol. 19, no. 4, pp. 513–521, Nov. 2007, doi: 10.1016/j.coms.2007.06.002.

[16] N. Shibuya and D. C. Jupiter, "Bone graft substitute," *Clin Podiatr Med Surg*, vol. 32, no. 1, pp. 21–34, Jan. 2015, doi: 10.1016/j.cpm.2014.09.011.

[17] A. Dukle, D. Murugan, A. Nathanael, L. Rangasamy, and T.-H. Oh, "Can 3D-printed bioactive glasses be the future of bone tissue engineering?," *Polymers (Basel)*, vol. 14, no. 8, p. 1627, Apr. 2022, doi: 10.3390/polym14081627.

[18] D. Savio and A. Bagno, "When the total hip replacement fails: A review on the stress-shielding effect," *Processes*, vol. 10, no. 3, p. 612, Mar. 2022, doi: 10.3390/pr10030612.

[19] A. Ferrández-Montero *et al.*, "Controlled SrR delivery by the incorporation of Mg particles on biodegradable PLA-based composites," *Polymers (Basel)*, vol. 13, no. 7, p. 1061, Mar. 2021, doi: 10.3390/polym13071061.

[20] C. M. Misch, "Autogenous bone is still the gold standard of graft materials in 2022," *J Oral Implantol*, vol. 48, no. 3, pp. 169–170, Jun. 2022, doi: 10.1563/aaid-joi-D-22-Editorial.4803.

[21] M. Rezapourian, N. Kamboj, I. Jasiuk, and I. Hussainova, "Biomimetic design of implants for long bone critical-sized defects," *J Mech Behav Biomed Mater*, vol. 134, p. 105370, Oct. 2022, doi: 10.1016/j.jmbbm.2022.105370.

[22] E. Brett, J. Flacco, C. Blackshear, M. T. Longaker, and D. C. Wan, "Biomimetics of bone implants: The regenerative road," *Biores Open Access*, vol. 6, no. 1, pp. 1–6, Dec. 2017, doi: 10.1089/biores.2016.0044.

[23] B. M. Nitschke, F. O. Beltran, M. S. Hahn, and M. A. Grunlan, "Trends in bioactivity: Inducing and detecting mineralization of regenerative polymeric scaffolds," *J Mater Chem B*, vol. 12, no. 11, pp. 2720–2736, 2024, doi: 10.1039/D3TB02674D.

[24] A. Dukle and M. R. Sankar, "3D-printed polylactic acid scaffolds for bone tissue engineering: Bioactivity enhancing strategies based on composite filaments and coatings," *Mater Today Commun*, vol. 40, p. 109776, Aug. 2024, doi: 10.1016/j.mtcomm.2024.109776.

[25] G. Turnbull *et al.*, "3D bioactive composite scaffolds for bone tissue engineering," *Bioact Mater*, vol. 3, no. 3, pp. 278–314, Sep. 2018, doi: 10.1016/j.bioactmat.2017.10.001.

[26] P. S. P. Poh, D. W. Hutmacher, M. M. Stevens, and M. A. Woodruff, "Fabrication and *in vitro* characterization of bioactive glass composite scaffolds for bone regeneration," *Biofabrication*, vol. 5, no. 4, p. 045005, Nov. 2013, doi: 10.1088/1758-5082/5/4/045005.

[27] H. F. Pereira, I. F. Cengiz, F. S. Silva, R. L. Reis, and J. M. Oliveira, "Scaffolds and coatings for bone regeneration," *J Mater Sci Mater Med*, vol. 31, no. 3, p. 27, Mar. 2020, doi: 10.1007/s10856-020-06364-y.

[28] J. Mitra, G. Tripathi, A. Sharma, and B. Basu, "Scaffolds for bone tissue engineering: Role of surface patterning on osteoblast response," *RSC Adv*, vol. 3, no. 28, p. 11073, 2013, doi: 10.1039/c3ra23315d.

[29] M. M. Sonekar and W. S. Rathod, "An experimental investigation on tribologial behavior of bio-implant material (SS-316 l & Ti6Al4V) for orthopaedic applications," *Mater Today Proc*, vol. 19, pp. 444–447, 2019, doi: 10.1016/j.matpr.2019.07.633.

[30] D. C. Greenspan, "Glass and medicine: The Larry Hench story," *Int J Appl Glass Sci*, vol. 7, no. 2, pp. 134–138, Jun. 2016, doi: 10.1111/ijag.12204.

[31] J. R. Jones, "Review of bioactive glass: From Hench to hybrids," *Acta Biomater*, vol. 9, no. 1, pp. 4457–4486, Jan. 2013, doi: 10.1016/j.actbio.2012.08.023.

[32] L. L. Hench and J. R. Jones, "Bioactive glasses: Frontiers and challenges," *Front Bioeng Biotechnol*, vol. 3, Nov. 2015, doi: 10.3389/fbioe.2015.00194.

[33] M. Pilia, T. Guda, and M. Appleford, "Development of composite scaffolds for load-bearing segmental bone defects," *Biomed Res Int*, vol. 2013, pp. 1–15, 2013, doi: 10.1155/2013/458253.

[34] S. Sharma, P. Sudhakara, J. Singh, R. A. Ilyas, M. R. M. Asyraf, and M. R. Razman, "Critical review of biodegradable and bioactive polymer composites for bone tissue engineering and drug delivery applications," *Polymers (Basel)*, vol. 13, no. 16, p. 2623, Aug. 2021, doi: 10.3390/polym13162623.

[35] Bai, X., Gao, M., Sun, Y., Zhu, X., Ma, X., & Guo, Q. (2018). *Bioactive hydrogels for bone regeneration*. Bioactive Materials, Elsevier. https://doi.org/10.1016/j.bioactmat.2018.05.006

[36] V. G. M. R. M. S. A. T. L. A. M. F. F. Veronesi, G. Giavaresi, "Bioactivity and bone healing properties of biomimetic porous composite scaffold: In vitro and in vivo studies," *J Biomed Mater Res A*, 2015,Volume 103, Issue 9 (2015), and the page range is pp. 2932–2941. doi: 10.1002/jbm.a.35433.

[37] E. F. G. O. A. N.-N. J. M. E. V. J. Barberi F. Baino, "Robocasting of SiO2-based bioactive glass scaffolds with porosity gradient for bone regeneration and potential load-bearing applications," *Materials*, 2019, 12(17), 2691. doi: 10.3390/ma12172691.

[38] M. N. R. A. P. T. Qiang Fu Eduardo Saiz, "Bioactive glass scaffolds for bone tissue engineering: State of the art and future perspectives," *Elsevier BV*, 2011, 31(3), 658–668. doi: https://doi.org/10.1016/j.msec.2011.04.022.

[39] H. Fu *et al.*, "In vitro evaluation of borate-based bioactive glass scaffolds prepared by a polymer foam replication method," *Materials Science and Engineering: C*, vol. 29, no. 7, pp. 2275–2281, Aug. 2009, doi: 10.1016/j.msec.2009.05.013.

[40] Y. L. G. T. R. C. J. W. G. M. L. G. C. Z. T. Z. Y. Z. Q. J. Xinran Tu Liyang Guo, "3D-printed gelatin/sodium alginate/58S bioactive glass scaffolds promote osteogenesis in vitro and in vivo," *J Biomater Appl*, 2023,38(3), 1–15. doi: 10.1177/08853282231152128.

[41] J. C. Chengtie Wu, "Mesoporous bioactive glasses: Structure characteristics, drug/growth factor delivery and bone regeneration application," *Royal Society*, 2012, doi: https://doi.org/10.1098/rsfs.2011.0121.

[42] D. L. M. Z. A. K. H. I. L. L. M. T. Deepak Raina Irfan Qayoom, "Guided tissue engineering for healing of cancellous and cortical bone using a combination of biomaterial based scaffolding and local bone active molecule delivery," *Elsevier BV*, 2018, doi: https://doi.org/10.1016/j.biomaterials.2018.10.004.

[43] P. F. Z. M. P. L. B. Y. J. D. Y. C. C. S. S. P. Chengde Gao Youwen Deng, "Current progress in bioactive ceramic scaffolds for bone repair and regeneration," *Multidisciplinary Digital Publishing Institute*, 2014, doi: https://doi.org/10.3390/ijms15034714.

[44] E. M. T. H. K. S. C. F. J. Ob. Elaine Quinlan Adolfo LpezNoriega, "Development of collagenhydroxyapatite scaffolds incorporating PLGA and alginate microparticles for the controlled delivery of rhBMP-2 for bone tissue engineering," *Elsevier BV*, 2014, doi: https://doi.org/10.1016/j.jconrel.2014.11.021.

[45] Z. E. G. B. S. R. J. B. S. Toosi H. Naderi-Meshkin, "Bioactive glass-collagen/poly (glycolic acid) scaffold nanoparticles exhibit improved biological properties and enhance osteogenic lineage differentiation of mesenchymal stem cells," *Front Bioeng Biotechnol*, 2022, 10, 963996. doi: 10.3389/fbioe.2022.963996.

[46] M. Laubach *et al.*, "The concept of scaffold-guided bone regeneration for the treatment of long bone defects: Current clinical application and future perspective," *J Funct Biomater*, vol. 14, no. 7, p. 341, Jun. 2023, doi: 10.3390/jfb14070341.

[47] M. Bahraminasab, "Challenges on optimization of 3D-printed bone scaffolds," *Biomed Eng Online*, vol. 19, no. 1, p. 69, Dec. 2020, doi: 10.1186/s12938-020-00810-2.

[48] Q. Zhang *et al.*, "High-strength hydroxyapatite scaffolds with minimal surface macrostructures for load-bearing bone regeneration," *Adv Funct Mater*, vol. 32, no. 33, Aug. 2022, doi: 10.1002/adfm.202204182.

[49] I. T. Ozbolat, W. Peng, and V. Ozbolat, "Application areas of 3D bioprinting," *Drug Discov Today*, vol. 21, no. 8, pp. 1257–1271, Aug. 2016, doi: 10.1016/j.drudis.2016.04.006.

[50] S. V Murphy and A. Atala, "3D bioprinting of tissues and organs," *Nat Biotechnol*, vol. 32, no. 8, pp. 773–785, Aug. 2014, doi: 10.1038/nbt.2958.

[51] P. S. Gungor-Ozkerim, I. Inci, Y. S. Zhang, A. Khademhosseini, and M. R. Dokmeci, "Bioinks for 3D bioprinting: An overview," *Biomater Sci*, vol. 6, no. 5, pp. 915–946, 2018, doi: 10.1039/C7BM00765E.

[52] R. Khajavi, M. Abbasipour, and A. Bahador, "Electrospun biodegradable nanofibers scaffolds for bone tissue engineering," *J Appl Polym Sci*, vol. 133, no. 3, Jan. 2016, doi: 10.1002/app.42883.

[53] A. Di Martino, L. Liverani, A. Rainer, G. Salvatore, M. Trombetta, and V. Denaro, "Electrospun scaffolds for bone tissue engineering," *Musculoskelet Surg*, vol. 95, no. 2, pp. 69–80, Aug. 2011, doi: 10.1007/s12306-011-0097-8.

[54] S. Pramanik, B. Pingguan-Murphy, and N. A. Abu Osman, "Progress of key strategies in development of electrospun scaffolds: Bone tissue," *Sci Technol Adv Mater*, vol. 13, no. 4, p. 043002, Aug. 2012, doi: 10.1088/1468-6996/13/4/043002.

[55] M. S. Kang, J.-H. Kim, R. K. Singh, J.-H. Jang, and H.-W. Kim, "Therapeutic-designed electrospun bone scaffolds: Mesoporous bioactive nanocarriers in hollow fiber composites to sequentially deliver dual growth factors," *Acta Biomater*, vol. 16, pp. 103–116, Apr. 2015, doi: 10.1016/j.actbio.2014.12.028.

[56] P. Wutticharoenmongkol, N. Sanchavanakit, P. Pavasant, and P. Supaphol, "Preparation and characterization of novel bone scaffolds based on electrospun polycaprolactone fibers filled with nanoparticles," *Macromol Biosci*, vol. 6, no. 1, pp. 70–77, Jan. 2006, doi: 10.1002/mabi.200500150.

[57] M. J. da S. Lima, E. F. de Melo, K. G. B. Alves, F. B. de Sá, and S. Alves Júnior, "Development of functionalized poly(ε-caprolactone)/hydroxyapatite scaffolds via electrospinning 3D for enhanced bone regeneration," *ACS Omega*, vol. 9, no. 45, pp. 45035–45046, Nov. 2024, doi: 10.1021/acsomega.4c05264.

[58] P. Kazimierczak, A. Benko, M. Nocun, and A. Przekora, "Novel chitosan/agarose/hydroxyapatite nanocomposite scaffold for bone tissue engineering applications: Comprehensive evaluation of biocompatibility and osteoinductivity with the use of osteoblasts and mesenchymal stem cells," *Int J Nanomedicine*, vol. 14, pp. 6615–6630, Aug. 2019, doi: 10.2147/IJN.S217245.

[59] R. Singhvi, G. Stephanopoulos, and D. I. C. Wang, "Effects of substratum morphology on cell physiology," *Biotechnol Bioeng*, vol. 43, no. 8, pp. 764–771, Apr. 1994, doi: 10.1002/bit.260430811.

[60] I. Łopianiak, M. Wojasiński, A. Kuźmińska, P. Trzaskowska, and B. A. Butruk-Raszeja, "The effect of surface morphology on endothelial and smooth muscle cells growth on blow-spun fibrous scaffolds," *J Biol Eng*, vol. 15, no. 1, p. 27, Dec. 2021, doi: 10.1186/s13036-021-00278-1.

[61] B. Boyan, "Surface roughness mediates its effects on osteoblasts via protein kinase A and phospholipase A2," *Biomaterials*, vol. 20, no. 23–24, pp. 2305–2310, Dec. 1999, doi: 10.1016/S0142-9612(99)00159-3.

[62] F. Romero-Gavilán *et al.*, "Roughness affects the response of human fibroblasts and macrophages to sandblasted abutments," *Biomed Eng Online*, vol. 23, no. 1, p. 68, Jul. 2024, doi: 10.1186/s12938-024-01264-6.

[63] I. Shivakoti, G. Kibria, R. Cep, B. B. Pradhan, and A. Sharma, "Laser surface texturing for biomedical applications: A review," *Coatings*, vol. 11, no. 2, p. 124, Jan. 2021, doi: 10.3390/coatings11020124.

[64] L. Tiainen *et al.*, "Novel laser surface texturing for improved primary stability of titanium implants," *J Mech Behav Biomed Mater*, vol. 98, pp. 26–39, Oct. 2019, doi: 10.1016/j.jmbbm.2019.04.052.
[65] V. M. Villapún, K. Man, L. Carter, P. Penchev, S. Dimov, and S. Cox, "Laser texturing of additively manufactured implants: A tool to programme biological response," *Biomaterials Advances*, vol. 153, p. 213574, Oct. 2023, doi: 10.1016/j.bioadv.2023.213574.
[66] V. Z. de Souza *et al.*, "Viability and collagen secretion by fibroblasts on titanium surfaces with different acid-etching protocols," *Int J Implant Dent*, vol. 5, no. 1, p. 41, Dec. 2019, doi: 10.1186/s40729-019-0192-4.
[67] Y. Zhang, S. E. Chen, J. Shao, and J. J. J. P. van den Beucken, "Combinatorial surface roughness effects on osteoclastogenesis and osteogenesis," *ACS Appl Mater Interfaces*, vol. 10, no. 43, pp. 36652–36663, Oct. 2018, doi: 10.1021/acsami.8b10992.
[68] Y. Liu *et al.*, "Characterization and evaluation of a femtosecond laser-induced osseointegration and an anti-inflammatory structure generated on a titanium alloy," *Regen Biomater*, vol. 8, no. 2, Mar. 2021, doi: 10.1093/rb/rbab006.
[69] M. Kumar, R. Kumar, and S. Kumar, "Coatings on orthopedic implants to overcome present problems and challenges: A focused review," *Mater Today Proc*, vol. 45, pp. 5269–5276, 2021, doi: 10.1016/j.matpr.2021.01.831.
[70] M. E. Lynge, R. van der Westen, A. Postma, and B. Städler, "Polydopamine—A nature-inspired polymer coating for biomedical science," *Nanoscale,* vol. 3, no. 12, p. 4916, 2011, doi: 10.1039/c1nr10969c.
[71] C.-T. Kao, C.-C. Lin, Y.-W. Chen, C.-H. Yeh, H.-Y. Fang, and M.-Y. Shie, "Poly(dopamine) coating of 3D printed poly(lactic acid) scaffolds for bone tissue engineering," *Materials Science and Engineering: C*, vol. 56, pp. 165–173, Nov. 2015, doi: 10.1016/j.msec.2015.06.028.
[72] X. Sun *et al.*, "Polydopamine-coated 3D-printed β-tricalcium phosphate scaffolds to promote the adhesion and osteogenesis of BMSCs for bone-defect repair: mRNA transcriptomic sequencing analysis," *J Mater Chem B*, vol. 11, no. 8, pp. 1725–1738, 2023, doi: 10.1039/D2TB02280J.
[73] E. Jimi, S. Hirata, K. Osawa, M. Terashita, C. Kitamura, and H. Fukushima, "The current and future therapies of bone regeneration to repair bone defects," *Int J Dent*, vol. 2012, pp. 1–7, 2012, doi: 10.1155/2012/148261.
[74] E. S. Thian and S. M. Best, "Materials viewpoints in bone regenerative medicine: Progress and prospects," *Materials Science and Technology*, vol. 24, no. 9, pp. 1027–1030, Sep. 2008, doi: 10.1179/174328408X341717.
[75] J. Maszybrocka, A. Stwora, B. Gapiński, G. Skrabalak, and M. Karolus, "Morphology and surface topography of Ti6Al4V lattice structure fabricated by selective laser sintering," *Bull Pol Acad Sci Tech Sci*, vol. 65, no. 1, pp. 85–92, Feb. 2017, doi: 10.1515/bpasts-2017-0011.
[76] L.-P. Yan, J. M. Oliveira, A. L. Oliveira, and R. L. Reis, "Current concepts and challenges in osteochondral tissue engineering and regenerative medicine," *ACS Biomater Sci Eng*, vol. 1, no. 4, pp. 183–200, Apr. 2015, doi: 10.1021/ab500038y.

[77] J. Li *et al.*, "3D printing for regenerative medicine: From bench to bedside," *MRS Bull*, vol. 40, no. 2, pp. 145–154, Feb. 2015, doi: 10.1557/mrs.2015.5.
[78] N. Yu, T. Nguyen, Y. D. Cho, N. M. Kavanagh, I. Ghassib, and W. V. Giannobile, "Personalized scaffolding technologies for alveolar bone regenerative medicine," *Orthod Craniofac Res*, vol. 22, no. S1, pp. 69–75, May 2019, doi: 10.1111/ocr.12275.
[79] K. Pushparaj *et al.*, "Out of box thinking to tangible science: A benchmark history of 3D bio-printing in regenerative medicine and tissues engineering," *Life*, vol. 13, no. 4, p. 954, Apr. 2023, doi: 10.3390/life13040954.
[80] I. Martin and R. Duhr, "Future of cellular therapies in orthopaedics: Different views, one common challenge," *J Orthop Res*, vol. 34, no. 1, pp. 10–11, Jan. 2016, doi: 10.1002/jor.23097.
[81] P. A. Povernov, L. S. Shibryaeva, L. R. Lusova, and A. A. Popov, "Modern polymer composite materials for bone surgery: Problems and prospects," *Fine Chem Technol*, vol. 17, no. 6, pp. 514–536, Jan. 2023, doi: 10.32362/2410-6593-2022-17-6-514-536.

Chapter 12

Challenges in bioimplant manufacturing

Deepak Kumar Naik, P. Sri Sai Krishna Aditya, Piyush Kumar, and C. Harsha Vardhan

12.1 INTRODUCTION

The manufacturing of bioimplants in itself is the most difficult step in the idea of using a foreign object in a human or an animal body for the purpose of aid. There are multiple factors like material compatibility, material availability, ease of manufacturing, ease of handling, performance, post manufacturing requirements, cost, etc., that affect this step. Some of the pre-fabrication, fabrication and post- fabrication commonly used in the present time are shown in Table 12.1.

Each bioimplant in itself is very unique—owing to the purpose it serves and the reaction of the host's body towards it. It is with a better understanding of both the human body, and the material response to in vivo conditions, and the outcomes of each process the implant material goes through, can we, in actuality, be able to manufacture an implant that would fulfil its purpose efficiently. Designing and manufacturing such an item is definitely a challenging job, owing to the fact that in every step of manufacturing, it has to be kept in mind that the process must not alter the material's nature in any adverse way which might render it unfit for being implanted in a host.

Ruling out the economic factor and adhering strictly to the manufacturing point of view, this chapter has been divided into three parts namely pre-processing, fabrication, and post-processing. Each of these sections introduce the challenges associated with these steps in the manufacturing processes they represent. The focus of these sections is to point out the exact places where these challenges arise from.

The flow chart has been prepared to show the stages involved in the manufacturing of the titanium-based bioimplant from its pre-fabrication to post-fabrication processes in Figure 12.1.

12.2 CHALLENGES IN PRE-FABRICATION PROCESS

Pre-Fabrication refers to all the steps that are involved in preparing the material for production or manufacturing of the implant. Based on the

DOI: 10.1201/9781003581192-12

Table 12.1 Different techniques used in different stages of the manufacturing of bioimplants

Pre-Fabrication Processes	*Fabrication Processes*	*Post-Fabrication Processes*
Material selection	Wrought and cast	Surface Coating
Design and modelling	Powder metallurgy	Surface Topography
Biocompatibility testing of the selected material	Additive manufacturing (EBM)	Surface finishing
Surface pre-treatment	Additive manufacturing (SLM)	Precision measurement

type of implant and the location of its implantation, the implant reveals some requirements which are mostly unique. To meet the requirements of such unique implants, extensive knowledge of materials and their behavior is essential. Knowledge of the material's response to the in vivo loading conditions, and biological tissues, and fluids plays a pivotal role in selecting the right material for the manufacturing of the implant. It is imperative that understanding and reviewing the properties of biomaterials is not only the base for selecting the material, but also deciding the manufacturing process that the material has to go through, in order to be able to obtain the best performance from the implant's side. The material characteristics being a detrimental factor in the long-term sustenance of the implant, establish that certain following requirements are to be met if the implant is to be utilized:

- In order to make sure that the implant is not toxic to the host's body and doesn't initiate any allergic reactions, the material should exhibit qualities like biocompatibility, bioinertness, osteoconductivity, osteoinductivity, and bioactivity as per the requirement of the host.
- To ensure that the implant serves its purpose for the intended duration, it has to be rendered resistant to both wear and corrosion, as the life span of the implants and recovery of host are directly determined by these. The debris from both these phenomena could lead to issues ranging from basic allergic reactions to the risk of tumors.
- Every implant that is to be implanted in the host has to be strong enough to be able to sustain the loading conditions that it has to face whilst in vivo conditions. Apart from strength, certain implants also rely on properties such as elasticity, a skin graft, and an arterial graft, for example. Hence, mechanical properties as such, tend to play a very important role in maintaining the functionality of the implants.
- Considering the economic point of view, in order for the implants to be available to all those in need, it is to be made sure that the manufacturing of the implants is economically valuable enough to sustain the industry and provide aid as well.

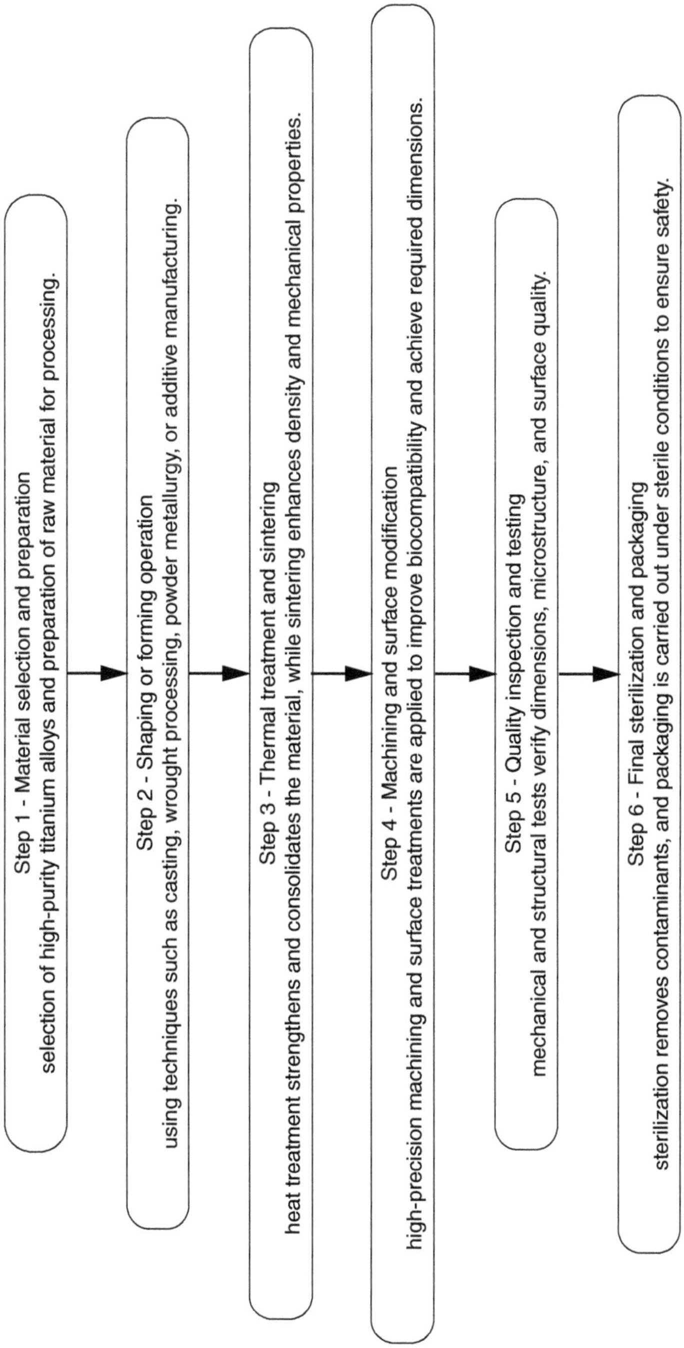

Figure 12.1 Complete manufacturing cycle of the bioimplants.

12.3 THE MATERIALS USED AS BIOMATERIALS

12.3.1 Stainless steel

Stainless steels are iron-base alloys with a minimum of 10.5%Cr as an alloying element that is needed to prevent the formation of rust. The austenitic 316L (18Cr–14Ni–2.5Mo) single-phase austenitic (FCC) stainless steel is the only category that is used for bioimplant applications [1,2]. This material exhibits really good corrosion resistance and toughness as well in vitro conditions. The superior control of the properties of the stainless steel have made it a material that can be manufactured easily [3]. Normal methods like casting cannot produce the part without non-metallic inclusions, which turn out to be highly brittle and further weaken the implant. Hence, special methods like VM and ESR are required to limit the above-stated as much as possible [3,4].

The mechanical working conditions inside a living body greatly differ from the external environment. A major drawback of the stainless steel implants is their low fatigue resistance, which renders them unfit for long term applications. Considering an average number of loading cycles, approximately 1×107 cycles [1], [5] being imposed on the implant, the implant has a high chance of failing —below its yield strength or ultimate tensile strength. Therefore, its application is limited to only short-term implants. It is also reported that the initiation of cracks from fatigues is generally initiated by pitting corrosion [6]. Ion leaching is also a phenomenon that has a high probability of occurrence in case of stainless steel implants, with Nickle ion [Nickel] being the ion that poses the highest risk in terms of inducing toxicity. But the enhanced bulk properties that Nickle provides are also something that cannot be sacrificed; therefore; to compensate by inducing higher amount of nitrogen and creating an ultra-fine grain structure, special methods of manufacturing are to be developed.

12.3.2 Cobalt-based alloys

Cobalt-based alloys is commonly seen in orthopedic applications, such as hip, knee, and shoulder prostheses. Partial implants like screws and plates are also made out of Cobalt alloys. These alloys exhibit excellent biocompatibility, a satisfactory resistance to corrosion in the chloride-rich environment by forming an oxide layer [7]. The strength of alloys based on cobalt tends to surpass the human cortical bones by 10 times. Owing to the outstanding mechanical properties of cobalt alloys, they are deemed fit for the manufacturing of orthopedic implantations. Cobalt alloys do show promising results in terms of their longevity, especially when compared to stainless steel [8].

While it may seem that the superior mechanical properties of cobalt and its alloys may be the solution for all the load bearing implants, but this gives rise to a severe complication by taking all the load on itself and denying the site around the implant from stimulus required for the remodeling of the bone, leading to a condition called bone atrophy. Casting is avoided in the manufacturing of implants using Co–Cr-based alloys as this method gives rise to large dendritic structure of the grains instead of a fine grain structure, resulting in lowered yield strength [9]. Powder metallurgical techniques have been proven helpful in getting the way around the above issue. This results in improved mechanical properties and corrosion resistance pertaining to the finer grain size. Another pressing issue with these alloys is that the so-formed oxide layer leaches ions and atoms of Cobalt, Molybdenum, Nickle, and chromium, which tends to increase the toxicity in the host's body if leached in excess quantities, leading to multiple organ failure.

12.3.3 Titanium-based alloys

The non-toxic and inert nature of Titanium makes it one of the best materials for the fabrication of implants [10]. Titanium surpasses stainless steel in its strength-to-weight ratio as they have been found to be about 25% stronger in terms of their ultimate tensile strength while having only 56% of the mass of the stainless steel. Owing to the lower elastic modulus of the Titanium-based alloys as compared to the cobalt alloys, Ti alloys further shield their surroundings from the much-required stress for the recovery [11]. The challenge being, no possible means eradicate this effect. The two most commercially used specifications for implants are Pure Ti (ASTM F67) and Ti 6Al-4V(ASTMF136) [12]. As previously mentioned, the superior mechanical properties of the alloys, their chemical stability, corrosion resistance due to its oxide layer, and bio inertness along with bio compatibility, have drawn a lot of attention towards these alloys and have enabled them to become the first choice when it comes to load bearing applications within the body [13]. When the corrosion resistance becomes the higher priority as compared to the mechanical strength, pure Titanium is preferred over its alloys. Traces of Aluminum and Vanadium in the alloy, which are added to act as phase stabilizers and to add to the strength and fracture toughness of the implants, tend to be leached into the body, leading to complications like osteomalacia (also called Rickets in children), peripheral neuropathy, and general allergy. To avoid this issue, usage of Molybdenum, Tantalum, Niobium, and Zirconium are being tested to replace Aluminum and Vanadium. However, there has been reports of extended healing periods and recovery times due to the low bioactive nature of the titanium alloy surface. The challenges on Titanium (Ti)-based implants is shown in Figure 12.2.

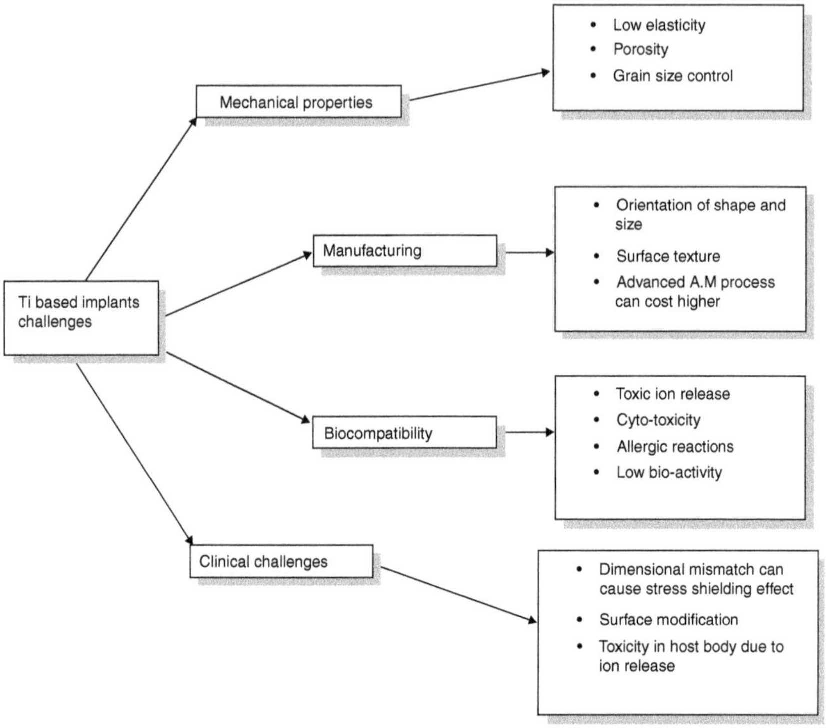

Figure 12.2 Challenges on titanium (Ti)-based implants.

12.3.4 Ceramics

Ceramics tend to exhibit a great set of properties which make them the class of materials that is highly "friendly" from the perspective of the human body. Their excellent biocompatibility has made them one of the most considered choices for the biocompatible coatings over metals, which tend to lack this property. Bioceramics are usually categorized into three types, namely, bioinert ceramics, bioactive ceramics, and bioresorbable ceramics.

- Bioinert
  As their name suggests, they are inert to the environment to which they are exposed to (i.e. the human body). This may be a result of formation of a thin non-adherent fibrous layer at the interface of ceramic and bone. Alumina and Zirconia are two well-known and used ceramics that fall under this class. Alumina can be seen to accompany the metallic femoral head as a dense layer which comes in contact with a polymeric acetabular cup in a replaced hip joint. The

inert type ceramics are fabricated densely for bearing in the joint replacement—to improve the strength of the material against wear and corrosion conditions. These types of implants are used in not just the above-mentioned applications but also as bone plates and screws, space fillings of diseased bone and vertebra prostheses and spacers, etc.

- Bio Active
  Bioactivity refers to the ability of the ceramic material to bond with the bone biologically and is meant for the purpose of enhancing the fixation —owing to its osteoconductive nature. Most commonly used bioactive ceramics are hydroxyapatite (Ca10(PO4)6(OH)2), bioglass (CaO- SiO2–P2O5–Na2O).
- Bioresorbable

As the name suggests, these materials are meant to degrade within the body in a gradual manner. This comes into use when the bones require a temporary fixation, and over time, the regenerated bone is to replace this implant, technically called biomaterial resorption and bone substitution. Ceramics like Calcite and Tricalcium Phosphate are some examples for ceramics under this class.

Despite having all the above-mentioned advantages and deemed as seemingly a great fit for implantation, ceramics pose a threat due to their inherent nature of being very brittle. In implants such as partial or complete hip replacements, there is usually a lot of wear between the femoral head and the acetabular cup. To avoid this wear or to minimize it, this ceramic coating is used as a thick layer, but the wear cannot be eliminated completely. Usually, the ceramics that are used for purposes like this are not bioresorbable. So, when debris is generated due to the wear, there are risks of damage to the surroundings. This wear might also induce corrosion on the femoral head, based on the material used for its manufacture.

12.3.5 Polymers

Given the fact that polymers have great manufacturability at comparatively lower costs, these materials show satisfactory mechanical properties, enough to be used in non-load bearing applications. The Biomedical sectors are witnessing an increasing usage of these materials for implantation purposes. One typical application of polymer in bioimplantology is as acetabular cups. Polymers like Collagen, Hyaluronic acid, and Chitosan are the ones which are mostly used and mostly heard of. Studies and reports reveal that the recently developed biodegradable polymer-based medical implants do not pose any poisonous or mutagenic effects on the host's body [14]. However, owing to their characteristics like hydrophobicity and crystallinity, they have potential to give rise to infections. Nevertheless, natural biopolymers have generated a better response as compared to synthetic ones. Their limited strength and stiffness raise a question on their reliability and longevity. Polymeric implants have been known to trigger reactions owing to their foreign nature, which is difficult to be manipulated with the help of ceramic or hard substance coating, also leading to responses that do not favor the tissues [15].

To summarize the pros and cons of polymer-based bioimplants, starting off with the best in them would be to introduce their capabilities, like their manufacturability into complex shapes and structures with easier handling, their physio mechanical properties varying over a wide range, and easy tunability of their surfaces.

Focusing on the challenges confronted while working with these materials include their ability of altering the surface chemistry of the surroundings by absorbing water and biomolecules. There may be a possibility of leaching of some compounds to the surroundings, breakdown or wear of the implant due to its limited strength, and also in some cases, they are difficult to sterilize.

12.3.6 Magnesium alloys

One of the most recent materials that are emerging and proving to be a viable material for bioimplants is Magnesium and its alloys. Owing to the inherent properties of Mg, like its natural biodegradability, close resemblance in bulk properties to those of a natural (cortical) bone, and also, a good strength-to-weight ratio, ensure a good weight-bearing capacity. When combined with rare earth elements like Calcium, Zinc, Yttrium, Zirconium, and Silver, these binary alloys are significantly used in orthopedic applications, for all the properties mentioned previously which help in bone conduction and also, induction, in some cases [16]. Magnesium is also considered to be a great fit for the orthopedic implants, as it has much lower values of elastic modulus. This indicates that the stress shielding effect in this case would also be very low than what we get to observe in case of other biometals. Based on the rate of degradation and corrosion, the cytocompatibility of Magnesium-based implants change. The rate of degradation of these alloys is usually very high, which poses two major threats to the host [17]: one being the reduced cytocompatibility and leaching effect, both of which result in high alkalinity which in turn proves to be unfavorable to cell proliferation and viability, while the other is the failure of the implant before its intended term of usage—leaving the surrounding underdeveloped and vulnerable to damage [18], [20]. Issues like gas embolism and impaired wound healing might occur due to the hydrogen gas released due to corrosion in chloride ion environment. To minimize this rapid degradation of the alloys, Magnesium is usually coated with other metals, bioactive ceramics, or polymers. Examples for such coating are polylactic acid

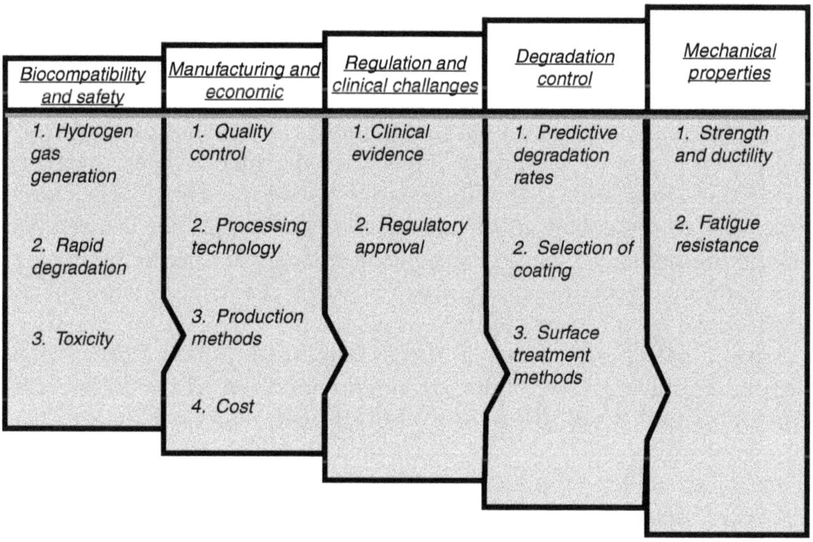

Figure 12.3 Challenges on magnesium (Mg)-based implants.

(PLA), polydopamine (PDA), and polycaprolactone (PCL), as well as bioactive ceramics like calcium phosphate (Ca-P) compounds are used. These challenges can be categorized into five broad areas: biocompatibility, mechanical properties, degradation, compliance, and cost factors. The challenges on Magnesium (Mg)-based implants is shown in Figure 12.3.

12.4 CHALLENGES IN FABRICATION PROCESSES

In recent years, significant developments have been made in the fabrication processes of bioimplants manufacturing, driven by advancements across various techniques. Each fabrication method brings unique challenges, impacting material properties of the material used for bioimplant, biocompatibility of the bioimplant, and bioimplant longevity. These processes are typically categorized into stages, with fabrication serving as the critical phase of forming and shaping. Most commonly-used methods, such as additive manufacturing, powder metallurgy, and EDM, have seen considerable improvements, yet they continue to encounter specific limitations that affect their suitability for bioimplant applications. State-of-the-art fabrication processes, while enabling precise customization and complex geometries, also bring forth challenges related to cost, production efficiency, and material consistency. The following sections will detail these fabrication challenges, with emphasis on specific methods essential to bioimplant development.

12.4.1 Casting

Casting and wrought are conventional methods of bioimplant manufacturing. These Techniques have long served as the basic and foundational techniques for bioimplant manufacturing. In the present time commercial orthopedic joints are majorly manufactured from wrought or casting [21]. Wrought products of Ti and its alloys are capturing 70% of the current market of bioimplants [24]. Whereas the casting is majorly used for the fabrication of the cobalt alloys such as Co-Cr-Mo [22,25]. Despite being well-established and capable of producing strong and durable bioimplants, these traditional processes bring forward specific challenges when applied to the particular requirements of these implants.

Major Challenges in wrought and casting are From an Economic perspective, Significant yield losses are often connected to the wrought and casting processes which affect the overall efficiency and profitability [26]. If consider working efficiency as a factor then wrought and casting processes require relatively long product cycle time and relatively more complex post treatments. Most importantly, wrought and casted metallic bioimplants possess much higher elastic modulus than living bones, which are liable to the stress shielding effect after implanting [27].

12.4.2 Powder metallurgy

Powder metallurgy is also very popular technique for the fabrication of Bioimplants. This process enables Bioimplant products to achieve fine Microstructure and uniform mechanical properties [28]. The advantage which makes it a very attractive technique for bioimplant fabrication is that it is nearly waste free shaping and forming techniques [26]. These techniques also offer the precision control and good mechanical strength to composite materials. The Bioimplant fabricated using the Powder Metallurgy Technique would realize a better integration than the bioimplants fabricated using casting and wrought Techniques. The Powder Metallurgy has been implemented on all the relevant metals and its alloys such as stainless steel (316L), Titanium and its alloys and cobalt alloys. Despite having these much advantages Powder Metallurgy also encounters some challenges that can impact the performance and Durability of Bioimplants.

Those challenges are Powder Metallurgy can only produce larger components due to restrictions in Press capacity. Additionally, compacting the metal powders can be costly and complex especially for the intricate shape. This factor makes it difficult to scale the process for large and complex implant shapes [29]. Creation of an alloy blend that is homogenous in nature is very challenging in Powder Metallurgy process. Specific Preparation methods are required for Pre alloyed Powders such as mechanical alloying and inert gas atomization, to achieve desired and consistent material properties that can increase complexity and cost to the Process.

12.4.3 Additive manufacturing

Additive manufacturing has significantly advanced the fabrication process of intricate, complex patient specific bioimplants. Additive manufacturing has shown so many advantages such as reduced waste material, this method has been proven to achieve the desired mechanical properties via controlling the product porosity. The two most used Additive manufacturing techniques are Electron Beam Melting (EBM) and Selective Laser Melting (SLM). This technique emerged in 1980s so it has arrived recently so this is still an area of research [30]. Despite being the new technology, this technique also encounters some challenges. The challenges in both EBM and SLM is explained below.

- For high temperature processes, EBM is considered advantageous, yet the process often results in rough surface finishes that may not meet the stringent biocompatibility standards for the bioimplants. This roughness can prevent the smooth integration of the bioimplant with the surrounding tissues inside the body. Due to high Temperatures in EBM, the Phase transformation can occur, and that can alter the mechanical properties of the bioimplant. Residual Stresses can be induced in the layers causing weak inter-layer bonding and increasing the risk of delamination. The setup used in this process, such as vacuum environment and high energy input, makes it an expensive process both in terms of initial as well as operational cost.
- SLM uses high power laser to fuse the metal powders layer by layer, this process is highly time consuming because precision is required at each stage of the fabrication. SLM processes often results in residual porosity within the structure, compromising implant's strength, wear and corrosion resistance, and overall performance in the biological environment. Sometimes, it can introduce defects like internal pores, cracks, and residual stresses, due to melt pool instability in the process. It also causes thermal distortion, specifically in the larger parts due to its heat intensive nature [31].

12.5 CHALLENGES IN THE POST- PROCESSING OF THE BIOIMPLANTS

Post processing, as the name suggests, is the last step in the manufacturing process of the bioimplants. This step plays a crucial role in determining the usability of the bioimplants. The bioimplant interacts with the host's body and its immune system only after it has been post-processed as per the requirements of the intended usage. Since most of the implants are metallic in nature, there is a high chance that the immune system senses it as a familiar foreign object and takes a step towards rejecting the implant. Non- metallic implants also tend to face the same fate as the metallic implants, but this is rare owing to the fact that the body is often exposed to metallic substrates in the form of jewelry, piercings, and surgical instruments. Such adverse response from the host's body is not favorable neither for the host nor for the implant itself. It is also to be noted that the implant has to face environments that are much harsher than mere atmospheric conditions and the inert conditions in which these implants are generally fabricated. The reaction between the implant and the bodily fluids and tissues of the host commences as soon as a contact is established between both. In long run, these implants, especially metallic, tend to leach their ions into the host's body, which may get transported to several other organs and accumulate. This may even lead to heavy and irreversible damage to those organs if not checked upon. These reaction between implants, especially Magnesium-based implants and the bodily fluids, also tend to liberate hydrogen gas which gets trapped in nearby regions forming gas cavities, which often tend to cause irritation, discomfort, and inflammation.

Even if the implant is accepted by the body, the recovery time of the host is a crucial aspect of the host's well-being. It is to be ensured that the surrounding tissues and the implant's interactions lead to the optimal recovery. Aspects such as porosity, surface roughness, adhesion, osteoinduction, and osteoconduction, play a very prominent role in determining the recovery of the host. All of the mentioned characteristics directly or indirectly depend on the post-processing of the implant. The surface of the implant, which directly interacts with the body, has to be optimized accordingly. Osteoconduction and Osteoinduction in particular, depend on the depth and roughness along with the chemical composition of the indents on the implant's surface. Achieving such qualities during the fabrication process itself is a very difficult task.

The implant's working life in vivo and in vitro conditions is determined by its bulk properties along with surface characteristics, especially when the implant is under cyclic loading. To ensure that events like fatigue failure do not take place before the intended duration, it is essential to strengthen the implant using post-processing methods like heat treatment. From the above-mentioned brief, it is evident that the post-processing is the detrimental step in the manufacturing of any bioimplant. It is such steps that we often tend to have major challenges with. Based on the above discussion, the further section has these challenges classified into five parts, as following:

- Challenges related to bulk properties of the implant
- Challenges related to the surface properties of the implant

- Challenges in surface finishing catering to better biomaterial interaction
- Challenges in inducing porosity for circulation and oxygenation
- Challenges related to the response of the host and the material

12.5.1 Challenges related to bulk properties of the implants

When implants are subjected to surface or any other type of treatment, it is to be made sure that the implant retains its desired mechanical properties if not attaining betterment. Material defects are a major challenge when studying implant performance and response in vivo and in vitro conditions. Alteration in the bulk nature and induced heterogeneity due to post-processing are one of the major causes for failure of the implants. Hence, limiting the parameters of post-processing to such extent that dual objective of attaining desired surface properties and retaining required bulk properties is of prime importance. Designers and process engineers are generally imposed of this challenge to optimize the manufacturing process of the implant—to ensure the above-mentioned.

12.5.2 Challenges related to surface properties of the implants

Surface properties like roughness, hardness, surface composition after surface treatment, wear resistance, and corrosion resistance play a dominant role in determining the longevity of the implant and the extent of interaction of the implant with the host cells. Cell adhesion, orientation, differentiation, and migration are directly linked with the surface patterns and finishing. Hence, it is of vital importance that the surface is molded in ways that facilitate the best possible growth and regeneration rate of new cells and tissues, whilst serving another purpose of reducing wear so that the debris will not be adrift within the host's body. Processes which intend to address the above mentioned come with their own set of challenges. These challenges are further divided into three sub sections as follows.

12.5.3 Challenges in surface finishing catering to better biomaterial interaction

It is evident that when the implant's material is biocompatible and bioactive, a greater surface area would only bring a better result in terms of cell growth. To achieve a greater surface area of interaction, grooving and indenting serve as the most valid strategies. Although there are multiple methods to perform the above, it is to be noted that each come with their own sets of pros and cons. Blasting of abrasive particles onto the surface of the implant is once such method, but it is required that the particles are of the same material as that of the implant. Usage of abrasives of other materials have reported a risk of change of the surface composition of the implant, and also, dissolution of such particles and release of ions might lead to inflammatory response in the body. Such is the case with chemical etching, as it has shown potential to weaken the mechanical properties despite having a good indenting capacity. In Titanium and its alloy-based implants, it also initiates hydrogen embrittlement of the surface, followed by micro cracks, and ultimately leading to the reduction in fatigue resistance of the implant. Modern technological application of Lasers at Ultraviolet wavelengths has shown promising results in promoting cell growth, but given the fact that high energy is used to achieve the above, micro cracks and heat affected zones have been seen in the grooves, ultimately putting the longevity of the implant at stake.

All the above issues indicate that there is no standard method with which the desired result can be obtained. Each material needs a tailor-made post-processing regime to ensure that it serves its purpose efficiently and effectively —when placed in the host's body.

12.5.4 Challenges in inducing porosity for circulation and oxygenation

In general, when coatings are to be applied by methods like sintering, the implant has to undergo compression at high temperatures. When the implant is intended to have a porous structure to support its biodegradability and compatibility, a process such as the one above will definitely reduce the porous nature of the implant like scaffolds, which ultimately hinder the osteogenesis intended. When dealing with degradable implants like the ones made of Magnesium, porosity plays a really important role in the controlled and even degradation of the implant. Nevertheless, the introduction of porosity also comes with a disadvantage of not being able to properly coat the exposed surfaces within the pores. This leads to uncontrolled degradation from the exposed sites.

12.5.5 Challenges related to host response and implant rejection

Being accepted by the host's body and not initiating any immunological defense is the most important aspect of a bioimplant's success. To achieve this, the host's immune system must be put under an illusion that the implant despite being a foreign object, is a part of the body. Simply put, the implant has to be Biocompatible. Post-processing steps must ensure that biocompatibility of the implant is realized while retaining the desired bulk properties and the surface properties, as mentioned in the previous sections.

If the implant material is inherently biocompatible, it is to be ensured that the post-processing steps do not alter its chemistry on the surface level. In either case where the implant has lost its biocompatibility due to the post-processing steps, or it inherently does not possess any bio compatible nature, it is required to make the implant's surface biocompatible. It is also to be ensured that the implant does not undergo corrosion upon interaction with body fluids and tissues. Keeping this aside, as already mentioned, ion leaching from the implant's surface is also to be eradicated. Taking all the above issues into account, the bioimplant has to be coated with a material that can provide a solution for the mentioned issues and also enhance the life of the implant.

Certain types of coatings like Hydroxyapatite (HA) and Calcium Phosphate (Ca-P) have been developed in this regard and have shown very promising results. But their performance in long-term in vivo conditions pose several problems. Issues such as resorption, degradation, and delamination of Ca-P coatings, ultimately lead to loss in implant fixation, formation of particulate debris, and in some cases, induce osteolysis as well. Methods such as sintering are difficult to control, given that they have to be performed at high temperatures, which may change the crystallinity and morphology of the coating completely. Most of these in vivo studies have been limited to animal bodies only, and not enough studies report anything related to human body conditions. Hence, the biocompatibility of the implant, along with the other issues mentioned, are yet to be studied completely and are far from being concluded.

12.6 CONCLUSION

The manufacturing of bioimplants presents challenges at every stage, from material selection to fabrication and post-fabrication. In the pre-fabrication stage, the choice of material is critical, requiring consideration of mechanical and biological properties, cost, and compatibility with the host body. Materials such as stainless steel, cobalt alloys, titanium alloys, magnesium alloys, polymers, and ceramics are commonly used —each offering unique advantages, limitations, and applications. Factors like the implant's shape, size, and purpose play a significant role in material selection. For instance, stainless steel is widely used for short-term implants due to its cost-effectiveness and ease of fabrication, while titanium alloys are preferred for long-term applications due to their superior biocompatibility and strength. Additionally, the cost of materials significantly impacts the feasibility of production, necessitating a balance between performance and affordability.

Fabrication processes, including casting, wrought techniques, powder metallurgy, and additive manufacturing (SLM and EBM), come with their own challenges, often tied to the selected material and design requirements. Key concerns include achieving the desired bulk and surface properties, such as mechanical strength, porosity, and biocompatibility. Each technique has specific advantages and limitations; for example, powder metallurgy is effective for manufacturing large implants, while additive manufacturing excels at intricate designs but is comparatively time-consuming. Post-fabrication processes are essential to address defects like poor surface finish, microstructural flaws, or insufficient surface roughness that may hinder implant integration with surrounding tissue. These processes, such as heat and chemical treatments, aim to improve properties like osteogenesis and osteoconduction. However, they must be carefully controlled to ensure bulk properties remain within acceptable limits and avoid compromising the implant's durability.

REFERENCES:

1. Kang, Cheng-Wei, and Feng-Zhou. State of the art of bioimplants manufacturing: Part I. *Advances in Manufacturing* **6** (2018): 20–40. https://doi.org/10.1007/s40436-017-0207-4
2. Khan, T., and Shabir Hussain Khahro. "Advancement in biomedical implant materials-A mini Review." *Frontiers in Bioengineering and Biotechnology* 12 (2024): 1400918.
3. Paital, Sameer R., and Narendra B. Dahotre. "Calcium phosphate coatings for bio-implant applications: Materials, performance factors, and methodologies." *Materials Science and Engineering: R: Reports* 66.1-3 (2009): 1–70.
4. Pilliar, Robert M. "Manufacturing processes of metals: The porcessing and properties of metal implants." *Metal and Ceramic Biomaterials* 1 (2018): 79–105.
5. Sumita, M., T. Hanawa, I. Ohnishi, et al. "Failure processes in biometallic materials." In: Milne I., Ritchie R., Karihaloo B. L. (eds) *IMOR Karihaloo, comprehensive structural integrity*, Pergamon, Oxford, pp 131–167. 2003.
6. Niinomi, Mitsuo. "Fatigue characteristics of metallic biomaterials." *International Journal of Fatigue* 29.6 (2007): 992–1000.
7. Karimi, Shima. *Corrosion behavior of metallic bio-implant alloys*. Diss. University of British Columbia, 2014.
8. Radenković, Goran, and Dušan Petković. "Metallic biomaterials." *Biomaterials in Clinical Practice: Advances in Clinical Research and Medical Devices* (2018): 183–224.
9. Sumayli, A. "Recent trends on bioimplant materials: A review." *Materials Today: Proceedings* 46 (2021): 2726–2731.
10. Shao, Longfei, Yiheng Du, Kun Dai, Hong Wu, Qingge Wang, Jia Liu, Yujin Tang, and Liqiang Wang. "β-Ti alloys for orthopedic and dental applications: A review of progress on improvement of properties through surface modification." *Coatings* 11 (2021).11(12), 1446. 1446.10.3390/coatings11121446
11. Naji, Fadia, Ahmed Abdullah, Qasim Murtaza, and M. S. Niranjan. "Challenges and opportunities in nano finishing of titanium alloys for biomedical applications: A review." *Precision Engineering* (2024).

12. Hazwani, Mohamad Rodzi Siti Nur, et al. "Fabrication of titanium-based alloys with bioactive surface oxide layer as biomedical implants: Opportunity and challenges." *Transactions of Nonferrous Metals Society of China* 32.1 (2022): 1–44.
13. Losic, Dusan. "Advancing of titanium medical implants by surface engineering: Recent progress and challenges." *Expert Opinion on Drug Delivery* 18.10 (2021): 1355–1378.
14. Abd Razak, Saiful Izwan, N. F. Ahmad Sharif, and W. A. W. Abdul Rahman. "Biodegradable polymers and their bone applications: A review." *International Journal of Basic and Applied Sciences* 12 (2012): 31–49.
15. Al-Shalawi, Faisal Dakhelallah, Azmah Hanim Mohamed Ariff, Dong-Won Jung, Mohd Khairol Anuar Mohd Ariffin, Collin Looi Seng Kim, Dermot Brabazon, and Maha Obaid Al-Osaimi. "Biomaterials as implants in the orthopedic field for regenerative medicine: Metal versus synthetic polymers." *Polymers* 15 (2023): 2601. https://doi.org/10.3390/polym15122601
16. Singh, Jashanpreet, et al. "Critical review on biodegradable and biocompatibility magnesium alloys: Progress and prospects in bio-implant applications." *Inorganic Chemistry Communications* (2024): **163**, 113111.
17. Kamrani, Sepideh, and Claudia Fleck. "Biodegradable magnesium alloys as temporary orthopaedic implants: A review." *Biometals* 32 (2019): 185–193.
18. Thomas, Kevin Koshy, Mah Noor Zafar, William G. Pitt, and Ghaleb A. Husseini. Biodegradable magnesium alloys for biomedical implants: Properties, challenges, and surface modifications with a focus on orthopedic fixation repair. *Applied Sciences* 14 (2024): 10. https://doi.org/10.3390/app14010010
19. Delavar, Hassan, Amirhossein Jabbari Mostahsan, and Hamdy Ibrahim. "Corrosion and corrosion-fatigue behavior of magnesium metal matrix composites for bio-implant applications: A review." *Journal of Magnesium and Alloys* 11.4 (2023): 1125–1161.
20. Kamrani, Sepideh, and Claudia Fleck. "Biodegradable magnesium alloys as temporary orthopaedic implants: A review." *Biometals* 32 (2019): 185–193.
21. Hussain, Muzamil, et al. "Advances in biodegradable materials: degradation mechanisms, mechanical properties, and biocompatibility for orthopedic applications." *Heliyon* 10, e26174. (2024).
22. Long, Marc, and H. J. Rack. "Titanium alloys in total joint replacement—A materials science perspective." *Biomaterials* 19.18 (1998): 1621–1639.
23. Murr, L. E., et al. "Microstructure and mechanical properties of open-cellular biomaterials prototypes for total knee replacement implants fabricated by electron beam melting." *Journal of the Mechanical Behavior of Biomedical Materials* 4.7 (2011): 1396–1411.
24. Murr, L. E., et al. "Microstructure and mechanical behavior of Ti–6Al–4V produced by rapid-layer manufacturing, for biomedical applications." *Journal of the Mechanical Behavior of Biomedical Materials* 2.1 (2009): 20–32.
25. Lampman, S. (1990). Wrought titanium and titanium alloys. In ASM Handbook, Volume 2: Properties and Selection: Nonferrous Alloys and Special-Purpose Materials, ASM International, pp. 592–633. https://doi.org/10.31399/asm.hb.v02.a0001081.

26. Alvarado, Jorge, et al. "Biomechanics of hip and knee prostheses." *Applications of Engineering Mechanics in Medicine, GED–University of Puerto Rico Mayaguez* (2003): 1–20.
27. Kang, Cheng-Wei, and Feng-Zhou Fang. "State of the art of bioimplants manufacturing: Part I." *Advances in Manufacturing* 6 (2018): 20–40.
28. Nagels, Jochem, Mariëlle Stokdijk, and Piet M. Rozing. "Stress shielding and bone resorption in shoulder arthroplasty." *Journal of Shoulder and Elbow Surgery* 12.1 (2003): 35–39.
29. Eisen, W. B., et al. (Eds.). (1998). *Powder Metal Technologies and* applications. In ASM Handbook, Volume 7, ASM International, Materials Park, Ohio.." (1998).
30. Dewidar, Montasser Marasy, Ho-Chel Yoon, and Jae Kyoo Lim. "Mechanical properties of metals for biomedical applications using powder metallurgy process: A review." *Metals and Materials International* 12 (2006): 193–206.
31. Bartolo, Paulo, et al. "Biomedical production of implants by additive electrochemical and physical processes." *CIRP Annals* 61.2 (2012): 635–655.

Chapter 13

Evaluating environmental and health impacts through a sustainable approach

Shrishti Sharma, R.S. Banshtu, and Adarsh Singh

INTRODUCTION

The city of Lucknow is situated at 26°51′N and 80°55′E. Lucknow has 2815033 residents as per the 2011 Census of India, and its current size is estimated to be 310 square kilometers. The second-largest city in North India, renowned for its extensive cultural history. Recently included on the national government's list of "Smart cities" for the advancement of lifestyle trends. A full-fledged international cricket stadium and a metro rail project are both in the works. Aeronautics, machine tools, distillery chemicals, furniture, and chikan embroidery are some of the prominent sectors in the Lucknow Urban Agglomeration. According to GDP, it is one of the top fifteen cities in India. Indoor levels of pollutants may be 2–5 times, and occasionally more than one hundred times higher than outdoor levels—stated by the US EPA. The third-highest risk factor in Southeast Asia, according to the Global Burden of Disease study, was indoor air pollution. We inhale 6–10 liters of air every minute (15–20 m3 per day); hence, dangerous compounds may be absorbed swiftly without our knowledge. The lungs are most harmed by inadequate IAQ since air contaminants initially come into touch with our respiratory system.

Let us start the study by looking at the factors that contribute to indoor air pollution in the environment [1]. The primary offenders are the gases and particles already existing in the area, which are further encouraged by the lack of sufficient ventilation seen in newer structures. Particles that are gathered indoors might be made up of a variety of things, such as carpet, furniture, dander from the residents, insects, fecal debris, smoking, cleaning products, and pollution from the outside. This prevents enough fresh air from the outside from entering the space, which would otherwise allow emissions already present in the indoor structure to be diluted. Due to this, certain pollutants may be present in higher concentrations due to rising temperatures and increased humidity [2]. The rate of external air supply that has been proven through experience to offer subjectively acceptable

DOI: 10.1201/9781003581192-13

interior air quality and to avoid the buildup of moisture in the building is adequate to keep the concentration of contaminants at healthily low levels.

Infiltration, natural ventilation, and mechanical ventilation are all ways that external air can enter or exit a structure. Infiltration is the process by which outside air enters structures through joints, apertures, and cracks in the walls, floors, and ceilings, as well as around windows and doors. When windows and doors are open, there is natural ventilation. Differences in air temperature between interior and outside air, as well as wind, are the main factors that contribute to infiltration and natural ventilation. Finally, there are a few mechanical ventilation devices, ranging from outdoor-vented fans that sporadically remove air from a single room, such as the bathroom or kitchen, to air handling systems that continuously remove indoor air while distributing filtered and conditioned outdoor air to key locations around the house using fans and ductwork.

SOURCES OF POLLUTION

Indoor air pollution comes from a variety of causes. These may incorporate:

- energy-consuming combustion devices
- tobacco items
- various furniture and building supplies, including—
  - worn-out insulation that contains asbestos
  - flooring, furniture, or carpet that has just been installed
  - furniture or cabinets constructed of certain pressed wood materials.
- products for maintaining and cleaning the home, for personal care, or for hobbies
- systems for central heating, cooling, and humidification
- moisture in excess
- external sources like-
  - radon
  - pesticides
  - outdoor air pollution.

The quantity and danger of any one source's emissions determine how significant it is in relation to other sources. In some circumstances, elements like the age of the source and whether it has been adequately maintained are crucial. An incorrectly set gas stove, for instance, might generate substantially more carbon monoxide than one that is correctly calibrated.

The discharge of contaminants can occur continually from some sources, including air fresheners, furniture, and building supplies. Other sources, including those connected to routine tasks like cleaning, redecorating, smoking, and engaging in hobbies, produce pollutants on a sporadic basis.

Higher and occasionally deadly quantities of pollutants can be released indoors by carelessly utilized items, broken equipment, or unvented appliances.

MONITORING AND MANAGEMENT LIMITS FOR INDOOR POLLUTANTS

Indoor air pollution has harmful consequences on human health, including an increased risk of respiratory diseases and asthma episodes, as well as irritation of the ears, nose, and throat. An essential initial step in controlling these substances' quantities is tracking the particles, chemicals, and gases. Here is a list of indoor air quality requirements along with the thresholds that are suggested by the EPA's Air Quality Index (AQI). IAQ can be affected by various chemicals, including gases (i.e., carbon monoxide, ozone, radon), volatile organic compounds (VOCs), particulate matter (PM) and fibers, organic and inorganic contaminants, and biological particles such as bacteria, fungi, and pollen [4]. Given the potential harm that VOCs, particulate matter including allergens and mildew, and combustion gases may cause to people's health and welfare, minimizing indoor air pollution is essential to achieving high performance. Some of these pollutants are known for causing flu-like symptoms, headaches, nausea, and irritation of the eyes, nose, and throat, in addition to their ability to start asthma or allergy episodes. The physical atmosphere of a school may also have a substantial impact, according to recent studies.

- Polycyclic Aromatic Hydrocarbons (PAHs): 10 ppm or less
- PM2.5 (Particulate matter): 0–12 ug/m3
- PM10 (Particulate Matter): 0 to 54 ug/m3
- Nitrogen Dioxide (NO2): 100 ppb- 1-hour standard
- Carbon Monoxide (CO): 8-hour workday with a 25-ppm maximum
- Carbon dioxide (CO2): 400 to 650 ppm
- Radon: no acceptable exposure limits
- Methylene chloride: A 250-ppm threshold for odor
- Volatile Organic Compounds (VOCs): 0–15 ppm
- Formaldehyde: 0–0.2 ppm

With the help of this study, we are here to dilate about a few pollutants on their origin and through which ways they enter the human body, their ill effects and how to prevent them.

Indoor Particulate Matter- The combination of solid particles in the air is known as particulate matter or particle pollution. While certain particles, such as dust, dirt, sand, and smoke, may be seen with the naked eye due to their size, other particles must be observed under a microscope. Although particulate matter can be released directly from a source, such as a beach or construction site, it frequently results through a complicated chemical interaction between contaminants released during the combustion of fuels. Several health problems, such as heart attacks, irregular heartbeats, worsening asthma, and worsened respiratory symptoms, can arise from prolonged exposure to particulate matter. People who already have respiratory conditions like asthma are more vulnerable to the negative effects of particulate matter. The Air Quality Index (AQI) is a reliable indication of pollution levels in the air and may be used to estimate the extent of exposure to this pollutant.

Particles of a diameter of 2.5 micrometers or less are known as PM2.5, or fine dust, and they are floating in the air. PM2.5 particles can be inhaled all the way into the lungs and are produced by internal processes or external air quality. To ensure that the thresholds are maintained, use the proper air filters for your system configuration.

PM10, or coarse dust particles with a diameter of 10 micrometers, are frequently referred to as such. Additionally present in the air, PM10 can be inhaled all the way to the lungs. These particles, like PM2.5, may be produced indoors or outside depending on the air quality. Thresholds can be maintained by using the appropriate air filters for your system configuration.[5]

Indoor PM levels rely on a number of variables, including outside levels, infiltration, the types of ventilation and filtration systems utilized, indoor sources, and residents' private activities. Indoor PM levels should be equal to or lower than outside levels in houses without smoking or other significant particle emitters.[6]

The source strengths for human activities were reported to vary from 0.1 and 1.4 mg.min.1 for PM10 and from 0.03 to 0.5 mg.min.1 for PM2.5.[7]

Additionally, these tiny particles have the potential to migrate from the kitchen to the living room and other rooms in the building, having a negative impact on the health of the residents.

Nitrogen dioxide (NO2): [8] One of the extremely reactive gases referred to as nitrogen oxides of nitrogen oxides is nitrogen dioxide (NO2) (NOx). The acids nitrous and nitric oxide are examples of additional nitrogen oxides. For the wider category of nitrogen oxides, NO2 is utilized as an indication. The main source of NO2 in the atmosphere is fuel combustion. Vehicles, lorries, buses, power plants, and off-road vehicles all emit NO2 as part of their emissions.

The human respiratory system's airways might get irritated when breathing air with a lot of NO2. Short-term exposures like these might exacerbate respiratory conditions, especially asthma, causing respiratory symptoms like coughing, wheezing, or breathing difficulties so bad that they might lead to hospital admissions and ER visits. Increased susceptibility to respiratory infections and the development of asthma may result from prolonged exposure to high NO2 concentrations. Children, the elderly, and those with asthma are often at higher risk for the negative effects of NO_2 on their health.

Particulate matter and ozone are created when NO_2 and other NO_x combine with other airborne molecules. Due to their detrimental effects on the respiratory system, both of these are dangerous when breathed.[9]

According to research, indoor NO_2 levels are impacted by both exterior and interior sources. As a result, high outdoor NO_2 levels from sources such as local traffic or combustion can have an impact on inside levels. According to a survey, the amount of effect that distance between buildings and traffic has on interior NO_2 levels is significant.

Carbon Dioxide (CO_2): is a trace quantity of an odorless, colorless gas that naturally exists in the atmosphere of the Earth. Increased CO_2 levels can result from densely inhabited spaces where many individuals are exhaling and inhaling the same air. These elevated levels have a major influence on comfort and productivity, leading to worker and staff weariness and a lack of concentration. By boosting ventilation, indoor CO_2 levels can be reduced, while fresh air levels are increased for occupant comfort. Displacement asphyxia is the method through which excessive amounts of CO_2 can cause harm. The presence of CO_2 and other gases displaces oxygen. Hyperventilation, diaphoresis, headache, bounding pulses, heated extremities, and eventually unconsciousness are the clinical signs of such exposures.

Since People within buildings exhale CO_2, indoor CO_2 levels are often greater than outside levels. Interior CO_2 levels are decreased via ventilation, which replaces indoor air with outdoor air. Therefore, elevated indoor CO_2 levels may be a sign that the air exchange rate is insufficient for the occupancy of the space.[10]

Due to the fact that people within buildings exhale CO_2, indoor CO_2 levels are often greater than outside levels. Interior CO_2 levels are decreased via ventilation, which replaces the air inside with the air outside.

As a result, increased carbon dioxide levels typically indicate inadequate ventilation. People who are inside high CO_2 buildings frequently complain of burning eyes, exhaustion, and headaches. These symptoms might be brought on by the interaction of carbon dioxide with the various other pollutants that are present in an insufficiently ventilated environment. Making sure that these buildings adhere to ASHRAE 62-1989's requirements is one step toward improving the interior air quality.

CONCLUSION

In this review the author has mentioned about how the indoor air pollutants emerge in the environment and has discussed a few pollutants which can be monitored with the latest technologies in the market. Due to its detrimental effects on health, which are similar to those of ambient air, indoor air has recently been a major source of worry. If exposed for an extended length of time, indoor air can potentially seriously injure human health. This paper lists out the major health effects of the pollutants discussed above. One of the main ways that these pollutants enter the human body is by air inhalation. Exposure to air pollution has been linked to a significant burden of disease and early mortality. Since air quality is rapidly declining in India due to the country's rapidly expanding urbanization, it has become a socially significant issue.

The best strategies to enhance the quality of the air inside your home are to lessen or eliminate the sources of pollution and to open windows to let in fresh air from outside. Research has also shown that filtration can be a useful adjunct to source control and ventilation. One may enhance indoor air quality by using a portable air purifier and/or replacing the air filter in your furnace or central heating, ventilation, and air-conditioning (HVAC) system. Air purifiers and air sanitizers are portable air cleaners that are intended to filter the air in a particular room or space. To clean the air in a whole house, central furnace or HVAC filters are used. Portable air purifiers and HVAC filters can lessen interior air pollution, but they cannot eliminate it.

REFERENCES

[1] Carbon dioxide in indoor air | National Collaborating Centre for Environmental Health | NCCEH – CCSNE. (n.d.). Retrieved December 5, 2022, from https://ncceh.ca/documents/field-inquiry/carbon-dioxide-indoor-air

[2] Cincinelli, A., & Martellini, T. (2017). *Indoor Air Quality and Health*. International Journal of Environmental Research and Public *Health* (Vol. 14, Issue 11, p. 1286). MDPI.

[3] Ferro, A. R., Kopperud, R. J., & Hildemann, L. M. (2004). Source Strengths for Indoor Human Activities that Resuspend Particulate Matter. *Environmental Science & Technology*, 38(6), 1759–1764. https://doi.org/10.1021/es0263893.

[4] Indoor Air Quality: Carbon Monoxide and Carbon Dioxide (AEN-125). (n.d.). *Department of Agricultural and Biosystems Engineering*. Retrieved December 5, 2022, from www.abe.iastate.edu/extension-and-outreach/indoor-air-quality-carbon-monoxide-and-carbon-dioxide-aen-125/.

[5] Kim, H., Kang, K., & Kim, T. (2018). Measurement of Particulate Matter (PM2.5) and Health Risk Assessment of Cooking-Generated Particles in the Kitchen and Living Rooms of Apartment Houses. *Sustainability*, 10(3), 843, Article 3. https://doi.org/10.3390/su10030843.

[6] Kodama, Y., Arashidani, K., Tokui, N., Kawamoto, T., Matsuno, K., Kunugita, N., & Minakawa, N. (2002). Environmental NO2 Concentration and Exposure in Daily Life along Main Roads in Tokyo. *Environmental Research*, 89(3), 236–244. https://doi.org/10.1006/enrs.2002.4350.

[7] US EPA, O. (2015, June 2). *Indoor Pollutants and Sources [Collections and Lists]*. www.epa.gov/indoor-air-quality-iaq/indoor-pollutants-and-sources.

[8] Wyon, D. P. (2004). The Effects of Indoor Air Quality on Performance and Productivity. *Indoor Air*, 14(7), 92–101.

[9] Yu, K.-P., Yang, K. R., Chen, Y. C., Gong, J. Y., Chen, Y. P., Shih, H.-C., & Candice Lung, S.-C. (2015). Indoor Air Pollution from Gas Cooking in Five Taiwanese Families. *Building and Environment*, 93, 258–266. https://doi.org/10.1016/j.buildenv.2015.06.024.

[10] Zhang, Y. (2005). *Indoor Air Quality Engineering*. CRC Press. Boca Raton, FL.

Chapter 14

AI-powered tailored PCOS treatment in a sustainable healthcare future

Neha Singh Raghuvanshi and Ashwani Kumar

14.1 INTRODUCTION

Polycystic ovary syndrome (PCOS) is a complex hormonal condition that impacts the reproductive system and metabolism of those affected. It is typically identified by disturbed menstrual cycles, raised androgen levels, and the detection of ovarian cysts. The fluctuation in menstrual cycles associated with PCOS often leads to difficulties with fertility in individuals of reproductive age. Furthermore, PCOS can occur with symptoms such as acne, excessive growth of facial and body hair and male-pattern baldness. Furthermore, a significant number of individuals with PCOS encounter insulin resistance, a condition in which their cells demonstrate decreased sensitivity to insulin, leading to rising insulin levels in the blood. This insulin resistance predisposes individuals to the onset of type 2 diabetes and metabolic syndrome. Additionally, PCOS increases the risk of obstructive sleep apnea and endometrial hyperplasia, a condition characterized by abnormal thickening of the uterine lining. Leveraging the power of artificial intelligence (AI), personalized nutrition plans can be meticulously crafted to address the specific needs and challenges faced by individuals with PCOS (Figure 14.1).

14.2 DATA COLLECTION AND ANALYSIS

AI algorithms can amalgamate data originating from a plethora of sources, comprising electronic health records, wearable devices, mobile applications, genetic tests, and patient-reported information. This amalgamation of diverse datasets empowers AI to foster a comprehensive comprehension of an individual's health status, encompassing hormonal levels, metabolic markers, dietary habits, activity levels, and symptoms associated with PCOS. Furthermore, AI methodologies, such as natural language processing (NLP), facilitate the analysis of unstructured data sources, including medical notes, patient diaries, and social media posts, to extract pertinent details regarding PCOS symptoms, treatment encounters, and lifestyle aspects.

DOI: 10.1201/9781003581192-14

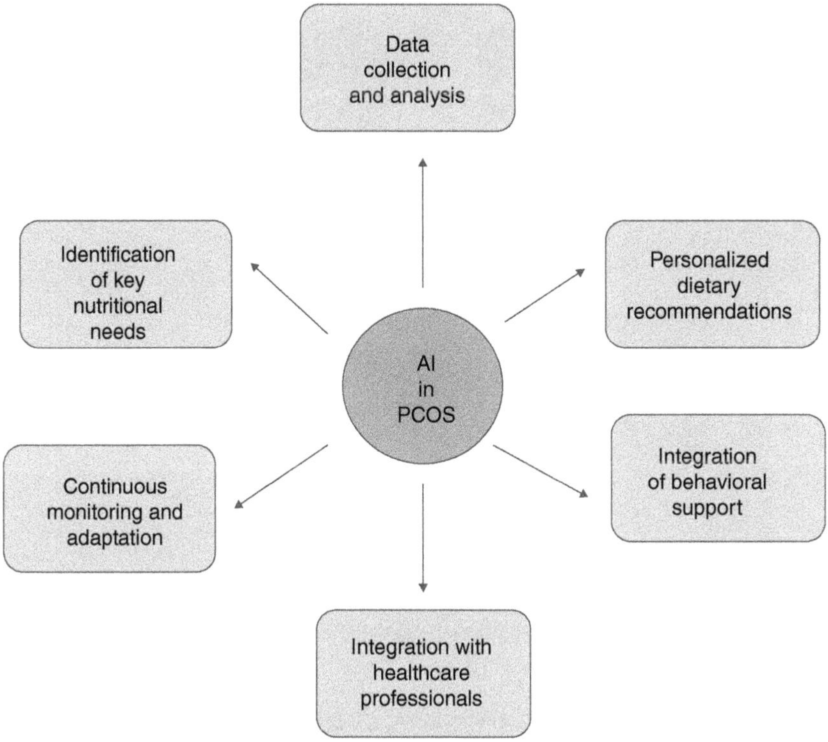

Figure 14.1 Application of AI in healthcare.

Such scrutiny aids in unveiling nuanced insights that might evade immediate detection solely through structured data, thereby enriching the depth and precision of the individual's PCOS profile. Additionally, AI algorithms demonstrate proficiency in pattern recognition and correlation analysis, enabling the discernment of subtle relationships between diverse variables linked with PCOS. Through the examination of expansive datasets, AI can unveil concealed patterns, such as correlations between specific dietary patterns, hormonal imbalances, and the severity of symptoms, thereby guiding the formulation of personalized nutrition recommendations. Employing AI-powered predictive analytics, it becomes feasible to forecast prospective health outcomes and risks predicated on the individual's PCOS profile and historical data (Figure 14.2).

Research suggests that Polycystic Ovary Syndrome (PCOS) often has a hereditary component, yet its precise etiology remains elusive. Given the lack of identifiable patterns in this medical condition, its onset is highly unpredictable, and no definitive cure exists. Both patients and healthcare

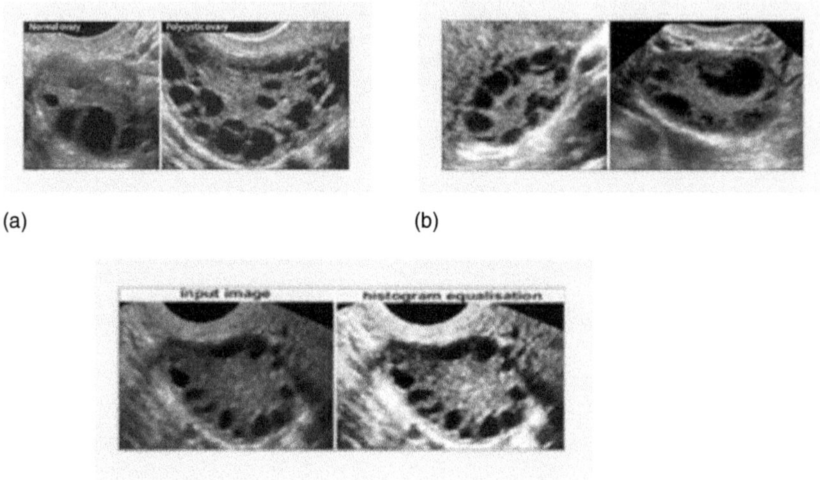

(a) (b) (c)

Figure 14.2 Images of ultrasound play a vital role in identifying follicles in patients with PCOS [1]. (a) Ultrasound image of normal; (b) Follicle detection image ovary and polycystic ovary; (c) Input image and histogram equalization.

providers grapple with the challenges of undergoing numerous medical tests and scans, which can be time-consuming and costly. Timely identification and intervention are crucial, as even minor lifestyle modifications can reduce the likelihood of encountering enduring health issues like type 2 diabetes and cardiovascular diseases.

Images of Ultrasound play a vital role in identifying follicles in patients with PCOS.[1] Manual detection of follicles is time-consuming and prone to problems such as inter- and intra-observer variability, which can adversely affect women's health. Hence, employing techniques and machinery for follicle detection becomes essential.

Also, using machine learning models, AI can anticipate the probability of developing complications such as insulin resistance, type 2 diabetes or cardiac related disease, allowing for proactive intervention and the application of risk reduction strategies. Furthermore, AI-facilitated monitoring systems possess the capacity to continuously amass real-time data from wearable devices, sensors, and other IoT (Internet of Things) devices, thereby furnishing instantaneous feedback on the individual's health status and adherence to treatment plans. This real-time monitoring facilitates prompt adjustments to the individual's care regimen and expedites intervention in the event of any deviations or emergent issues (Table 14.1). AI systems must accord top priority to privacy and security measures to safeguard

Table 14.1 Techniques used for studying the PCOS related issues [2]

Authors	*Technique*	*Objective*	*Year*
Cheng et al.	Rule based classifier and Gradient boosted Tree classifiers	PCOS determination from Ultrasound Images	2016
Dewi, R.M. and Wisesty	Gabor wavelet based feature extraction and CNN	PCOS determination from Ultrasound Images.	2018
Mehrotra et al,	2 sample-test, Bayesian and Logistic Regression (LR) classifier	PCOS determination from clinical and metabolic parameters.	2011
Sachdev et al.	Prospective observational study: Obese nonobese PCOS	Obese PCOS patients have a higher risk of adverse outcomes.	2019
Zhang et al	Machine-learning algorithms	PCOS prediction from identification of new PCOS genes.	2019
Joham et al	Logistic regression on data from cross-sectional analysis of a longitudinal cohort	Examination of factors associated with infertility and use of fertility treatment.	2015
K. Meena, M. Manimekalai and S. Rethinavalli	Information Gain Subset. Evaluation and Neuro Fuzzy methods of feature selection and Decision Tree classifier	Framework for Filtering the PCOS Attributes	2015

sensitive health data obtained from individuals with PCOS. Implementing robust encryption, anonymization techniques, and access controls ensures compliance with data protection regulations and upholds patient confidentiality [2].

14.3 IDENTIFICATION OF KEY NUTRITIONAL NEEDS

Polycystic ovary syndrome (PCOS) presents unique challenges in nutritional management due to its heterogeneous nature. Artificial intelligence (AI) plays a crucial role in identifying key nutritional needs in PCOS patients by analyzing diverse data sets and generating personalized recommendations. This case study demonstrates how AI facilitates the identification of nutritional needs in PCOS patients, leading to tailored dietary interventions.

Mustafa et al. [3] introduced iDietScoreTM—a meal-suggesting system tailored for players and individuals, considering factors such as training cycle, age, food preferences, and sports category. Initially, interviews with sports nutritionists or dieticians informed the system's design by understanding athletes' macronutrient needs. A protocol-based system was crafted, aligning a patient's nutrition requirements with the database of meal plans, ultimately offering personalized meal recommendations. Salloum and Tekli

[4] developed a unique flowchart for nutritional meal suggestions. Their framework included modules for weight assessment, caloric intake, exercise recommendations, and progress testing, integrating fuzzy logic for enhanced functionality. The evaluation involved 50 patients and 11 nutritionists.

Sefa-Yeboah et al. [5] designed a genetic algorithm-supported AI application to gauge a patient's energy equilibrium and estimate energy consumption for obesity management, tailoring meal recommendations based on user input and health data. Shen et al. [6] introduced an ML model for meal image recognition to aid healthy diet maintenance and obesity control, leveraging a CNN model fine-tuned with augmentation and multi-crop technology. Kumar et al. [7] suggested a multilayer perceptron model for nutrition type classification and energy estimation, offering tailored food lists for obesity management, outperforming SVM in calorie prediction accuracy. These methods collectively offer avenues for early obesity identification and management through ML techniques, emphasizing the importance of healthy nutrition planning based on individual needs to mitigate obesity-related health risks.

The study employs several supervised algorithms (GB, BME, XGB, SVM, RF, KNN) for obesity prediction, and unsupervised nearest-neighbor method for meal recommendations based on individual nutrient needs. Two datasets are used: one predicts obesity using physical symptoms and food habits, while the other recommends meals categorized by time. The evaluation dataset, from UCI ML repository, contains 16 attributes with 2111 records. Another dataset with 13 attributes is created, including physical characteristics and eating habits, labeled with obesity levels. Attributes cover age, weight, height, gender, family obesity history, meal frequency, high-calorie food consumption, vegetable intake, smoking, alcohol, etc. (Table 14.2).

Table 14.2 Data with attributes descriptions and values [10]

Attribute (obesity Data set)	*Values*
Gender	[M,F]
Age	[16, 18]
Height	[1.44, 1.93] in mts
Weight	[38,133] in kgs
Family history	[Y,N]
Intake of high calorie food	[Y,N]
Intake of vegetables	[2,3]
Count of main meals	[2,3]
Intake of food between meals	[None, seldom, every-day, Regularly]
Daily water intake	[3,4]
Intake of alcohol	[None, seldom, every-day, Regularly]
Obesity Level	Normal, Overweight-I, Overweight-I I, Obesity-I, Obesity-II, Underweight

The ML models are assessed with varying data ratios (90:10, 80:20, 70:30, 60:40) for training/testing. The nutrition scheduling dataset comprises 93 meal plans, divided into breakfast, morning snacks, lunch, snacks, and dinner, with total calorie and macronutrient breakdown. The focus lies in predicting adult obesity levels using ML algorithms, leveraging physical attributes and dietary habits for training. Pre-processing involves selecting attributes related to physical characteristics and eating behaviors for model training (Figure 14.3). Calorie needs are determined from fundamental data like age, weight, and height using Basal Metabolic Rate, and meals with detailed macronutrient content are suggested accordingly (Table 14.3) [10].

Several pre-processing steps are undertaken on the collected dataset, including the elimination of outliers, addressing imbalanced classes, and evaluating attribute correlation levels. In this dataset, numerous feature variants are categorized and are consequently transformed into continuous variables to comply with the requirement of ML models, which solely accept numerical data (Figure 14.4).

The pre-processed dataset undergoes normalization with Standard Scaler to range between 0 and 1. Bagging, a technique generating multiple training sets by random sample selection, is deployed alongside boosting and other ML models (Figure 14.5). Boosting sequentially enhances weak learners to form a robust prediction model. Six models (GB, XGB, BME, SVM, RF, KNN), each with specific parameter configurations, predict obesity levels. Gradient Boosting and XGBoost employ multiple trees with adjustable

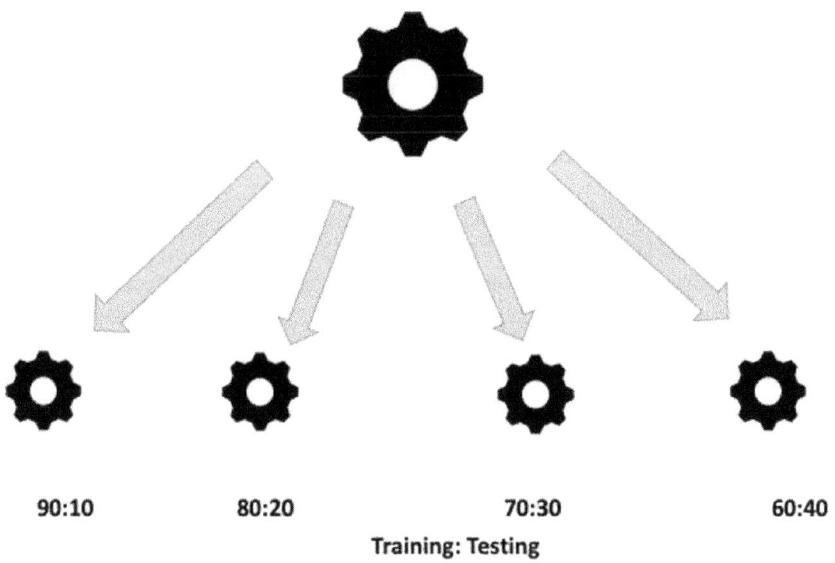

Figure 14.3 Segregation of data for training and testing [10].

Table 14.3 Sample meal plan

Meal	
Breakfast	2 Veg Pancake, 1/4 bowl Blackberries, 1 tsp Peanut butter -290 calories
Morning snacking	3/4 boiled Green Peas — 145 Calories
Lunch	Bean and avocado with 1 bread, 1 bowl cucumber — 240 calories
Evening Snacking	1 Plum — 29 Calories
Dinner	Salad with 1 pita bread -495 Calories

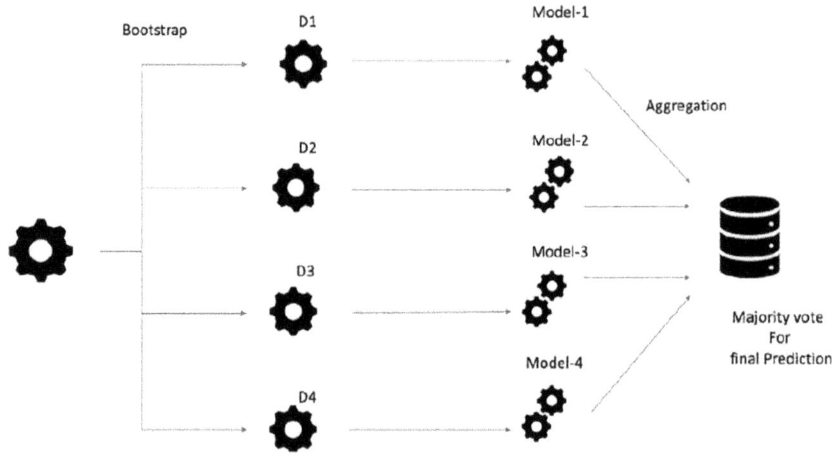

Figure 14.4 Bagging approach to produce the final result.

parameters, while Random Forest controls overfitting with bootstrap subsamples. With a 95.7% accuracy, Random Forest excels, while Bagging Classifier, utilizing decision trees, outperforms SVM as a base estimator in ensemble meta-estimation.

Furthermore, SVM operates as a supervised learning technique that employs a separating hyperplane to perform precise classifications. In essence, the model provides an optimal hyperplane for categorizing new samples based on trained labeled data. Lastly, KNN is used to determine the nearest neighbors for object classification.

14.4. PERSONALIZED DIETARY RECOMMENDATIONS

AI is using machine learning techniques to generate personalized nutrition plans designed to the individual's unique PCOS profile and health goals by recommending specific macronutrient distribution, portion sizes, meal

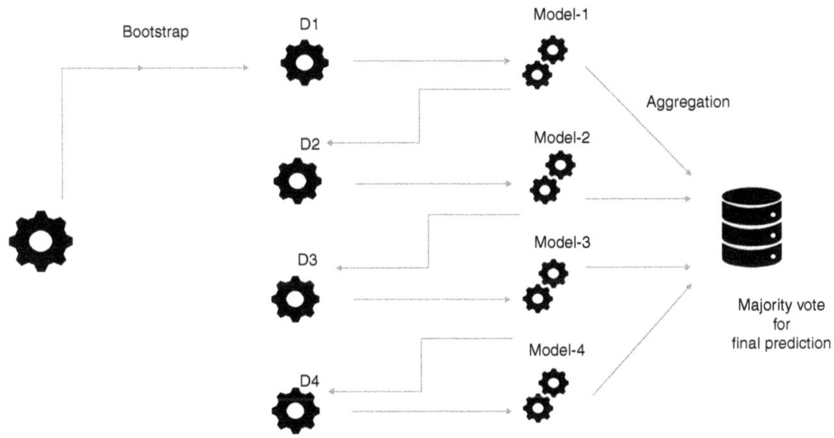

Figure 14.5 Boosting algorithms to produce the final result.

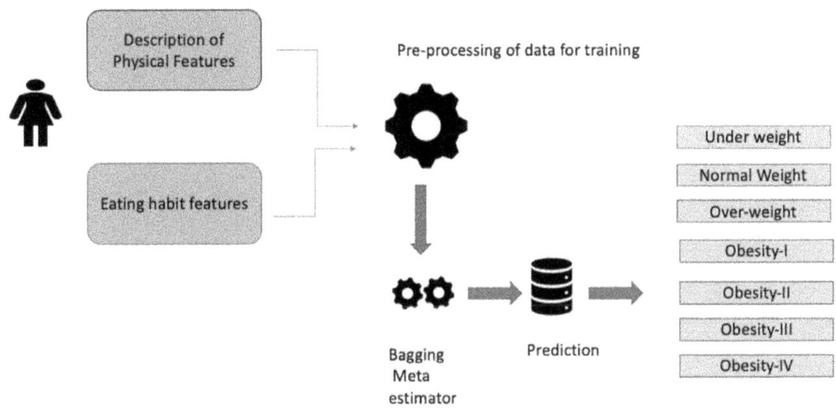

Figure 14.6 Obesity prediction ML model work flow.

timing, and food choices to address the individual's nutritional needs and promote hormonal balance. Managing nutrition and achieving weight loss are fundamental aspects of addressing overweight and obesity in individuals (Figures 14.6 and 14.7).

In the proposed project, a model is developed to aid dietitians or healthcare providers in forecasting meal plans tailored to individuals' calorie needs to support healthy weight maintenance and combat obesity. This model is employed to determine individual weight status, ranging from underweight to obese. Initially, user input including height, weight, and age is utilized to calculate the daily calorie intake requirement. Distinct calorie requirements

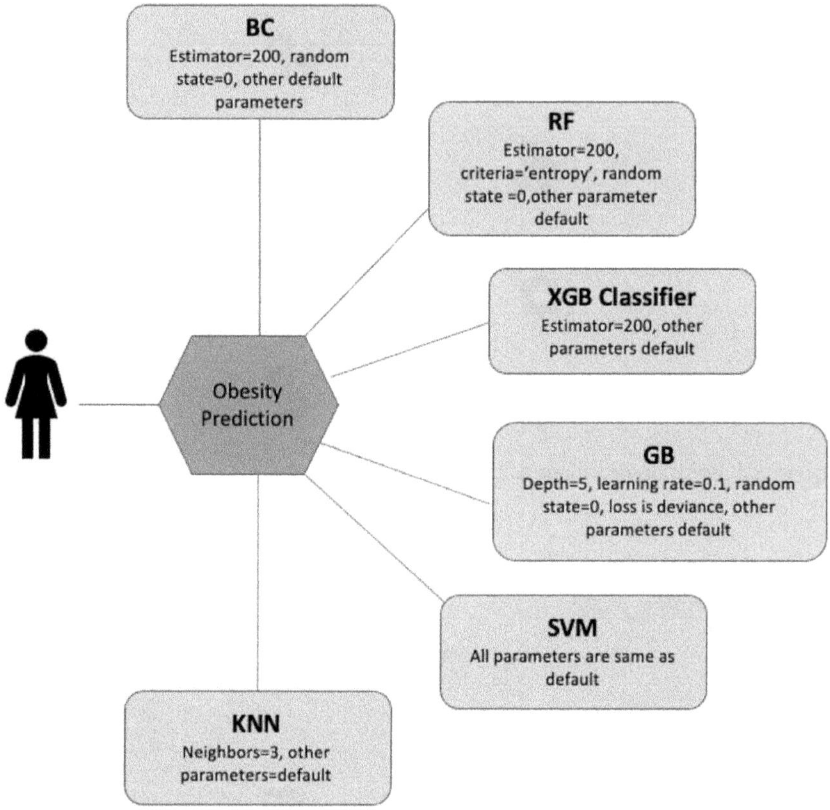

Figure 14.7 Models parameters to predict obesity.

for males and females are determined using the Harries–Benedict equation as outlined in Eqs. (a) and (b) [10].

Total calorie calculation for women = 655+9.5 x weight + 1.84 x height – 4.6 x age ----- (a)

Total calorie calculation for men = 66.4 +13.75 x weight + 5.00 x height – 6.7 x age ----- (b)

Based on the individual's calorie requirements, a nutrition plan comprising five sub-meals (breakfast, morning snacks, lunch, evening snacks, and dinner) is recommended using the Nearest Neighbors learning approach, illustrated in Figure 14.8. This method operates as an unsupervised technique for determining neighbors, where 'k' represents the number of neighbors. For instance, if a user needs 1200 calories daily, this method will generate approximately 'k' number of meals totaling 1200 calories. The experimental setup specifies parameters such as the number of neighbors, the

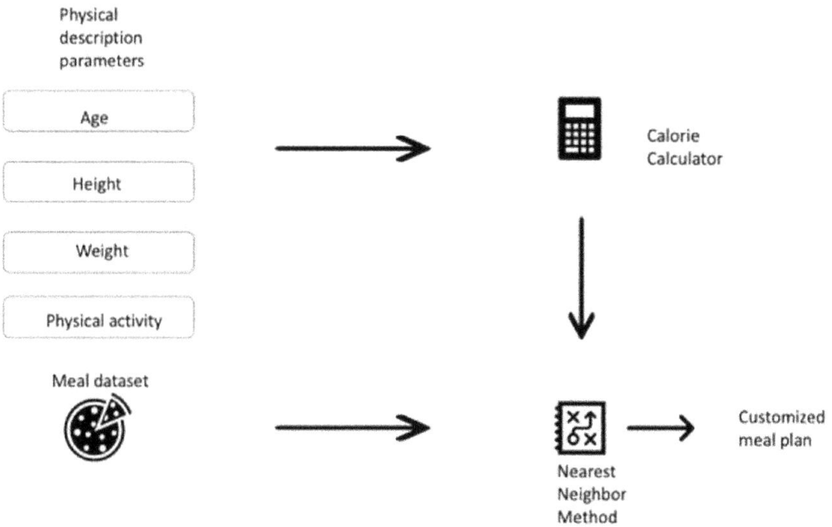

Figure 14.8 An ML model to predict meals as per caloric requirements [10].

algorithm for neighbor search, the metric parameter set to Euclidean, and retaining default settings for other search method parameters (Figure 14.8).

In the involved research endeavor, obesity levels are anticipated using six machine learning (ML) algorithms, and personalized meal suggestions are provided based on individuals' calorie requirements. The outcomes of all obesity calculation and meal planning models are elaborated upon in the "Performance Analysis Metrics" section [10]. Here, obesity levels are predicted involving six ML algorithms, and personalized meal recommendations are provided to individuals based on their calorie requirements. The consequences of all obesity prediction and meal planning models are discussed in the "Performance analysis metrics" section (Tables 14.4 and 14.5).

Performance metrics (Tables 14.4 and 14.5) including precision, recall, F-1 score, and accuracy are obtained from the confusion matrix and calculated by engaging given equations. A confusion matrix provides a structured representation for analyzing the performance of each class by computing the true positive, true negative, false positive, and false negative instances of the prediction model. It serves as a useful tool in evaluating the effectiveness and quality of the classification model.

In this proposed study, the models are assessed using the obesity dataset, employing performance metrics such as precision, recall, and F-1 score. Table 14.4 displays that all models exhibit very similar accuracy levels, with the GB and XGB classifier models demonstrating superior performance,

Table 14.4 Performance evaluation metrics and comparison of classifiers

Algorithm	*Accuracy %*	*Weighted avg precision%*	*Weighted avg. recall %*	*Weighted avg F-1 Score %*
RF	95.74	96	**96**	96
weBagging Classifier	95.90	96	96	96
XGB Classifier	**97.79**	**98**	**98**	**98**
GB classifiers	**97.16**	**97**	**97**	**97**
SVM	87.7	88	88	88
KNN	82.3	82	83	82

Table 14.5 Data split ratio effect on the percentage

ML classification model	*90-10%*	*80-20%*	*70-30%*	*60-40%*
RF	96.23%	95.74%	95.74%	95.5%
Bagging Classifier	95.75%	95.75%	95.9%	95.05%
XGB Classifier	97.64%	97.87%	97.79%	96.45%
GN classifiers	98.11%	97.87%	97.16%	96.33%
SVM	87.7%	88.18%	87.7%%	87.34%
KNN	82.3%	82.03%	82.33%	81.42%

exhibiting a 0.16% difference in accuracy compared to others. Conversely, SVM and KNN algorithms exhibit comparatively poorer performance. Notably, the accuracy gap between the top-performing models (XGB and GB) and the least effective model (KNN) is approximately 15%. Table 14.5 presents a comprehensive overview of performance metrics calculated on both training and testing data, partitioned into 70% and 30%, respectively [11].

Individuals who are overweight face an increased likelihood of developing various severe conditions such as diabetes, hypertension, stroke, cancer, and more. Detecting and forecasting these ailments in their early phases is crucial to prevent their progression to advanced stages. Machine learning (ML) and ensemble learning techniques have proven to be efficient in the realm of disease diagnosis and prediction.

14.5 INTEGRATION OF BEHAVIORAL SUPPORT

The study examines secondary outcomes of a 3-month single-blind, metformin-stratified, parallel-group randomized controlled trial (RCT) focusing on pulse-based and TLC diets' effects on cardiometabolic risk in women with PCOS (Figure 14.9). Participants were assigned either a pulse-based or TLC diet for 16 weeks without energy restrictions. The pulse-based diet included standard meals containing split peas, chickpeas, or lentils,

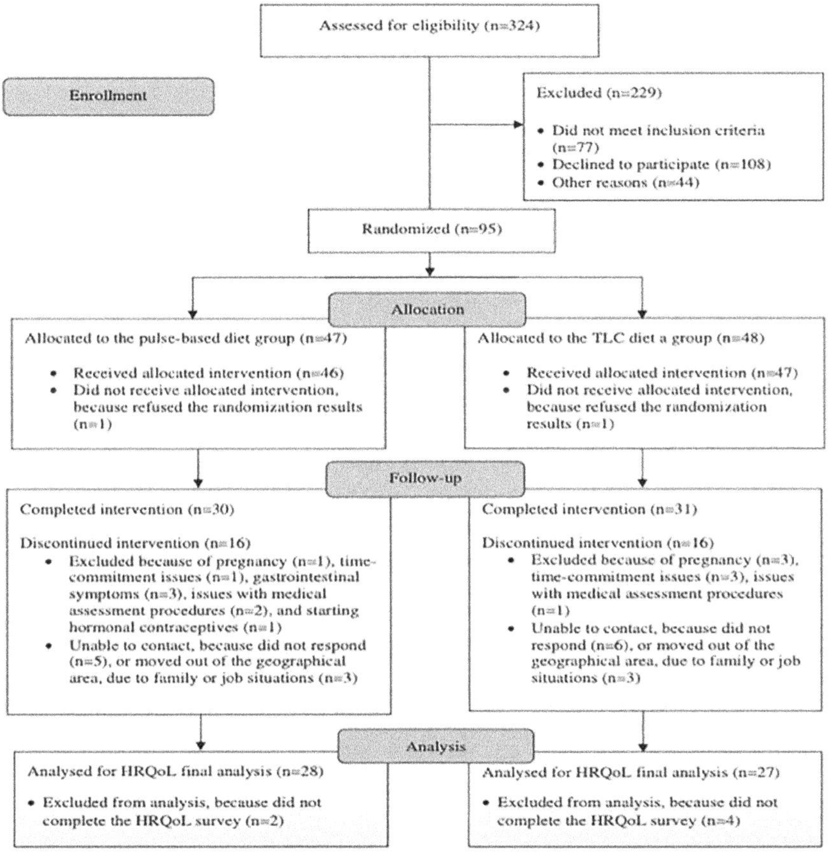

Figure 14.9 Flow chart of study [12].

while TLC diet adhered to TLC guidelines. All participants underwent low-impact aerobics training five days a week for 45 minutes, alongside PCOS counselling. Monthly individualized health counselling and continuous monitoring were provided. Assessments included hirsutism, acne severity, and endocrine measures. Insulin resistance was evaluated using HOMA-IR [12]. Participants' health-related quality of life (HRQoL) was assessed using a PCOS-specific survey with 82 items across five domains: healthcare satisfaction, health concerns, PCOS knowledge, healthy lifestyle behaviors, and feelings about participation. Additionally, feelings regarding PCOS diagnosis were evaluated separately. The survey included open-ended questions for qualitative feedback, rated on Likert scales. Thirty participants in the pulse-based group and 31 in the TLC group completed the 16-week intervention, with 90% completing pre- and post-intervention surveys. Baseline characteristics, including metformin use, were similar between groups. No notable differences were observed in baseline characteristics or HRQoL domain scores between completers and dropouts.

14.6 CONTINUOUS MONITORING AND ADAPTATION

Artificial Intelligence (AI) assumes a pivotal role in the ongoing surveillance and adjustment of treatment approaches for individuals afflicted with Polycystic Ovary Syndrome (PCOS), presenting personalized and proactive healthcare solutions. PCOS, a multifaceted endocrine disorder characterized by hormonal imbalances, irregular menstruation, and ovarian cysts, poses challenges necessitating tailored and adaptable treatment modalities, which AI-driven technologies adeptly facilitate. In terms of Continuous Monitoring, AI-enabled platforms facilitate the continual tracking of various physiological parameters linked to PCOS, enabling timely symptom detection, disease progression tracking, and treatment optimization. These platforms leverage wearable devices, mobile applications, and connected sensors to gather real-time data on menstrual cycles, hormone levels, physical activity, dietary patterns, and other pertinent health metrics. Through data aggregation and analysis, AI algorithms discern patterns, trends, and anomalies indicative of PCOS exacerbations or treatment inefficiencies. For instance, fluctuations in hormone levels or menstrual irregularities trigger prompt, personalized interventions like medication adjustments or lifestyle modifications. Additionally, AI-driven virtual health assistants employ natural language processing to engage with patients, eliciting symptom reports and furnishing real-time guidance and support.

Adaptive Treatment Strategies are made possible by AI algorithms, which customize treatment regimens based on individual patient data, treatment response, and evolving disease status. Leveraging machine learning and predictive modeling, AI platforms forecast the likelihood of PCOS-associated complications such as insulin resistance, cardiovascular disease, and infertility. Continual patient data monitoring and risk assessment empower AI algorithms to propose personalized interventions aimed at averting future health risks and optimizing treatment outcomes. For example, AI-driven decision support systems scrutinize medical imaging scans like ovarian ultrasound images to discern PCOS characteristic features and gauge disease severity. This analysis informs tailored treatment plans, encompassing hormone level regulation prescriptions or lifestyle modification recommendations to enhance metabolic health.

Illustrating AI's role in PCOS management is a Case Study featuring Sarah, a 28-year-old PCOS patient grappling with symptom management and fertility enhancement. Sarah's healthcare provider recommends integrating AI-driven technologies into her treatment regimen to facilitate continuous monitoring and adaptive interventions. Equipped with a wearable device, Sarah tracks her menstrual cycles, hormone levels, and physical activity —synchronizing data to a mobile application linked to an AI-powered platform. This platform conducts real-time data analysis, identifying PCOS exacerbation indicators and furnishing personalized recommendations for lifestyle modifications, medication adjustments, and follow-up appointments. Moreover, Sarah benefits from virtual health coaching sessions with an AI-driven virtual assistant, receiving guidance on nutrition, exercise, stress management, and medication adherence. Over time, Sarah's treatment regimen adapts based on treatment response, disease evolution, and personalized risk assessment, resulting in improved symptom management, metabolic health, and fertility outcomes.

Notwithstanding the potential benefits of AI in PCOS management, several challenges must be addressed for optimal effectiveness and scalability. These encompass data privacy concerns, interoperability issues, algorithmic bias, and regulatory oversight imperatives. Additionally, AI-driven interventions must integrate seamlessly into existing healthcare workflows and be supported by robust clinical evidence to ensure patient safety and efficacy. Future research endeavors should focus on developing AI algorithms capable of analyzing multi-modal data streams, integrating patient preferences and values into treatment decision-making, and assessing the long-term impact of AI-driven interventions on patient outcomes and healthcare costs.

In conclusion, AI stands poised to revolutionize the continuous monitoring and adaptation of treatment strategies for females afflicted with PCOS, furnishing personalized and proactive healthcare solutions. By harnessing AI-driven platforms, healthcare providers can conduct real-time disease surveillance, tailor treatment plans to individual patient needs, and optimize outcomes through adaptive interventions. While challenges persist, sustained innovation and collaboration among clinicians, researchers, and technology developers hold promise for enhancing the quality of care and life for PCOS patients globally.

14.7 INTEGRATION WITH HEALTHCARE PROFESSIONALS

The incorporation of Artificial Intelligence (AI) into the collaboration between healthcare professionals for the management of Polycystic Ovary Syndrome (PCOS) patients represents a transformative advancement, providing improved diagnosis, treatment, and patient care. AI acts as a valuable ally to healthcare professionals, enhancing their abilities, streamlining processes, and enhancing patient outcomes through individualized and data-driven interventions. AI-powered remote monitoring solutions empower healthcare professionals to oversee the health status and treatment adherence of PCOS patients beyond conventional clinical settings. Equipped with AI algorithms, wearable devices, mobile applications, and telehealth platforms enable real-time data collection and analysis, allowing proactive intervention in response to changing symptoms or treatment responses. Healthcare professionals can remotely oversee patients' physiological parameters, medication compliance, and lifestyle habits, delivering timely guidance and assistance as necessary [13].

AI-driven decision support tools provide healthcare professionals with immediate clinical insights and actionable recommendations during patient consultations. Through natural language processing algorithms, electronic health records, medical literature, and patient-reported data are analyzed—aiding healthcare professionals in clinical decision-making. AI-powered diagnostic assistance systems interpret medical imaging scans and laboratory results, facilitating the interpretation of intricate data and enhancing diagnostic accuracy. AI-driven virtual health assistants offer personalized education, support, and self-management resources to PCOS patients, fostering health literacy and encouraging active patient involvement in their care. Healthcare professionals leverage AI-driven chatbots and virtual coaches to engage patients in ongoing conversations, delivering evidence-based information, and promoting adherence to treatment plans and lifestyle changes. By nurturing patient empowerment and self-efficacy, AI enhances patient engagement and long-term health outcomes.

In conclusion, the integration of AI with healthcare professionals significantly enhances the management of PCOS patients by enabling precise diagnosis, personalized treatment, continuous monitoring, decision support, and patient engagement. Leveraging the capabilities of AI-driven technologies, healthcare professionals can provide more efficient, effective, and patient-centered care —ultimately enhancing the quality of life for individuals grappling with PCOS.

REFERENCES

1. A. Agrawal, R., Ambad, R. Lahoti, P. Muley, P.S. Pande, Role of artificial intelligence in PCOS detection. *J. Datta Meghe Inst. Med. Sci. Univ.* 17(2), pp. 491–494, Apr–Jun 2022.
2. A. Denny, A. Raj, A. Ashok, C.M. Ram, R. George, i-HOPE: Detection and prediction system for polycystic ovary syndrome (PCOS) using machine learning techniques. *TENCON 2019 – 2019 IEEE Region 10 Conference (TENCON), Kochi, India*, 2019, pp. 673–678.
3. N. Mustaf, A.H. Abd Rahman, N.S. Sani, M.I. Mohamad, A.Z. Zakaria, A. Ahmad, N.H. Yatiman, R.A. Talib, P.B. Koon, N.S. Safii, iDietScoreTM: Meal recommender system for athletes and active individuals. *Int. J. Adv. Comput. Sci. Appl.* 11(12), 176–183 (2020).
4. G. Salloum, J. Tekli, Automated and personalized nutrition health assessment, recommendation, and progress evaluation using fuzzy reasoning. *Int. J. Hum. Computer Stud.* 151, 102610 (2021).
5. Z. Shen, A. Shehzad, S. Chen, H. Sun, J. Liu, Machine learning based approach on food recognition and nutrition estimation. *Procedia Computer Sci.* 174, 448–453 (2020).

6. R.D. Kumar, E.G. Julie, Y.H. Robinson, S. Vimal, S. Seo, Recognition of food type and calorie estimation using neural network. *J. Supercomputing.* 77(8), 8172–8193 (2021).
7. D.C. Frankenfield, E.R. Muth, W.A. Rowe, The Harris-Benedict studies of human basal metabolism: History and limitations. *J. Am. Dietetic Assoc.* 98(4), 439–445 (1998).
8. F.M. Palechor, A. de la Hoz Manotas, Dataset for estimation of obesity levels based on eating habits and physical condition in individuals from Colombia, Peru and Mexico. *Data Br.* 25, 104344 (2019). https://doi.org/10.1016/j.dib.2019.1043449.
9. EatingWell, "Diet Meal Plan to Lose *Weight.*" *EatingWell*, n.d. Available at: EatingWell. Accessed July 2022.
10. R. Kaur, R. Kumar, M. Gupta, Predicting risk of obesity and meal planning to reduce the obese in adulthood using artificial intelligence. *Endocrine.* 78, 458–469 (2022).
11. M. Kazemi, L.E. McBreairty, D.R. Chizen, et al., A comparison of a pulse-based diet and the therapeutic lifestyle changes diet in combination with exercise and health counselling on the cardio-metabolic risk profile in women with polycystic ovary syndrome: A randomized controlled trial. *Nutrients.* 10(10), 1387 (2018).
12. C. Ju, R. Zhao, J. Sun, X. Wei, B. Zhao, Y. Liu, H. Li, T. Chen, X. Zhang, D. C. Ju, R. Zhao, J. Sun, X. Wei, B. Zhao, Y. Liu, H. Li, T. Chen, X. Zhang, D. Gao, B. Tan, H. Yu, Y. Jin, "Privacy-preserving technology to help millions of people: Federated prediction model for stroke prevention," *arXiv preprint* arXiv:2006.10517 (2020).

Index

For Product Safety Concerns and Information please contact our EU
representative GPSR@taylorandfrancis.com
Taylor & Francis Verlag GmbH, Kaufingerstraße 24, 80331 München, Germany

www.ingramcontent.com/pod-product-compliance
Ingram Content Group UK Ltd.
Pitfield, Milton Keynes, MK11 3LW, UK
UKHW021505240926
475702UK00035B/451

* 9 7 8 1 0 3 2 9 4 6 7 7 1 *